HOLISTIC HEALTHCARE

VOLUME 2

Possibilities and Challenges

HOLISTIC HEALTHCARE

VOLUME 2

Possibilities and Challenges

Edited by

Anne George, MD

Snigdha S. Babu

M. P. Ajithkumar, PhD

Sabu Thomas, PhD

AAP | APPLE
ACADEMIC
PRESS

Apple Academic Press Inc.
3333 Mistwell Crescent
Oakville, ON L6L 0A2, Canada

Apple Academic Press, Inc.
1265 Goldenrod Circle NE
Palm Bay, Florida 32905, USA

© 2019 by Apple Academic Press, Inc.

First issued in paperback 2021

No claim to original U.S. Government works

ISBN 13: 978-1-77463-405-9 (pbk)
ISBN 13: 978-1-77188-715-1 (hbk)

Library and Archives Canada Cataloguing in Publication

Holistic healthcare. Volume 2 : possibilities and challenges / edited by Anne George, MD, Snigdha S. Babu, M. P. Ajithkumar, PhD, Sabu Thomas, PhD.
Includes bibliographical references and index.
Issued in print and electronic formats.
ISBN 978-1-77188-715-1 (hardcover).--ISBN 978-0-42948-780-4 (PDF)
1. Integrative medicine. 2. Holistic medicine. I. George, Anne, 1961-, author, editor II. Babu, Snigdha S., editor III. M. P., Ajithkumar IV. Thomas, Sabu, editor

| R733.H64 2017 | 615.5 | C2016-907938-4 | C2016-907939-2 |

Library of Congress Cataloging-in-Publication Data

Title: Holistic healthcare. Volume 2: possibilities and challenges / edited by Anne George, MD, Snigdha S. Babu, Ajithkumar M.P., PhD, Sabu Thomas, PhD.
Names: George, Anne, 1961- editor. | Babu, Snigdha S., editor. | M. P., Ajithkumar, editor. | Thomas, Sabu, editor.
Description: Includes bibliographical references and index.
Identifiers: Canadiana (print) 20190042575 | Canadiana (ebook) 20190042605 | ISBN 9781771887151 (hardcover) | ISBN 9780429487804 (PDF)
Subjects: LCSH: Integrative medicine. | LCSH: Holistic medicine.
Classification: LCC R733 .H642 2019 | DDC 615.5—dc23

Apple Academic Press also publishes its books in a variety of electronic formats. Some content that appears in print may not be available in electronic format. For information about Apple Academic Press products, visit our website at **www.appleacademicpress.com** and the CRC Press website at **www.crcpress.com**

ABOUT THE EDITORS

Anne George, MD

Anne George, MD, MBBS, DGO, Dip Acupuncture, is an Associate Professor in the Department of Anatomy at the Government Medical College, Kottayam, Kerala, India. She has organized several international conferences, is a fellow of the American Medical Society, and is a member of many international organizations. Dr. George has worked in several different international labs, which include the laboratories at Laval University, Quebec, Canada; Faculty of Medicine, University of Vienna, Vienna, Austria; and the Department of Immunology, Katholieke University of Leuven, Leuven, Belgium. Dr. George has edited many books and published research articles and reviews in international journals and has presented many papers at international conferences. Her major research interests are human anatomy, polymeric scaffolds for tissue engineering, diabetes, nature cures, diet, and human health. She received her MBBS, Bachelor of Medicine, and her Bachelor of Surgery from Trivandrum Medical College, University of Kerala, India. She acquired a DGO (Diploma in Obstetrics and Gynecology) from the University of Vienna, Austria; a Diploma of Acupuncture from the University of Vienna; and her MD from Kottayam Medical College, Mahatma Gandhi University, Kerala, India.

Snigdha S. Babu

Snigdha S. Babu is pursuing her PhD at the International and Inter University Centre for Nanoscience and Nanotechnology, Mahatma Gandhi University, India. She has research experience in the field of biotechnology, polymer science, and nanotechnology. Her specialization is in microbiological applications of nanomaterials.

M. P. Ajithkumar, PhD

M. P. Ajithkumar, PhD, is a postdoctoral fellow of the International and Inter University Centre for Nanoscience and Nanotechnology, Mahatma Gandhi University, Kottayam, India. He pursued his PhD in Chemistry from Manipal University, India. He has more than 8 years of research experience in the area of chemistry and is an expert in polymer synthesis and materials chemistry. His current research is focused on developing carbon dots and graphene materials for imaging, sensing, and energy applications.

Sabu Thomas, PhD

Sabu Thomas, PhD, is currently the Pro-Vice Chancellor of Mahatma Gandhi University and Professor of Polymer Science and Engineering at the School of Chemical Sciences of Mahatma Gandhi University, Kottayam, Kerala, India. He is the Founder and Director of the International and Inter University Centre for Nanoscience and Nanotechnology, a center that was established to carry out intense research in the field of nanotechnology. He is an outstanding leader with sustained international acclaim for his work in polymer science and engineering, polymer nanocomposites, elastomers, polymer blends, interpenetrating polymer networks, polymer membranes, green composites and nanocomposites, nanomedicine, and green nanotechnology. Dr. Thomas's groundbreaking inventions in polymer nanocomposites, polymer blends, green bionanotechnological, and nano-biomedical sciences have made transformative differences in the development of new materials for the automotive, space, housing, and biomedical fields. Professor Thomas has received a number of national and international awards, which include Fellowship of the Royal Society of Chemistry, London, MRSI medal, Nano Tech Medal, CRSI medal, Distinguished Faculty Award, and Sukumar Maithy Award for the best polymer researcher in the country. He is in the list of most productive researchers in India and holds the No. 5 position. Very recently, Professor Thomas has been conferred Honoris Causa (DSc) by the University of South Brittany, Lorient, France and Universite de Lorraine, France. Professor Thomas has published over 750 peer-reviewed research papers, reviews, and book chapters. He has coedited 50 books and is the inventor of 5 patents. He has supervised 73 PhD theses and his h-index is 81 with nearly 31,574 citations. Professor Thomas has delivered over 300 Plenary/ Inaugural and Invited lectures in national/international meetings over 30 countries. He has established a state of the art laboratory at Mahatma Gandhi University in the area of polymer science and engineering and nanoscience and nanotechnology.

CONTENTS

LIST OF CONTRIBUTORS

Kanika Aggarwal
Department of Zoology and Environmental Sciences, Punjabi University, Patiala 147002, Punjab, India

Snigdha S. Babu
International and Inter University Centre for Nanoscience and Nanotechnology, Mahatma Gandhi University, Kottayam 686560, Kerala, India

Binoy Surendra Babu
Directorate of Health Services, Trivandrum 695312, Kerala, India

Sukhwinder Bhullar
Department of Mechanical Engineering, Bursa Technical University, Bursa, Turkey
St. Boniface Hospital Albrechtsen Research Centre, Winnipeg, Manitoba, Canada

Shilpa Bisht
Laboratory for Molecular Reproduction and Genetics, AIIMS, New Delhi 110029, India

D. S. Bormane
AISSMS COE, Savitribai Phule Pune University, Pune 411033, India

Rima Dada
Department of Anatomy, Laboratory for Molecular Reproduction and Genetics, All India Institute of Medical Sciences (AIIMS), New Delhi 110029, India

Parnika Dicholkar
Department of Pharmacology, Shobhaben Pratapbhai Patel School of Pharmacy & Technology Management, SVKM's NMIMS, Vile Parle (West), Mumbai 400056, Maharashtra, India

Ann Holaday
Anglia Polytechnic, Cambridge University, Cambridge, UK

Mihir Invally
Department of Pharmacology, Shobhaben Pratapbhai Patel School of Pharmacy & Technology Management, SVKM's NMIMS, Vile Parle (West), Mumbai 400056, Maharashtra, India

Tejal G. Joshi
CEO, Shree Garbhsanskar Centre

Nandakumar Kalarikkal
International and Inter University Centre for Nanoscience and Nanotechnology, Mahatma Gandhi University, Kottayam 686560, Kerala, India
School of Pure and Applied Physics, Mahatma Gandhi University, Kottayam 686560, Kerala, India

Ginpreet Kaur
Department of Pharmacology, Shobhaben Pratapbhai Patel School of Pharmacy & Technology Management, SVKM's NMIMS, Vile Parle (West), Mumbai 400056, Maharashtra, India

Seema Kedar
JSPM's Rajarshi Shahu College of Engineering, Savitribai Phule Pune University, Pune 411033, India

Vrajeshkumar G. Khambholja
Managing Director, Shree Garbhsanskar Centre

Shiv B. Kumar
Laboratory for Molecular Reproduction and Genetics, AIIMS, New Delhi 110029, India

G. Kumaravel
Vikram Sarabhai Space Centre, Thiruvananthapuram 695024, India

Robin L. LaBarbera
Department of Special Education, School of Education, Biola University, 13800 Biola Ave.,
La Mirada, CA 90639, USA

K. L. Meena
Department of Basic Principles, National Institute of Ayurveda, Jaipur, Rajasthan, India

Klimenko M. Mikhailovich
Academy of Medical Technology, OOO Scientific Industrial Enterprise "Exergy," Lenina Prospect
Bld. 120, Apt. 131, 650023 Kemerovo, Russia

Hiral Mistry
Department of Pharmacology, Shobhaben Pratapbhai Patel School of Pharmacy & Technology
Management, SVKM's NMIMS, Vile Parle (West), Mumbai 400056, Maharashtra, India

Ronnie G. Moore
School of Public Health, Physiotherapy and Sports Science and School of Sociology, University
College Dublin, Dublin 4, Ireland

Govind Pareek
Department of Basic Principles, National Institute of Ayurveda, Jaipur, Rajasthan, India

Satish G. Patil
Department of Physiology, BLDE University's Shri B.M. Patil Medical College, Hospital &
Research Centre, Vijayapura 586103, Karnataka, India

Shankargouda S. Patil
Department of Medicine, BLDE University's Shri B.M. Patil Medical College, Hospital & Research
Centre, Vijayapura 586103, Karnataka, India

E. K. Radhakrishnan
School of Biosciences, Mahatma Gandhi University, Kottayam 686560, Kerala, India

K. Ranjithkumar
Division of Health Management, School of Medical Education, Mahatma Gandhi University,
Kottayam 686008, Kerala, India

S. Regi Ram
Division of Health Management, School of Medical Education, Mahatma Gandhi University,
Kottayam 686008, Kerala, India

Rajesh Sagar
Department of Psychiatry, All India Institute of Medical Sciences (AIIMS), New Delhi 110029, India

Jitendar Sharma
Division Health Care Technology and Innovations, National Health System Resource Centre, New
Delhi, India
Andhra Pradesh Medtech Zone, Visakhapatnam, Andhra Pradesh, India

Devinder Singh
Department of Zoology and Environmental Sciences, Punjabi University, Patiala 147002, Punjab, India

Maneesha Solanki
Dhondumama Sathe Homoeopathic Medical College, Pune, Maharashtra, India

Vibha Sood
Department of Basic Principles, National Institute of Ayurveda, Jaipur, Rajasthan, India

Sabu Thomas
International and Inter University Centre for Nanoscience and Nanotechnology, Mahatma Gandhi University, Kottayam 686560, Kerala, India
School of Chemical Sciences, Mahatma Gandhi University, Kottayam 686560, Kerala, India

Madhuri Tolahunase
Department of Anatomy, Laboratory for Molecular Reproduction and Genetics, All India Institute of Medical Sciences (AIIMS), New Delhi 110029, India

LIST OF ABBREVIATIONS

5HT	serotonin
8-OHdG	8-hydroxy-2-deoxyguanosine
AChE	acetyl cholinesterase
ACP	acid phosphatase
ADHD	attention-deficit hyperactivity disorder
AE	adverse effect
AKT	autokinesiotherapy
ALS	advanced life support
ANOVA	analysis of variance
ART	assisted reproductive technology
BDI	Beck Depression Inventory
BLS	basic life support
BP	blood pressure
BSA	bovine serum albumin
CAM	complementary and alternative medicine
CCHR	Citizen's Commission on Human Rights
CGI	clinical global impression
CHD	chronic heart disease
CM	*Commiphora mukul*
CNS	central nervous system
CPF	chlorpyrifos
CPR	cardiopulmonary resuscitation
CV	cardiovascular
CVS	cardiovascular system
DASH	dietary approaches to stop hypertension
DBP	diastolic blood pressure
DD	depressive disorder
DHFWS	District Health & Family Welfare Samiti
DM	diabetes mellitus
DMO	Duty Medical Officer
DPD	dynamic pain display
EC	education control
EMRI	Emergency Management and Research Institute

EMS	emergency medical services
EQ-5D	EuroQol 5D
ERS	emergency response services
GAF	Global Assessment of Functioning
GR	glutathione reductase
HADS	Hospital Anxiety and Depression Scale
HDRS	Hamilton Depression Rating Scale
HPA	hypothalamic–pituitary–adrenal
ICSI	intracytoplasmic sperm injection
IPD	in patient department
ISH	isolated systolic hypertension
IVF	in vitro fertility
LDH	lactate dehydrogenase
LPO	lipid peroxidation
LTP	long-term potentiation
MADRS	Montgomery–Asberg Depression Rating Scale
MDD	major depressive disorder
MDE	major depressive episode
MGI	massage and gymnastic instrument
NAD	nothing abnormal detected
NE	norepinephrine
NO	nitric oxide
NRHM	National Health Rural Mission
OP	organophosphate
OPD	outpatient department
OS	oxidative stress
PA	physical activity
PFC	prefrontal cortex
PHQ	Patient Health Questionnaire
PIH	pregnancy-induced hypertension
PK	pancha karma
PMR	passive muscle relaxation
PMS	premental syndrome
PP	pulse pressure
PtMS	postmitochondrial supernatant
PTSD	posttraumatic stress disorder
PUFA	polyunsaturated fatty acid
Rb	retinoblastoma

RBC	red blood cells
RCT	randomized controlled trial
RKS	Rogi Kalyan Samitis
ROS	reactive oxygen species
RR	respiratory rate
RS	respiratory system
SBP	systolic blood pressure
SEM	scanning electron microscope
SF-36	short form 36
SNS	sympathetic nervous system
SOD	superoxide dismutase
SSRI	selective serotonin reuptake inhibitor
SVM	support vector machine
TCA	tricyclic antidepressant
TEM	transmission electron microscope
TM	transcendental meditation
TMS	transcranial magnetic stimulation
VAS	visual analogue scale

PREFACE

Holistic medicine aims to bring about optimal health by perceiving an individual as a composite of his/her physical, mental, psychological, emotional, social, and spiritual aspects. This branch of medicine involves detailed examination, diagnosis, and treatment of all these elements. Holistic medicine's combinatorial strategy will also help in alleviating the high levels of side effects and allergies brought about by the conventional medication regimes.

This book is a compilation of contributions from scientists, healthcare experts, and doctors working actively to bring about wholesome healing to every individual. The Sixth International Conference on Holistic Medicine, held on September 9, 2016, proved to be a great platform for experts specializing in traditional medicine, diabetes, yoga/body, mind/applied physiology, medicinal plants/herbal medicine, new developments in medicinal research and animal modeling, complementary/holistic medicine, homeopathy, meditation/spirituality/heath, and Unani/Tabiyat, which constitutes the cutting edge of holistic therapies. This book hopes to preserve the finest essence of the conference for generations to come. Here, chapters that deal with improving general health of people in various walks of life to treating some very challenging diseases have been included. Various schools of treatments, exercise regimes, and meditations are discussed in the following chapters. The chapters will shed light and hopefully help in spreading awareness and popularity of this wonderful and wholesome branch of medicine. We hope that this book will cater to the needs of researchers, pharmaceutical experts, and medical practitioners worldwide.

—The Editors

PART I
Yoga in Holistic Healthcare

CHAPTER 1

BENEFITS OF MEDITATION AND YOGA IN CLINICALLY DEPRESSED PATIENTS

MADHURI TOLAHUNASE[1], RAJESH SAGAR[2*], and RIMA DADA[1]

[1]*Department of Anatomy, Laboratory for Molecular Reproduction and Genetics, All India Institute of Medical Sciences (AIIMS), New Delhi 110029, India*

[2]*Department of Psychiatry, All India Institute of Medical Sciences (AIIMS), New Delhi 110029, India*

Corresponding author. E-mail: rima_dada@rediffmail.com

ABSTRACT

Approximately one in six individuals suffers from depression. The prevalence of depression appears to have increased over the past few decades. Several factors in the modern lifestyle significantly contribute to this rise. Many of these factors can potentially be modified, yet they receive little consideration in the treatment of depression. First-line management of depression primarily comprises psychotherapy and pharmacological treatment. For treatment-resistant patients, several invasive and noninvasive options are emerging. Empirical evidence is limited for most of these treatments. Yoga is the well-known modifier of lifestyle, but not yet fully explored and adopted in the management of depression. It constitutes a major element of upcoming "lifestyle medicine." Meditation and yoga are important components in this nexus between clinical treatments and public health promotion that involve the application of social, environmental, biological, somatic, and psychological principles to enhance physical and mental wellbeing. Large-scale adoption of yoga as a lifestyle may also provide opportunities for general health promotion and potential prevention of depression. In this chapter, we provide a narrative discussion of causes, principles of management, and details of yoga as these relate to depression.

1.1 INTRODUCTION

Depression is a complex heterogeneous disorder comprising phenotypes with varying degrees of liability for affective, cognitive, neurovegetative, and psychomotor alterations. It is associated with an increased risk of developing chronic noncommunicable disease conditions such as diabetes mellitus, heart disease, and stroke.[1] In addition, patients with depression are almost 20-fold more likely to die by suicide than the general population.[2] According to new estimates by the World Health Organization, depression is the largest disability worldwide with the number of people living with depression increasing by over 18% between 2005 and 2015. Depression is twice as common in female as in men.[3] Depression has been estimated to have a prevalence in children of 2.5% and in adolescents of 4–8%.[4] There is a broad spectrum of depressive disorders (DDs) characterized by the presence of sad, empty, or irritable mood and varying degrees of other somatic and cognitive changes. According to the *American Diagnostic and Statistical Manual of Mental Disorders*, 5th edition,[5] disturbance of mood is the predominant feature of mood disorders. They are further divided into major DD (MDD), disruptive mood dysregulation disorder (for children aged up to 18 years), persistent DD (dysthymia; DD), premenstrual dysphoric disorder, substance-induced DD, DD due to another medical condition, as well as other and unspecified DD categories for subsyndromal cases that do not fulfill the criteria for MDD or DD. MDD is characterized by one or more major depressive episodes (MDEs)—a discrete period during which an individual experiences clear-cut changes in affect, cognition, and neurovegetative functions to a moderate degree for 2 weeks or longer with a diminution of their previous level of functioning. MDD is a highly prevalent disorder. The most recent global estimates of the prevalence were 16.2% for lifetime and 6.6% for the 12 months before the survey.[6]

1.2 CAUSES OF DEPRESSION

Dualistic theories separating mind and brain are being replaced with more integrated models that consider the biological, psychological, and social influences that produce depression. Kandel's understanding of mind–brain interactions provides a model for understanding the nature and possible causes of depression,[7] particularly:

- all mental processes derive from the brain;
- genes and their protein products determine neuronal connections and functioning;
- life experiences influence gene expression and psychosocial factors feed back to the brain;
- altered gene expression that produces changes in neuronal connections contributes to maintaining abnormalities of behavior;
- psychotherapy produces long-term behavior change by altering gene expression.

Therefore, both genetic and environmental factors are implicated in the etiology and treatment of depression.[8,9] Recent advances in the study of the genetic basis of depression have produced interesting findings, such as a functional polymorphism of the serotonin (5HT) transporter gene, which can be used to predict selective 5HT reuptake inhibitor (SSRI) response in the context of life stress.[10] Thus, depression can be understood to be the consequence of life stress interacting with heritable genetic and personality vulnerabilities that produce physiological and psychological dysfunction.

The prolonged exposure to stress produces characteristic alterations in brain neurotransmitter function often described as a "chemical imbalance."[11] This refers to alterations in the major chemical messenger systems responsible for neuronal transmission: 5HT, norepinephrine (NE), and dopamine. Depression has been associated with reductions in neurotransmission in these systems, and currently available antidepressant medications are thought to work by reversing these deficits. The alterations in these neuronal systems produce the characteristic psychological and somatic symptoms characteristic of depression. Recently, glutamate has been proposed as a mediator of neuronal and synaptic repair in emerging treatments for depression like ketamine.[12]

From among the other theories of the etiology of depression, one very interesting model has been proposed by Brown et al.[13] (Fig. 1.1), who describe mechanisms responsible for the onset, provocation, and perpetuation of depression. A "severe life event" can provoke the onset of an MDE. Proximal risk factors mediate the onset of the depressive episode, and distal risk factors both mediate the proximal risk factors and foster the perpetuation of a chronic illness course.

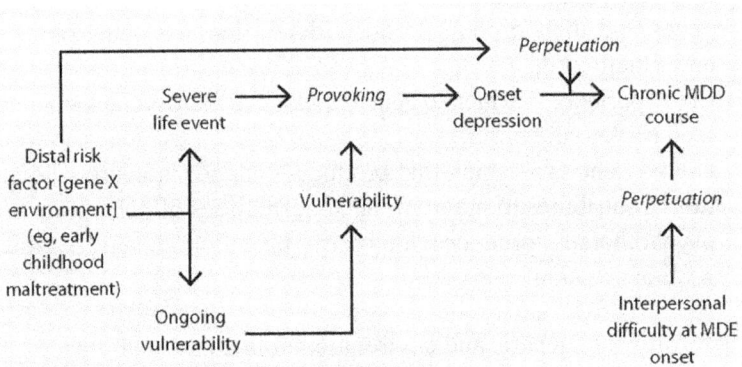

FIGURE 1.1 Modeling onset and course of depressive episodes. This model proposes mechanisms that are responsible for the onset, provocation, and perpetuation of depression. A "severe life event" can provoke the onset of a major depressive episode (MDE). Proximal risk factors (e.g., a poor-quality interpersonal relationship) mediate the onset of the depressive episode. Distal risk factors (e.g., early childhood maltreatment) both mediate the proximal risk factors (life events and ongoing vulnerabilities) and foster the perpetuation of a chronic illness course. MDD, major depressive disorder. Reproduced with permission from Brown et al., 2009.[13] ©Elsevier.

In addition, there are many medical diseases that commonly manifest with symptoms of depression, and many drugs can also produce depressive symptoms as adverse effects. Several other psychiatric diseases can also present with symptoms of depression, including schizophrenia, anxiety disorders, eating disorders, and substance abuse.

1.3 PRINCIPLES OF THERAPY

The essential principle in the effective treatment of depression is optimizing treatment on an individual basis. A variety of observer-rated and self-report measures is available to assess both severity and outcome after treatment,[14,15] and some of the most common[16] are listed in Table 1.1.

TABLE 1.1 Commonly Used Outcome Measures.

Outcome	Measure	Comment
Observer rated		
Symptoms	Hamilton Depression Rating Scale (HDRS)	The HDRS has a greater emphasis on somatic symptoms compared with the MADRS. The CGI is a single overall assessment of illness severity
	Montgomery–Asberg Depression Rating Scale (MADRS)	
	Clinical Global Impression (CGI)	
Adverse effects (AEs)	Spontaneous report	Although categorization of AEs has been standardized, systematically elicited assessment is rare
Function	Global Assessment of Functioning (GAF)	GAF is a composite measure of symptom severity and function
Self-rated		
Symptoms	Beck Depression Inventory (BDI)	BDI is widely used and covers the range of depressive symptoms
	Hospital Anxiety and Depression Scale (HADS)	HADS includes anxiety assessment and omits somatic symptoms
	Patient Health Questionnaire (PHQ-9)	PHQ-9 rates how often depressive symptoms have been present rather than severity
Adverse effects	Global AE questionnaires not commonly used	Questionnaires for specific AEs are sometimes used (e.g., for sexual AEs)
Function	Medical Outcomes Study Short Form 36 (SF-36)	The SF-36 assesses functioning and health status
Quality of life	EuroQol 5D (EQ-5D)	A simple global health measure used in for health economic analyses

Reproduced with permission from Freidman et al. *Handbook of Depression*, 2nd edition © Springer; 2014.

1.3.1 ALLOSTATIC LOAD

The complex processes in the brain identify and characterize what is stress. Stress response involves two-way communication between the brain and the cardiovascular, immune, metabolic, and other systems via the nervous system, endocrine system, and hypothalamic–pituitary–adrenal (HPA) axis. Homeostasis refers to the mechanisms that keep the parameters of an organism's internal milieu within the ranges necessary for survival. Maintaining a state of optimal homeostasis demands incurring the least possible long-term costs while an organism addresses the immediate needs. McEwen[17] (Fig. 1.2) proposes that allostasis is the adaptive process of maintaining stability during conditions that are outside of the usual homeostatic range. Allostatic load is the cost to the body for maintaining this stability during deviations from the usual homeostatic range, often reflected in pathophysiological conditions and disease progression. Physiologic systems activated by stress can both protect the body in the short term and damage the body in the long term, especially when stress becomes chronic and an allostatic load is incurred. For example, in response to a real or perceived threat, elevated blood pressure and heart rate due to increased sympathetic nervous system (SNS) activity is beneficial in the short term for survival. But a state of sustained high SNS activity, often due to sustained stress response, has diverse long-term effects with increased risk of cardiovascular and other chronic disorders.

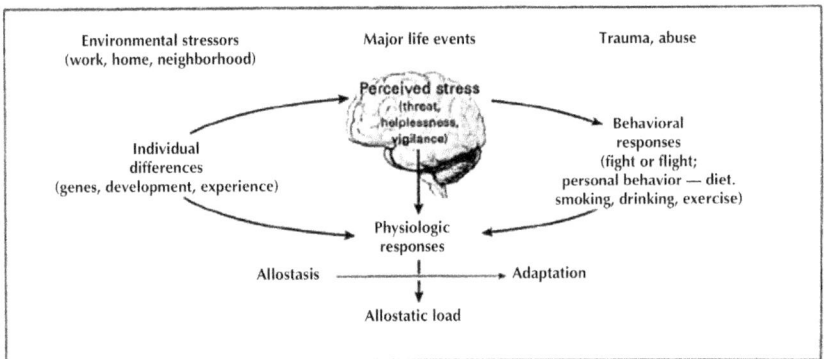

FIGURE 1.2 The stress response and development of allostatic load are illustrated. Reproduced with permission from McEwen © 2000 Nature Publishing Group.[17]

In stress, exacerbated disorders like depression, stress from psychological, physically external, and physically internal sources result in allostatic load. Various interventions for depression include pharmacotherapy; psychotherapy, physical therapy, and various mind–body therapies including yoga; and noninvasive and invasive surgical therapies. Ideal interventions reduce allostatic load and shift the regulatory systems toward optimal homeostasis.

1.4 MANAGEMENT OF DEPRESSION

In the management of depression options include, pharmacotherapy, psychotherapy, exercise, yoga, and other mind–body therapies, and several emerging treatments. Patient preferences and prior treatment history should always be taken into account. The commonly adopted stepped-care model proposes that the least intrusive, most effective intervention is provided first. If the initial intervention shows no benefit or if the individual declines an intervention, an appropriate intervention from the next step should be offered.

1.4.1 PHARMACOTHERAPY

1.4.1.1 MONOAMINE-BASED ANTIDEPRESSANT DRUGS

Narrow focus, over the last three decades, on increasing monoamine levels in the synaptic cleft (by blocking reuptake or degradation of monoamines) was overly simplistic. Monoaminergic neurotransmission is extremely complex and includes several neurotransmitters, presynaptic and postsynaptic receptors, transporters, and enzymes that determine the availability and the effects of the specific monoaminergic transmitter. The exact mechanism by which antidepressants exert their effects remains incompletely understood. Still pharmacologic modulation of monoamines is the first line of treatment and includes SSRIs and 5HT–noradrenaline reuptake inhibitors.

1.4.1.2   TOLERABILITY AND EFFICACY

All of the monoamine-based antidepressant drugs, regardless of their pharmacological class, have fundamentally modest efficacy, with response rates around 50%, and show a characteristic delayed (typically more than several weeks) response to treatment. In addition, they are associated with long-term adverse effects including weight gain, sexual dysfunction, and sleep disturbances.

1.4.2   PSYCHOTHERAPY

Psychotherapy for depression comes in many different forms. These different paradigms rely on different conceptual models and prescribe techniques that vary to some degree in their focus and methods. The most classical, cognitive–behavioral therapy teaches the patient with depression to identify negative, distorted thinking patterns that contribute to depression and provides skills to test and challenge these negative thoughts, replacing them with more accurate positive ones. Psychotherapy produces effects that are mostly equivalent to pharmacotherapy. Although it is clearly effective, many people have barriers to access, including time constraints, lack of available services, and cost.

1.4.3   PHYSICAL EXERCISE AND MIND–BODY THERAPIES

Exercise: Regular exercise is important for maintaining good physical and mental health.[18] Exercise is generally classified as aerobic (e.g., running or walking), resistance (e.g., weight training), or mindfulness based (e.g., yoga or qigong).

Yoga: Yoga is used in the treatment of depression in various contexts. Evidence is available that yoga can provide remission from depression in both naïve depression patients[19] and in depressed patients who are taking antidepressant medications but who are only in partial remission.[20]

1.4.4   COMPLEMENTARY AND INTEGRATIVE HEALTH TREATMENTS

Complementary and integrative health treatments have been used either alone or in combination with conventional therapies in patients with depression. They include

- dietary supplements (nutraceuticals)—*S*-adenosylmethionine,[21]
- herbs—St John's-wort, *Rhodiola rosea*, Saffron, and others,[22]
- folate,[23–25]
- acupuncture,
- omega-3 fatty acids, and
- hormones—dehydroepiandrosterone.

1.4.5 EMERGING TREATMENTS FOR DEPRESSION

1.4.5.1   ANTIDEPRESSANT DRUGS THAT ARE NOT MONOAMINE BASED

These are being developed to decrease untoward side-effects. Compounds that are under development include

- neurokinin-1 antagonists,
- glutamatergic system modulators,
- anti-inflammatory agents,
- opioid tone modulators and opioid-κ antagonists,
- hippocampal neurogenesis-stimulating treatments, and
- antiglucocorticoid therapies.

The degree of advancement in the development process varies across these different mechanisms, although all of these types of compounds have shown some degree of promise in the treatment of depression.

1.4.5.2   NOVEL PHARMACOLOGICAL APPROACHES

Novel approaches are being considered, which improve neuroplasticity and other biological mechanisms.

- Parenteral or intranasal administration of the glutamatergic drugs ketamine or esketamine, which are antagonists of N-methyl-d-aspartate.
- Intravenous scopolamine.
- The opioid modulator ALKS 5461.

Their efficacy is not well established yet for these treatments.

1.4.5.3   INVASIVE AND NONINVASIVE NEUROLOGICAL INTERVENTIONS

These treatments are commonly used in treatment resistant depression. They include

- electroconvulsive therapy,
- repetitive transcranial magnetic stimulation (TMS),
- deep TMS,
- transcranial direct current stimulation,
- low-field magnetic stimulation,
- vagus nerve stimulation, and
- deep brain stimulation.

They are providing new clues into biological mechanisms in depression and some of them may be used as first-line treatment in future.

1.4.6   COMBINED PHARMACOTHERAPY AND NONPHARMACOLOGICAL TREATMENTS

Several studies have shown that initiating treatment with both psychotherapy and pharmacotherapy produces significantly better outcomes than either treatment alone.

1.4.7 TECHNOLOGY-SUPPORTED CARE

Depression intervention technologies, which use computers, tablets, and phones to manage depression,[26] are effective at reducing symptoms of depression, when applied correctly. The rapid rate at which technology advances means that technology-based interventions will continue to grow and evolve rapidly. An emerging area of technology is digital phenotyping, which harnesses the growing availability of data generated continuously in the course of daily lives to create behavioral markers related to depression. Harnessing personal sensing platforms has the potential to shift our treatment tools from episodic to continuous, from reactive to proactive and from provider-centered to patient-centered.

1.5 SCIENTIFIC BASIS FOR THE BENEFITS OF YOGA

Yoga is one of the commonest forms of complementary and alternative medicine therapies, which is increasingly being practiced worldwide.[27] It is an ancient Indian practice based on the principles of mind–body medicine. The word "yoga" comes from the Sanskrit "yuj," meaning "yoke" or "union." Among the many forms of yoga, Rajyoga is commonly adopted in modern yoga-based interventions and is practiced through multiple steps, guided by Patanjali's Ashtanga (eight limbs) principles,[28] comprising of *yama* (moral codes, self-control), *niyama* (self-purification and process for maintaining morality), *asana* (posture), *pranayama* (breath control), *pratyahara* (governing sense), *dharana* (concentration), *dhyana* (meditation), and *samadhi* (supreme contemplation and meditation).

Yoga has been used to treat a variety of conditions including neurological and psychiatric disorders. Evidence emerging from the multiple studies on the beneficial effects of yoga on these diverse conditions suggests numerous mechanisms of its action. Effects of yoga in medical conditions like depression with overlapping pathophysiologies can be explained based on the principle that yoga practices reduce allostatic load in stress response systems and restore optimal homeostasis. Reduction in allostatic load, associated with pathogenesis of depression, by yoga can be understood by analyzing the effects at the level of modifications in pathophysiological processes. Despite advances in our understanding of the neurobiology of depression, currently no established mechanism can explain all facets of the disease. Accordingly, we restrict our description of the mechanism of benefits of yoga to pathophysiological models of depression that are supported by findings from clinical studies. Yoga has both physical and mental components, and benefits from yoga are derived from the unique integration of changes in both mind and body.

Physical activity (PA) and exercise component of yoga: Modernity has formalized exercise undertaken by the average person and reduced the amount of work- and leisure-time PA. Our lifestyles are increasingly sedentary, with the resultant side-effect of lifestyle related chronic and complex medical conditions like depression and obesity, currently recognized as a major health problems worldwide. While adequate PA (based on clinical guidelines) is associated with fewer depressive symptoms, insufficient PA is a risk factor for DDs. Large systematic reviews suggest that exercise improves depression. Any form of PA is known to increase neuroplasticity in the brain.[29] PA in any form increases resilience to stress.[30] Exercise lowers cortisol, alters neurotransmitter function, and even promotes growth of the hippocampus, a phenomenon also seen after prolonged antidepressant use.[31] The positive impact of exercise on depression is mainly attributed to an increase in 5HT, NE, and endorphins in the brain. Numerous other studies support the benefits of moderate aerobic exercise on depression in various populations.[32,33] This risk factors may be best modified in early development, as regular PA since childhood reduces the risk of developing depression in adulthood. Yoga- and meditation-based lifestyle intervention is relatively safe and has been shown to provide a range of additional health benefits. Yoga also increases self-efficacy and self-esteem (via activity scheduling and attainment of goals) which are important psychological issues among people who are depressed.[34]

Meditation, mindfulness, and mental component of yoga: Meditative practices have an application in improving mood and preventing the tumescence of a depressive episode. A key aspect of meditation practice involves self-awareness (mindfulness), which arises through paying attention in the present moment, and nonjudgmentally. The use of meditation commonly involves both mindful awareness during yoga practice and mindfulness during everyday situations and social interactions, which may be relatively perceived as stressful. Meditative practices can be readily incorporated into people's lives and requires only basic training. Meditation regulates the emotional responses and improves the cognitive functioning by several mechanisms. Electroencephalographic studies have

revealed a significant increase in alpha and theta activity during meditation. Meditation has shown elevations in whole blood 5HT levels.[35] An
increase in melatonin and decrease in cortisol have been associated with
the meditative component of yoga.[36] Each of these factors contributes to
maintain optimum homeostasis. For example, a rise in melatonin promotes
circadian rhythms like sleep and improves mind–body communications by
appropriately modifying immune system and stress response. Numerous
studies have suggested that decreasing sustained levels of cortisol may
decrease depression symtoms.[37,38]

Yoga and stress reduction: There is a cyclic relationship in neurological
mechanisms involved in depression and stress responsivity. Therefore,
there is a "kindling" effect in the chronic nature of depression, such that
every episode of depression increases the likelihood of recurrence.[38] There
is a strong link between stress and depression, and increased stress levels
can significantly affect the severity of depression. Stress is considered
to be one of the most significant predictors of health and depression is
a leading contributor to global burden of disease and increased risk of
mortality. Research indicates that yoga can reduce stress in depression and
associated conditions[39] and is fundamental to treatment of depression.

Early-life adverse events and yoga in early life: The HPA axis is at the
center of the comprehensive neurobiological model that seeks to explain
the long-lasting consequences of stress. Early-life stress produces persistent increases in the activity of corticotropin-releasing hormone-containing
neural circuits. Individuals who suffer from adverse life events in childhood show, as adults, a markedly enhanced activity of the HPA axis when
exposed to stressors. Indeed, glucocorticoid receptor function is reduced in
these individuals (so-called glucocorticoid resistance). These individuals
also show increased activation of the inflammatory system, which is under
physiological inhibitory control by cortisol. Indeed, glucocorticoid resistance, HPA axis hyperactivity and increased inflammation are all evident in
depression. Practitioners of yoga show resilience to stress and don't show
decreased levels of cortisol and inflammatory markers. Yoga interventions
in depression have shown to decrease cortisol and inflammatory markers.
Therefore, to decrease the impact of childhood adversity on the health
and wellbeing of the individual and prevent depression in adulthood, yoga
may be adopted from the earliest point of life possible.

Improvements in the markers of cellular aging: Stress and depression
are associated with increased risk of other chronic medical illnesses, and

increased morbidity and mortality. This correlation between depression and aging-related illnesses suggests that depression may be related to accelerated cellular aging.[40,41] The connection between depression and accelerated cellular aging involve several pathways, including stress response and inflammation. For example, inflammation is linked to telomere shortening and the cytokines that are involved in intercellular signaling for the regulation of infection and injury may be responsible for this link. Inflammation causes oxidative stress, which in turn leads to DNA damage and telomere shortening.

Evidence indicates that yoga intervention can slow-down accelerated aging and may improve following biomarkers of cellular aging in both apparently healthy[42,43] and clinically depressed patients.[38]

a.   Increase in telomere length and telomerase enzyme levels. Telomere length decreases due to aging, which is also seen in depression. Yoga reverses these changes.

b.   Reduction in oxidative stress.

c.   Reduction in inflammatory biomarkers like interleukin-6 (IL-6).

d.   Reduction in stress induced markers like cortisol.

Improvements in the markers of neuroplasticity: Yoga has been shown to moderate a range of biological pathways including neuroplasticity. Yoga stimulates the central nervous system release of endorphins, monoamines, and brain-derived neurotrophic factor in the hippocampus.[34,42] Evidence from several imaging studies indicate that regular practice of meditation and yoga a wide range of effects like alterations in gray matter morphology, increased cortical thickness in the prefrontal cortex (PFC) and right anterior insula,[44] increased oxygenated hemoglobin in the anterior PFC.[45,46] These findings suggest that yoga can increase neuroplasticity and decrease neurodegeneration associated with MDD. Yoga can not only provide remission from clinical depression, it can help prevent relapses in remitted patients. Yoga can also help development and adaptations of the brain to make individual stress resilient and prevent development of depression.

1.6 OUTLOOK FOR THE FUTURE OF YOGA IN DEPRESSION

It is important to consider yoga while giving due importance to other major components of lifestyle medicine, which include PA or exercise, dietary modification, adequate relaxation/sleep and social interaction, and the reduction of addictive habits such as smoking, drugs, and alcohol. One should also consider the influence of other lifestyle factors that have substantial potential to affect health, such as environmental issues (e.g., urbanization and pollution), and the increasing human interface with technology. While data supports that yoga (and other interventions) is a modifier of overall mental and physical health, rigorous research needs to address the long-term application of yoga for depression prevention and management. Critically, studies exploring lifestyle modification involving multiple lifestyle elements including yoga are needed. While the judicious use of medication and psychological techniques are still advocated, considering the complexity of human depression, regular yoga and lifestyle modification should be used as a routine part of treatment and preventative efforts.

KEYWORDS

- depression
- yoga
- meditation
- cellular aging
- neuroplasticity
- monoamine hypothesis
- allostatic load

REFERENCES

1. Bauer, U. E.; Briss, P. A.; Goodman, R. A.; Bowman, B. A. Prevention of Chronic Disease in the 21st Century: Elimination of the Leading Preventable Causes of Premature Death and Disability in the USA. *Lancet* **2015,** *384*(9937), 45–52.
2. Chesney, E.; Goodwin, G. M.; Fazel, S. Risks of All Cause and Suicide Mortality in Mental Disorders: A Meta-Review. *World Psychiatry* **2014,** *13*, 153–160.

3. Seedat, S. Cross-National Associations Between Gender and Mental Disorders in the World Health Organization World Mental Health Surveys. *Arch. Gen. Psychiatry* **2009**, *66*, 785–795.

4. Bromet, E. Cross-National Epidemiology of DSM-IV Major Depressive Episode. *BMC Med.* **2011**, *9*, 90.

5. Vahia, V. N. Diagnostic and Statistical Manual of Mental Disorders 5: A Quick Glance. *Indian J. Psychiatry* **2013**, *55*(3), 220–223.

6. Vos, T. Global, Regional, and National Incidence, Prevalence, and Years Lived with Disability for 301 Acute and Chronic Diseases and Injuries in 188 Countries, 1990–2013: A Systematic Analysis for the Global Burden of Disease Study 2013. *Lancet* **2015**, *386*, 743–800.

7. Kinderman, P. A Psychological Model of Mental Disorder. *Harv. Rev. Psychiatry* **2005**, *13*(4), 206–217.

8. Geschwind, D. H.; Flint, J. Genetics and Genomics of Psychiatric Disease. *Science* **2015**, *349*, 1489–1494.

9. Kessler, R. C. The Effects of Stressful Life Events on Depression. *Ann. Rev. Psychol.* **1997**, *48*, 191–214.

10. Margoob, M.; Mushtaq, D.; Murtza, I.; Mushtaq, H.; Ali, A. Serotonin Transporter Gene Polymorphism and Treatment Response to Serotonin Reuptake Inhibitor (Escitalopram) in Depression: An Open Pilot Study. *Indian J. Psychiatry* **2008**, *50*(1), 47.

11. Dean, J.; Keshavan, M. The Neurobiology of Depression: An Integrated View. *Asian J. Psychiatr.* **2017**, *27*, 101–111.

12. Murrough, J. W.; Abdallah, C. G.; Mathew, S. J. Targeting Glutamate Signalling in Depression: Progress and Prospects. *Nat. Rev. Drug Discov.* **2017**, *16*(7), 472–86.

13. Brown, D. W.; Anda, R. F.; Tiemeier, H.; Felitti, V. J.; Edwards, V. J.; Croft, J. B.; Giles, W. H. Adverse Childhood Experiences and the Risk of Premature Mortality. *Am. J. Prev. Med.* **2009**, *37*(5), 389–396.

14. Kamenov, K.; Cabello, M.; Nieto, M.; Bernard, R.; Kohls, E.; Rummel-Kluge, C.; Ayuso-Mateos, J. L. Research Recommendations for Improving Measurement of Treatment Effectiveness in Depression. *Front. Psychol.* **2017**, *8*, 356.

15. Lam, R. W.; Parikh, S. V.; Michalak, E. E.; Dewa, C. S.; Kennedy, S. H. Canadian Network for Mood and Anxiety Treatments (CANMAT) Consensus Recommendations for Functional Outcomes in Major Depressive Disorder. *Ann. Clin. Psychiatry* **2015**, *27*(2), 142–149.

16. Anderson, I. M. Principles of Therapy. In *Handbook of Depression*; Friedman, E. S., Anderson, I. M., Eds.; Springer Healthcare Ltd.: Tarporley, 2014; pp 33. Figure 4.2.

17. McEwen, B. S. Allostasis and Allostatic Load: Implications for Neuropsychopharmacology. *Neuropsychopharmacology* **2000**, *22*(2), 108–124.

18. Blumenthal, J. A.; Babyak, M. A.; Moore, K. A.; Craighead, W. E.; Herman, S.; Khatri, P.; Waugh, R.; Napolitano, M. A.; Forman, L. M.; Appelbaum, M.; Doraiswamy, P. M.; Krishnan, K. R. Effects of Exercise Training on Older Patients with Major Depression. *Arch. Intern. Med.* **1999**, *159*(19), 2349–2356.

19. Prathikanti, S.; Rivera, R.; Cochran, A.; Tungol, J. G.; Fayazmanesh, N.; Weinmann, E. Treating Major Depression with Yoga: A Prospective, Randomized, Controlled Pilot Trial. *PLoS One* **2017**, *12*(3), e0173869.

20. Shapiro, D.; Cook, I. A.; Davydov, D. M.; Ottaviani, C.; Leuchter, A. F.; Abrams, M. Yoga as a Complementary Treatment of Depression: Effects of Traits and Moods on Treatment Outcome. *Evid. Based Complement. Alternat. Med.* **2007**, *4*(4), 493–502.

21. Bottiglieri, T. *S*-Adenosyl-l-methionine (SAMe): From the Bench to the Bedside— Molecular Basis of a Pleiotrophic Molecule. *Am. J. Clin. Nutr.* **2002**, *76*(5), 1151s–1157s.

22. Shelton, R. C. St John's Wort (Hypericum Perforatum) in Major Depression. *J. Clin. Psychiatry* **2009**, *70*(Suppl 5), 23–27.

23. Farah, A. The Role of l-Methylfolate in Depressive Disorders. *CNS Spectr.* **2009**, *14*(1 Suppl 2), 2–7.

24. Morris, D. W.; Trivedi, M. H.; Rush, A. J. Folate and Unipolar Depression. *J. Altern. Complement. Med.* **2008**, *14*(3), 277–285.

25. Stahl, S. M. Novel Therapeutics for Depression: l-Methylfolate as a Trimonoamine Modulator and Antidepressant-Augmenting Agent. *CNS Spectr.* **2007**, *12*(10), 739–744.

26. Mohr, D. C.; Burns, M. N.; Schueller, S. M.; Clarke, G.; Klinkman, M. Behavioral Intervention Technologies: Evidence Review and Recommendations for Future Research in Mental Health. *Gen. Hosp. Psychiatry* **2013**, *35*, 332–338.

27. McCall, M. C.; Ward, A.; Roberts, N. W.; Heneghan, C. Overview of Systematic Reviews: Yoga as a Therapeutic Intervention for Adults with Acute and Chronic Health Conditions. *Evid. Based Complement. Alternat. Med.* **2013**, 945895.

28. Satchidananda, S. S. *The Yoga Sutras of Patanjali*; Integral Yoga Publications: Yogaville, Virginia, US, 2010.

29. Hötting, K.; Röder, B. Beneficial Effects of Physical Exercise on Neuroplasticity and Cognition. *Neurosci. Biobehav. Rev.* **2013**, *37*(9, Part B), 2243–2257.

30. Agudelo, L. Z.; Femenía, T.; Orhan, F.; Porsmyr-Palmertz, M.; Goiny, M.; Martinez-Redondo, V.; Correia, J. C.; Izadi, M.; Bhat, M.; Schuppe-Koistinen, I.; Pettersson, A. T.; Ferreira, D. M. S.; Krook, A.; Barres, R.; Zierath, J. R.; Erhardt, S.; Lindskog, M.; Ruas, J. L. Skeletal Muscle PGC-1α1 Modulates Kynurenine Metabolism and Mediates Resilience to Stress-Induced Depression. *Cell* **2014**, *159*(1), 33–45.

31. Lucassen, P. J.; Meerlo, P.; Naylor, A. S.; van Dam, A. M.; Dayer, A. G.; Fuchs, E.; Oomen, C. A.; Czeh, B. Regulation of Adult Neurogenesis by Stress, Sleep Disruption, Exercise and Inflammation: Implications for Depression and Antidepressant Action. *Eur. Neuropsychopharmacol.* **2010**, *20*(1), 1–17.

32. Dunn, A. L.; Trivedi, M. H.; Kampert, J. B.; Clark, C. G.; Chambliss, H. O. Exercise Treatment for Depression: Efficacy and Dose Response. *Am. J. Prev. Med.* **2005**, *28*(1), 1–8.

33. Richardson, C. R.; Avripas, S. A.; Neal, D. L.; Marcus, S. M. Increasing Lifestyle Physical Activity in Patients with Depression or Other Serious Mental Illness. *J. Psychiatr. Pract.* **2005**, *11*(6), 379–388.

34. Mathersul, D. C.; Rosenbaum, S. The Roles of Exercise and Yoga in Ameliorating Depression as a Risk Factor for Cognitive Decline. *Evid. Based Complement. Alternat. Med.* **2016**, *2016*, 4612953.

35. Yu, X.; Fumoto, M.; Nakatani, Y.; Sekiyama, T.; Kikuchi, H.; Seki, Y.; Sato-Suzuki, I.; Arita, H. Activation of the Anterior Prefrontal Cortex and Serotonergic System

is Associated with Improvements in Mood and EEG Changes Induced by Zen Meditation Practice in Novices. *Int. J. Psychophysiol.* **2011**, *80*(2), 103–111.

36. Tooley, G. A.; Armstrong, S. M.; Norman, T. R.; Sali, A. Acute Increases in Night-Time Plasma Melatonin Levels Following a Period of Meditation. *Biol. Psychol.* **2000**, *53*(1), 69–78.

37. Thirthalli, J.; Naveen, G. H.; Rao, M. G.; Varambally, S.; Christopher, R.; Gangadhar, B. N. Cortisol and Antidepressant Effects of Yoga. *Indian J. Psychiatry* **2013**, *55*(Suppl 3), S405–S408.

38. Kinser, P. A.; Lyon, D. E. Major Depressive Disorder and Measures of Cellular Aging: An Integrative Review. *Nurs. Res. Pract.* **2013**, *2013*, 469070.

39. Riley, J. Estimates of Regional and Global Life Expectancy, 1800–2001. *Popul. Dev. Rev.* **2005**, *31*(3), 537–543.

40. Lin, J.; Epel, E.; Blackburn, E. Telomeres and Lifestyle Factors: Roles in Cellular Aging. *Mutat. Res.* **2012**, *730*(1–2), 85–89.

41. Verhoeven, J. E.; Revesz, D.; Epel, E. S.; Lin, J.; Wolkowitz, O. M.; Penninx, B. W. Major Depressive Disorder and Accelerated Cellular Aging: Results from a Large Psychiatric Cohort Study. *Mol. Psychiatry* **2014**, *19*(8), 895–901.

42. Tolahunase, M.; Sagar, R.; Dada, R. Impact of Yoga and Meditation on Cellular Aging in Apparently Healthy Individuals: A Prospective, Open-Label Single-Arm Exploratory Study. *Oxid. Med. Cell. Longev.* **2017**, *2017*, 9.

43. Epel, E. S.; Puterman, E.; Lin, J.; Blackburn, E. H.; Lum, P. Y.; Beckmann, N. D.; Zhu, J.; Lee, E.; Gilbert, A.; Rissman, R. A.; Tanzi, R. E.; Schadt, E. E. Meditation and Vacation Effects have an Impact on Disease-Associated Molecular Phenotypes. *Transl. Psychiatry* **2016**, *6*, e880.

44. Hölzel, B. K.; Carmody, J.; Vangel, M.; Congleton, C.; Yerramsetti, S. M.; Gard, T.; Lazar, S. W. Mindfulness Practice Leads to Increases in Regional Brain Gray Matter Density. *Psychiatry Res. Neuroimaging* **2011**, *191*(1), 36–43.

45. Singh, K.; Bhargav, H.; Srinivasan, T. M. Effect of Uninostril Yoga Breathing on Brain Hemodynamics: A Functional Near-Infrared Spectroscopy Study. *Int. J. Yoga* **2016**, *9*(1), 12–19.

46. Deepeshwar, S.; Vinchurkar, S. A.; Visweswaraiah, N. K.; Nagendra, H. R. Hemodynamic Responses on Prefrontal Cortex Related to Meditation and Attentional Task. *Front. Syst. Neurosci.* **2014**, *8*, 252.

CHAPTER 2

RETINOBLASTOMA: A DISEASE FOR CONCERN, ROLE OF YOGA, AND MEDITATION-BASED LIFESTYLE INTERVENTION IN REDUCING THE CHILDHOOD DISEASE BURDEN

SHILPA BISHT, SHIV B. KUMAR, and RIMA DADA*

Laboratory for Molecular Reproduction and Genetics, AIIMS, New Delhi 110029, India

Corresponding author. E-mail: rima_dada@rediffmail.com

ABSTRACT

Retinoblastoma is the most common childhood intraocular malignancy and ranks fourth in the list of mortalities in Indian children. Oxidative stress (OS) and oxidative DNA damage cause peroxidative damage to the sperm plasma membrane, DNA fragmentation in sperm nuclear/ mitochondrial genome, and dysregulation in levels of mRNAs/transcripts. OS-induced sperm DNA damage is associated with pathologies such as male infertility, recurrent pregnancy loss, congenital malformations, and high frequency of childhood disorders including childhood cancers. The etiology of childhood cancer and increased disease burden is linked to OS and oxidative DNA damage in sperm of their fathers. OS is predominantly caused by a host of lifestyle-related factors, the majority of which are modifiable by adoption of simple lifestyle interventions. Yoga and meditation cause significant decline in OS and oxidative DNA damage and aid in regulating OS levels such that reactive oxygen species-meditated signal transduction, gene expression, and several other physiological functions are not disrupted. Yoga and meditation-based interventions help in improving sperm DNA integrity thereby reducing the sperm-associated pathologies and childhood disorders including childhood cancers in the next generations.

2.1   INTRODUCTION

Retinoblastoma (Rb) is the most common neoplasm of the eye in childhood, accounting for about 3% of all the childhood cancers.[1] Rb affects the children at a very younger age with about two-thirds of the cases diagnosed before 2 years of age, and more than 90% of the cases are diagnosed before the age of 5 years. The worldwide incidence of Rb is reported to be around 1 case in every 15,000–20,000 live births which corresponds to about 9000 newly diagnosed Rb cases every year.[2] The basis for Rb development was first explained by *Alfred G. Knudson's Two-hit hypothesis which explains that* "Two mutational events are rate limiting for the development of Retinoblastoma and all cases of Retinoblastoma develops as a result of loss-of-function of both the copies of *RB1* tumor-suppressor gene."[3] *RB1* was the first identified tumor-suppressor gene located on 13q14.2, and its discovery has set the paradigm for the discovery of novel tumor-suppressor and oncogenes that play an important role in tumor invasion and metastasis.[4] Rb is clinically distinguished into two forms: bilateral or multifocal, heritable form which accounts for about 40% of all the cases and associated with biallelic inactivation of *RB1* gene where the first hit is constitutional, and the second hit occurs somatically in one or more retinal cells. The unilateral or unifocal form of Rb is nonheritable in nature and accounts for about 60% of all the cases where both *RB1* alleles are damaged only in the developing retina, but 15% of the unilateral cases also carry a heritable constitutional mutation in the *RB1* gene.[5] In case of children with bilateral heritable disease, a constitutional *RB1* mutation is already present that predisposes to Rb and one additional hit damages the second *RB1* allele and initiates Rb or may initiate other cancers later in life such as lung, bladder, bone, skin, and brain cancer. In the developing countries, the mean age at diagnosis is 27 months for unilateral Rb and 15 months for bilateral Rb. Genetic testing in unilateral cases is essential as preliminary investigation for Rb because in the absence of a positive family history, unilateral cases may involve the germ line *RB1* mutation and, thus, are capable of being transmitted to the next generation.[6]

In 2013, Gallie et al. discovered a new subset of unilateral nonfamilial Rb tumors characterized by no detectable *RB1* mutations (*RB1*[+/+]), high-level *MYCN* oncogene amplification (28–121 copies), distinct aggressive histological features, poor prognosis, and very early age of diagnosis, that is, 4.5 months as compared with 27 months for children with nonfamilial unilateral (*RB1*[−/−]) Rb. These *RB1*[+/+]/*MYCN*[A] cases constitute 1% of all Rb tumors. This new subset of Rb has challenged the dogma that this cancer is always initiated by the loss-of-function of both the copies of *RB1* gene.[7] The role of *MYCN* in Rb pathogenesis needs to be further investigated as it may act as a tumor driver in the absence of nonmutated *RB1* gene.

Oxidative stress (OS) which is caused by an imbalance in the production of reactive oxygen species (ROS) and antioxidant defenses in the cell is associated with damage in the cellular components, inactivates essential metabolic enzymes, and disrupts signal transduction pathways.[8] OS is also associated with peroxidative damage to the sperm plasma membrane, DNA fragmentation in sperm nuclear/mitochondrial genome and causes dysregulation in levels of mRNAs/transcripts.[9] OS-induced sperm DNA damage is associated with male infertility, recurrent pregnancy loss, congenital malformations, and high frequency of childhood disorders including childhood cancers.[10] Parental age, particularly advanced paternal age (>40 years), is associated with differential methylation patterns in the paternal sperm DNA which may lead to de novo germ line mutations and, hence, increased disease risk in the next progeny.[11]

Yoga is a comprehensive philosophical system that seeks to bring into balance all the disparate aspects of body, mind, and personality. The practice of yoga has a strong historical and cultural significance in India which has emerged as one of the leading countries for studies on yoga interventions.[12] Yoga is currently gaining prominence as an alternative for improving physical and mental wellbeing even in western societies.[13] Yoga system comprises of collection of asanas (postures), pranayama (breathing exercises), and dhyana (meditation). Yoga is practiced to reduce stress and to treat anxiety, high blood pressure, and musculoskeletal conditions. Simple lifestyle interventions involving "yoga" and "meditation" improve muscle function, body composition, peak oxygen consumption, peak power output, and exercise tolerance.[14] With many reviews and guidelines published within the last couple of years, evidence of the effectiveness of yoga in alleviating adverse effects of primary cancer therapy and in improving the quality of life is emerging.[15] However, till date, no report on effect of yoga and meditation on nuclear genome has been reported. Adoption of mind–body exercise such as yoga has an impact on muscular activity with internally directed focus, producing a temporary self-contemplative mental state. It also triggers neurohormonal mechanisms that bring about health benefits, evidenced by the suppression of sympathetic activity.[16] Rb is the most common childhood cancer in prevalence, and its incidence is increasing in the developing countries. In addition to exposure to environmental pollutants (air and water borne), insecticides and pesticides which took toll on human health, one of the targets is the male germ cell, a cell most vulnerable to various environmental insults. This has led to significant reduction in quality of sperm, though the sperm may possess normal motility with normal morphology. The various external environmental factors and internal milieu may adversely affect sperm mitochondrial and nuclear genome, and loss of genome integrity may lead to adverse health outcome of offspring by increasing mutagenic load in sperm and by affecting its epigenome. Studies from our lab has shown that yoga and meditation can not only decrease the mutagenic load in a cell but also affect epigenome by increasing expression levels of antioxidant genes and by decreasing levels of inflammatory cytokines.[17] This has highly significant impact on the health of next generations and, thus, may reduce disease burden. Paternal sperm DNA damage may be one of the causative factors for initiating cancers and other birth defects or neuropsychiatric disorders in their children during early childhood. Lifestyle interventions like "yoga" and "meditation" may help in reducing OS and thus, may result in improving quality of paternal sperm DNA, and this may help in reducing the burden of childhood cancers or other diseases in the next progeny.

2.2 PATERNAL SPERM DNA DAMAGE AND INCREASING INCIDENCES OF CHILDHOOD CANCERS

DNA damage, largely owing to OS, is a major cause of defective sperm function and has been correlated with adverse clinical outcomes including impaired fertilization, disrupted preimplantation, low rates of implantation, increased incidences of miscarriages, high rate of morbidity, and childhood disorders in the offspring including childhood cancers and diminished fertility.[18] OS not only disrupts the integrity of sperm DNA but also limits its fertilizing potential as a result of collateral damage to proteins and lipids in the plasma membrane of sperm. The origins of such OS appear to involve the sperm mitochondria, which have a tendency to generate high levels of superoxide anion as a prelude to entering the intrinsic apoptotic pathway.[19] The factors responsible for inducing sperm DNA damage are many ranging from unhealthy lifestyle-related factors, such as smoking, excessive alcohol intake, high intake of saturated food, obesity, advanced age, and physical or environmental factors, such as heat, air pollution, and electromagnetic radiation, as well as a range of various xenobiotic compounds, chemotherapeutic agents, abnormalities of lipid metabolism, etc. These all factors together contribute to OS in the human spermatozoa causing sperm DNA damage and fragmentation.[20] It is clini- cally evidenced that damage to human sperm DNA may adversely affect reproductive outcomes and that spermatozoa of infertile men possess substantially more DNA damage than do spermatozoa of fertile men which further increase the burden of childhood diseases including childhood cancers in the next progeny.[21]

Recent studies from our lab have documented increased incidence of childhood cancers born to fathers with advanced paternal age and men who smoke and consume tobacco in any form.[22] Epigenome is a continu- ously changing entity affected both by internal and external factors. OS up-regulate the levels of DNA methyltransferases and, thus, seminal OS may lead to epigenetic alterations, and a recent study has reported that paternal sperm DNA methylation is associated with early signs of autism.[11] Alterations in the sperm epigenome may cause hypermethylation of tumor suppressor genes and hypomethylation of repetitive elements which is may be the underlying pathology in oncogenesis and increased risk of child- hood cancers in the next generation.[23] Assisted reproductive technologies (ARTs) such as in vitro fertilization and intra cytoplasmic sperm injection (ICSI) have been currently utilized with a pace to overcome the problems associated with advanced maternal age and male factor infertility.[24] When ARTs are used to address defective sperm function, the natural selection process that occurs during fertilization is bypassed and might result in an increased risk of birth defects and genetic and/or epigenetic abnormalities in the child.[25] An increase in incidence of cancer has also been reported in children conceived by ARTs.[26] Recent studies have also investigated an increase in the hospitalization of ARTs offspring in infancy and early childhood compared with children who are conceived spontaneously,

whereas other investigations have revealed abnormal retinal vasculariza-
tion and an eightfold increase in the incidence of undescended testicles in
boys conceived by ICSI.[27]

Paternal cigarette smoking is another risk factor for increasing incidences of childhood cancers in the next progeny.[28] The gaseous as well
as particulate contents of cigarette smoke, which include several notable
carcinogens, such as cadmium, radioactive polonium, benzopyrenes,
dimethylbenzanthracene, naphthalene, methylnaphthalene, and, among
others, polycyclic aromatic hydrocarbons, have a profound negative effect
on sperm parameters (including the motility, morphology, and sperm
count), cause OS, and therefore have negative effects on reproductive
outcomes.[29] Antioxidant enzymes and small molecular mass free radical
scavengers are also generated in the male tract and are major constituents
of the antioxidant protection afforded to the spermatozoa by seminal
plasma. The most important of these scavengers are vitamin C, uric acid,
tryptophan, spermine, and taurine.[30] If antioxidants such as ascorbate are
depleted, for example, by heavy smoking, the result is OS within the male
reproductive tract and DNA damage to the spermatozoa.[31] Men who are
heavy smokers have shown increased levels of oxidative DNA base adduct
8-hydroxy-2'deoxyguanosine (8-OHdG), high chromatin fragmentation,
and low concentrations of antioxidant vitamins in their semen ejaculates.[22]
As a consequence, DNA-damaged spermatozoa from heavy smokers are
able to engage in the process of fertilization, with consequences for the
ultimate health and well-being of the embryo. Thus, the offspring of heavy
smokers are four to five times more likely to develop childhood cancer
than the children of nonsmoking fathers.[32] Furthermore, some studies have
shown that possible mutagenic–promutagenic effects of smoking on DNA
integrity in the male germ line has been reinforced that 15% of all childhood cancers are directly attributable to paternal smoking.[33]

2.3   HUMAN SPERM DNA AND CHROMATIN STRUCTURE

Unlike the relatively loose structure of chromatin (DNA and nuclear
histone proteins) in somatic cells, human sperm chromatin is often poorly
compacted and frequently contains DNA strand breaks.[34] In addition, the
likelihood of damage to the mitochondrial genome during the differentiation and functional lifespan of a spermatozoon is so great that these

structures are ubiquitinated and destroyed in the oocyte after fertilization, to overcome the risk of them contributing to the embryonic mitochondrial pool.[9] During spermatogenesis, the spermatid nucleus is remodeled and condensed, which is associated with the displacement of histones by transition proteins and then by protamines. The DNA strands are tightly wrapped around the protamine molecules (about 50 kb of DNA per prot-amine), forming tight and highly organized loops.[35] Such a high level of condensation of the sperm nucleus aids in maintenance of the hydrody-namic shape, which aids both in sperm motility and its transit through the male and female reproductive tract and vital for maintenance of genomic integrity maintaining the epigenetic imprints.[36] Inter and intramolecular disulfide cross-links between the cysteine-rich protamines are responsible for the compaction and stabilization of the sperm nucleus. Protamines are highly basic (rich in arginine) and are the most abundant nuclear proteins in many species, including mammals, and provide extensive packaging of the sperm genome.[37] It is thought that this nuclear compaction is important to protect the sperm genome from external stresses such as oxidation or temperature elevation. The current understanding is that sperm chromatin is tightly packaged by protamines, but up to 15% of the DNA remains packaged by histones at specific DNA sequences (i.e., there is a nonrandom association between histones and DNA sequences). The histone-bound DNA sequences are less tightly compacted and include the telomeres and promoters of genes that are involved in fertilization and early embryo development.[38] The retained histones are associated with the nuclear periphery and with telomeres. Although the bulk of the sperm DNA is in the nucleus, a small fraction is of mitochondrial origin (within the sperm midpiece). The sperm mitochondrial DNA is a small, circular DNA that is not bound to proteins. Mitochondria are the source as well as the targets of ROS-induced damage and free-radical oxidation to the spermatozoa, and mitochondrial DNA exhibits a high rate of mutation because of the absence of histone protection and very limited capacity for DNA damage repair due to a complete lack of nucleotide-excision repair mechanism.[39] Sperm motility is related to the mitochondrial volume within the sperm midpiece, and mutations or deletions in the mitochondrial DNA have been associated with reduced sperm motility. The mutation rate of mitochondrial DNA is estimated to be two orders of magnitude higher than that of nuclear DNA and mitochondria harboring mutations produce more free radicals and less ATP than their fully functional counterparts.[40]Although inheritance of mitochondrial DNA is primarily maternal, but paternal transmission of mitochondrial DNA mutations have also been reported.[41]

2.4 CAUSES OF SPERM DNA DAMAGE

OS induces fragmentation in both nuclear and mitochondrial DNA and affects sperm motility by peroxidative damage to axoneme and depletion in intracellular ATP and also results in impairment in development and differentiation of microtubule apparatus. Spermatozoa with tremendously higher levels of DNA damaged due to chromatin fragmentation as a result of elevated OS have very low potential for natural fertility.[42] It is essential to explore the factors that cause decline in sperm function which disrupt genomic integrity and factors which aid in its maintenance. Defective sperm function is encompassed by multifaceted causal factors including genetic, epigenetic, age, environment, and lifestyle which work individually or in consortium to exert their detrimental impact on sperm function.[43] Unhealthy lifestyle-related factors such as smoking, excessive alcohol intake, a diet rich in saturated fats and proteins, a sedentary lifestyle, psychological stress, obesity and advanced paternal age (>40 years of age) all contribute to the risk of elevated OS and, hence, sperm DNA damage. Furthermore, environmental factors such as exposure to air pollution or to persistent organic pollutants, exposure to high temperatures, plasticizers, metals (particularly transition metals such as cadmium, lead, iron, and copper), chemotherapeutic agents, environmental toxicants (acrylamide, endosulfan, bisphenol A, and phthalates), electromagnetic radiation, systemic and testicular infection, and varicocele can all increase the levels of OS in spermatozoa.[44]

During early development, apoptosis plays a major role in the ontogeny of the germ line as a means of regulating the germ cell: Sertoli cell ratio, which ultimately defines the extent of male fertility.[45] The theory that sperm DNA damage is may be due to apoptosis (programmed cell death) has been challenged. Apoptosis during normal spermatogenesis results in the destruction of up to 75% of potential spermatozoa. The selective apoptosis of these early germ cells prevents over proliferation of the cells and selectively aborts abnormal sperm forms.[33] Advancing age and gonadotoxins (e.g., cancer therapies) have been associated with reduced levels of germ cell apoptosis in the testicle and an increased percentage of ejaculated spermatozoa with DNA damage, which suggests that in these men both spermatogenesis and apoptosis have been disrupted.[46] A majority of factors, including unhealthy lifestyles, exposure to electromagnetic radiation, exposure to environmental toxins, use of chemotherapeutic agents such as cisplatin, exposure to bisphenol A and deletions in spermatogenesis regulatory genes, in both human and experimental animals, might also lead to induction of apoptosis. All these factors can promote the generation of OS, which has adverse effects on spermatogenesis and generates spermatozoa with poorly remodeled chromatin.[47] Physiological strand breaks are a possible cause of DNA damage in the male germ line. DNA fragmentation in spermatozoa is a result of unresolved strand breaks created during the normal process of spermiogenesis in order to relieve the torsional stress involved in packaging a very large amount of DNA into a very small sperm head.[48] Normally, these "physiological" strand breaks are corrected by a complex process involving H2Ax phosphorylation and the subsequent activation of nuclear poly(adenosine diphosphate-ribose) polymerase and topoisomerase. However, if spermiogenesis has been disrupted for some reason, then the restoration of these cleavage sites might be impaired and the spermatozoa, lacking any capacity for DNA repair in their own right, would be released from the germinal epithelium still carrying their unresolved strand breaks.[49] The majority of the DNA damage encountered by spermatozoa is caused by oxidative stress. The effects of OS are compounded by the physical architecture of human spermatozoa, which prevents nucleases from entering the sperm nuclear DNA and inducing fragmentation. The apoptotic cascade, which is initiated as a result of excessive generation of ROS and OS, impedes essential sperm function, thus rendering the sperm inactive and immotile. Thus, the development of therapies that ameliorate or inhibit oxidative-stress-induced apoptosis in sperm cells is an immediate requirement.[30]

2.5   OXIDATIVE STRESS IN THE MALE GERM LINE

One of the major contributory factors to defective sperm function is OS. The human spermatozoa have the capacity to generate ROS such as superoxide anion and have the proven ability of ROS-induced DNA damage.[50] There exists a strong correlation between DNA strand breaks on the one hand and the presence of 8-hydroxy-2′-deoxyguanosine

8-OHdG adducts on the other.[51] 8-OHdG is a sensitive marker of oxidative attacks on DNA and is a clear indicator that OS is central to the etiology of DNA damage in the male germ line. OS could arise as a consequence of excess exposure to ROS and might be a consequence of deficiencies in the antioxidant strategies that the male tract puts in place to protect the spermatozoa from free radical attack.[10] The spermatozoon is particularly susceptible to OS because it possesses abundant targets for oxidation in the form of polyunsaturated fatty acids (PUFAs) (50% of the fatty acid inhuman spermatozoa is docosahexaenoic acid with six double bonds per molecule) and the DNA present in the sperm nucleus and mitochondria. Furthermore, the carbon–hydrogen dissociation energies of PUFAs are the lowest in the bis-allylic methylene position, thus rendering these lipids particularly vulnerable to oxidation. The lipid peroxidation cascade, which is initiated by oxidation of nicotinamide adenine dinucleotide phosphate (NADPH), leading to hydrogen abstraction, generates carbon-centered lipid radicals, which combine with oxygen to produce peroxyl or alkoxyl radicals, which then sequester hydrogen from the adjacent carbon atoms in order to stabilize.[52] The sperm cells also possess little in the way of intrinsic antioxidant defenses, because they have shed a majority of their cytoplasm and, hence, possess only low levels of cytoplasmic antioxidant enzymes such as glutathione peroxidase (GPx), catalase, and superoxide dismutase.[53] Moreover, whatever cytoplasm they do possess is largely confined to one compartment of this cell, the midpiece. There is very little the spermatozoon can do to protect the large area of plasma membrane overlying the sperm head and tail. There is also very little that the cell can do to actively protect its DNA other than to compact it with protamines. However, the latter brings with it its own problems because the tightly compacted, almost crystalline DNA present in the sperm head is not amenable to DNA repair. Rather, DNA damage just accumulates in these cells over their life span for eventual repair within the oocyte after fertilization.[54] The oxidative DNA damage observed in spermatozoa includes single-strand and double-strand breaks, DNA fragmentation, the introduction of abasic sites, purine, pyrimidine, and deoxyribose modifications and DNA cross-linking, which can result in arrest or induction of gene transcription, induction of signal transduction pathways, accelerated telomeric DNA attrition, replication errors, genomic instability, and GC to TA transversions. These changes are also observed during carcinogenesis and might explain the link between infertility and cancer.[51] The only real protection that these cells possess is to be found in the extracellular antioxidants provided by the secretions of the male reproductive tract. The epididymis, for example, produces highly specialized enzymes in the form of extracellular superoxide dismutase and a specific form of selenocysteine independent GPx, GPx5.[55] When the latter was knocked out, the animals developed an age-related phenotype associated with the induction of oxidative DNA damage in the spermatozoa and the appearance of birth defects in the offspring including congenital malformations, complex neuropsychiatric disorders, and childhood cancers in children fathered by men with defective sperm cells.[56]

2.6 ROLE OF YOGA AND MEDITATION IN REDUCING THE DISEASE BURDEN

OS in the male germ line is caused by a host of lifestyle related which are modifiable by adoption of simple lifestyle interventions like yoga and meditation.[57] Antioxidant regimens and lifestyle modifications could both be plausible therapeutic approaches that enable the burden of OS-induced sperm DNA damage and associated burden of childhood disorders including cancers.

Lifestyle interventions including yoga and meditation can substantially improve the integrity of sperm DNA by reducing levels of oxidative DNA damage, regulating OS and by increasing the expression of genes responsible for DNA repair, cell-cycle control, and anti-inflammatory effects.[17] Antioxidant supplementation is helpful in relieving the OS injury to the spermatozoa, but there are plenty of evidences which suggests that indiscriminate or long-term usage of antioxidants for the treatment of sperm associated pathologies such as male infertility or male factor associated recurrent spontaneous abortions can result in a state of "reductive stress" which is rather harmful and interferes with the physiological ROS levels causing enhanced ROS generation by mitochondria leading to oxidative injury to the sperm cell.[9] Complementary and alternative medicine therapies, such as yoga and meditation, are being increasingly used as an adjunct to modern medicine and might reduce incidences of OS-induced sperm DNA damage and associated pathologies such as childhood cancers in the next generation. In an ongoing study in our laboratory, we have documented the reduction in seminal ROS levels as well as sperm DNA fragmentation index levels following a short-term yoga and meditation intervention. Thus, simple lifestyle interventions like yoga and meditation may significantly reduce oxidative damage to sperm DNA and thereby may reduce burden of childhood morbidity, cancer, and autism in the next generation. Further, we are also investigating if reversal of OS (reduced free radical levels) due to this intervention may reverse the aberrant methylation pattern in the sperm DNA. We have documented significant reduction in OS, DNA fragmentation index, seminal ROS levels, oxidative DNA damage, and 8-OHdG levels and a significant improvement in DNA quality and total antioxidant capacity followed by 6 months practice of yoga and meditation in fathers of children affected with nonfamilial sporadicnheritable Rb.[58]

2.7 CONCLUSION

Recent studies have shown important role of sperm genome damage in several childhood diseases (cancer, neuropsychiatric diseases, and autism), infertility, recurrent spontaneous abortions, and congenital malformations. Sperm genome is highly vulnerable to OS-induced damage and mutated at a much higher rate by virtue of cell and oxidative damage. Thus, it is important to detect if single lifestyle intervention can minimize oxidative damage to sperm genome and mutation load and thereby reduce disease burden in the offspring. Lifestyle interventions like "yoga" and "meditation" may help in reducing oxidative damage to paternal genome and normalize dysregulated transcripts and, thus, reduce mutagenic load and disease burden in children. Majority of autism spectrum disorder and several childhood cancers, few psychological disorders are believed to be paternal in origin. The sperm is most vulnerable to poor lifestyle habits and environmental toxicants. Therefore, simple lifestyle interventions like yoga and meditation can minimize oxidative damage to paternal genome which will improve quality of paternal sperm DNA and thus may help in reducing the incidences of childhood cancers including Rb.

KEYWORDS

- retinoblastoma
- childhood cancer
- oxidative stress
- oxidative DNA damage
- yoga

REFERENCES

1. Dimaras, H.; Kimani, K.; Dimba, E. A.; Gronsdahl, P.; White, A.; Chan, H. S.; Gallie, B. L. Retinoblastoma. *Lancet* **2012,** *379* (9824), 1436–1446.
2. Kivelä, T. *The Epidemiological Challenge of the Most Frequent Eye Cancer: Retinoblastoma, An Issue of Birth and Death*; BMJ Publishing Group Ltd., 2009.
3. Knudson, A. G. Mutation and Cancer: Statistical Study of Retinoblastoma. *Proc. Natl. Acad. Sci.* **1971,** *68* (4), 820–823.
4. Saxena, P.; Kaur, J. Differential Expression of Genes in Retinoblastoma. *Clin. Chim. Acta* **2011,** *412* (23), 2015–2021.
5. (a) Cavenee, W. K.; Hansen, M. F.; Nordenskjold, M.; Kock, E.; Maumenee, I.; Squire, J. A.; Philips, R. A.; Gallie, B. L. Genetic Origin of Mutations Predisposing to Retinoblastoma. *Science* **1985,** *228,* 501–504; (b) Lohmann, D. R.; Gallie, B. L. Retinoblastoma: Revisiting the Model Prototype of Inherited Cancer. In *American Journal of Medical Genetics Part C: Seminars in Medical Genetics*; Wiley Online Library: 2004; pp 23–28; (c) Thériault, B. L.; Dimaras, H.; Gallie, B. L.; Corson, T. W. The Genomic Landscape of Retinoblastoma: A Review. *Clin. Exp. Ophthalmol.* **2014,** *42* (1), 33–52.
6. Richter, S.; Vandezande, K.; Chen, N.; Zhang, K.; Sutherland, J.; Anderson, J.; Han, L.; Panton, R.; Branco, P.; Gallie, B. Sensitive and Efficient Detection of RB1 Gene Mutations Enhances Care for Families with Retinoblastoma. *Am. J. Hum. Genet.* **2003,** *72* (2), 253–269.
7. Rushlow, D. E.; Mol, B. M.; Kennett, J. Y.; Yee, S.; Pajovic, S.; Thériault, B. L.; Prigoda-Lee, N. L.; Spencer, C.; Dimaras, H.; Corson, T. W. Characterisation of Retinoblastomas without RB1 Mutations: Genomic, Gene Expression, and Clinical Studies. *Lancet Oncol.* **2013,** *14* (4), 327–334.
8. Schieber, M.; Chandel, N. S. ROS Function in Redox Signaling and Oxidative Stress. *Curr. Biol.* **2014,** *24* (10), R453–R462.
9. Bisht, S.; Dada, R. Oxidative Stress: Major Executioner in Disease Pathology, Role in Sperm DNA Damage and Preventive Strategies. *Front. Biosci. (Scholar edition)* **2017,** *9,* 420.
10. Bisht, S.; Faiq, M.; Tolahunase, M.; Dada, R. Oxidative Stress and Male Infertility. *Nat. Rev. Urol.* **2017,** *14* (8), 470–485.

11. Feinberg, J. I.; Bakulski, K. M.; Jaffe, A. E.; Tryggvadottir, R.; Brown, S. C.; Goldman, L. R.; Croen, L. A.; Hertz-Picciotto, I.; Newschaffer, C. J.; Fallin, M. D. Paternal Sperm DNA Methylation Associated With Early Signs of Autism Risk in an Autism-Enriched Cohort. *Int. J. Epidemiol.* **2015,** *44* (4), 1199–1210.

12. Feuerstein, G. The Yoga Tradition: It's History, Literature, Philosophy and Practice (Kindle Locations 11801–11803). Hohm Press. Kindle Edition. He is Specifically Associated with the Kaula Sect of the Siddha Movement, Within Which He May Have Founded the Yoginî-Kaula Branch: 2013.

13. Barnes, P. M.; Bloom, B.; Nahin, R. L. *Complementary and Alternative Medicine Use Among Adults and Children: United States, 2007*; US Department of Health and Human Services, Centers for Disease Control and Prevention, National Center for Health Statistics Hyattsville, MD, 2008.

14. Briegel-Jones, R. M.; Knowles, Z.; Eubank, M. R.; Giannoulatos, K.; Elliot, D. A Preliminary Investigation into the Effect of Yoga Practice on Mindfulness and Flow in Elite Youth Swimmers. *Sport Psychol.* **2013,** *27* (4), 349–359.

15. Demark-Wahnefried, W.; Jones, L. W. Promoting a Healthy Lifestyle Among Cancer Survivors. *Hematol. Oncol. Clin. N. Am.* **2008,** *22* (2), 319–342.

16. Sengupta, P. Health Impacts of Yoga and Pranayama: A State-of-the-Art Review. *Int. J. Prev. Med.* **2012,** *3* (7), 448–458.

17. Tolahunase, M.; Sagar, R.; Dada, R. Impact of Yoga and Meditation on Cellular Aging in Apparently Healthy Individuals: A Prospective, Open-Label Single-Arm Exploratory Study. *Oxid. Med. Cell. Longev.* **2017.**

18. Evgeni, E.; Charalabopoulos, K.; Asimakopoulos, B. Human Sperm DNA Fragmentation and Its Correlation with Conventional Semen Parameters. *J. Reprod. Infertility* **2014,** *15* (1), 2.

19. Aitken, R. J.; Smith, T. B.; Jobling, M. S.; Baker, M. A.; De Iuliis, G. N. Oxidative Stress and Male Reproductive Health. *Asian J. Androl.* **2014,** *16* (1), 31.

20. Kumar, S.; Murarka, S.; Mishra, V.; Gautam, A. Environmental & Lifestyle Factors in Deterioration of Male Reproductive Health. *Indian J. Med. Res.* **2014,** *140* (7), 29.

21. Hwang, K.; Walters, R. C.; Lipshultz, L. I. Contemporary Concepts in the Evaluation and Management of Male Infertility. *Nat. Rev. Urol.* **2011,** *8* (2), 86–94.

22. Kumar, S. B.; Chawla, B.; Bisht, S.; Yadav, R. K.; Dada, R. Tobacco Use Increases Oxidative DNA Damage in Sperm-Possible Etiology of Childhood Cancer. *Asian Pac. J. Cancer Prev.* **2015,** *16* (16), 6967–6972.

23. Guerrero-Bosagna, C.; Weeks, S.; Skinner, M. K. Identification of Genomic Features in Environmentally Induced Epigenetic Transgenerational Inherited Sperm Epimutations. *PLoS One* **2014,** *9* (6), e100194.

24. Bakos, H. W.; Thompson, J. G.; Feil, D.; Lane, M. Sperm DNA Damage is Associated With Assisted Reproductive Technology Pregnancy. *Int. J. Androl.* **2008,** *31* (5), 518–526.

25. Høst, E.; Lindenberg, S.; Smidt-Jensen, S. The Role of DNA Strand Breaks in Human Spermatozoa used for IVF and ICSI. *Acta Obstet. Gynecol. Scand.* **2000,** *79* (7), 559–563.

26. Reigstad, M. M.; Larsen, I. K.; Myklebust, T. Å.; Robsahm, T. E.; Oldereid, N. B.; Brinton, L. A.; Storeng, R. Risk of Cancer in Children Conceived by Assisted Reproductive Technology. *Pediatrics* **2016,** *137* (3), e20152061.

27. (a) Ericson, A.; Nygren, K.; Olausson, P. O.; Källén, B. Hospital Care Utilization of Infants Born after IVF. *Hum. Reprod.* **2002,** *17* (4), 929–932; (b) Källén, B.; Finnström, O.; Nygren, K.-G.; Olausson, P. O. In Vitro Fertilization in Sweden: Child Morbidity Including Cancer Risk. *Fertil. Steril.* **2005,** *84* (3), 605–610.

28. Pang, D.; McNally, R.; Birch, J. Parental Smoking and Childhood Cancer: Results from the United Kingdom Childhood Cancer Study. *Br. J. Cancer* **2003,** *88* (3), 373–381.

29. Richthoff, J.; Elzanaty, S.; Rylander, L.; Hagmar, L.; Giwercman, A. Association between Tobacco Exposure and Reproductive Parameters in Adolescent Males. *Int. J. Androl.* **2008,** *31* (1), 31–39.

30. Greco, E.; Iacobelli, M.; Rienzi, L.; Ubaldi, F.; Ferrero, S.; Tesarik, J. Reduction of the Incidence of Sperm DNA Fragmentation by Oral Antioxidant Treatment. *J. Androl.* **2005,** *26* (3), 349–353.

31. Aitken, R. J.; Roman, S. D. Antioxidant Systems and Oxidative Stress in the Testes. *Oxid. Med. Cell. Longev.* **2008,** *1* (1), 15–24.

32. Ji, B.-T.; Shu, X.-O.; Zheng, W.; Ying, D.-M.; Linet, M. S.; Wacholder, S.; Gao, Y.-T.; Jin, F. Paternal Cigarette Smoking and the Risk of Childhood Cancer among Offspring of Nonsmoking Mothers. *J. Natl. Cancer Inst.* **1997,** *89* (3), 238–243.

33. Sorahan, T.; Prior, P.; Lancashire, R.; Faux, S.; HultÃ, M. Childhood Cancer and Parental use of Tobacco: Deaths from 1971 to 1976. *Br. J. Cancer* **1997,** *76* (11), 1525.

34. Ioannou, D.; Miller, D.; Griffin, D. K.; Tempest, H. G. Impact of Sperm DNA Chromatin in the Clinic. *J. Assist. Reprod. Genet.* **2016,** *33* (2), 157–166.

35. Aoki, V. W.; Carrell, D. T. Human Protamines and the Developing Spermatid: Their Structure, Function, Expression and Relationship with Male Infertility. *Asian J. Androl.* **2003,** *5* (4), 315–324.

36. Oliva, R. Protamines and Male Infertility. *Hum. Reprod. Update* **2006,** *12* (4), 417–435.

37. Oliva, R.; Dixon, G. H. Vertebrate Protamine Genes and the Histone-to-Protamine Replacement Reaction. *Prog. Nucleic Acid Res. Mol. Biol.* **1991,** *40,* 25–94.

38. Kosower, N. S.; Katayose, H.; Yanagimachi, R. Thiol-Disulfide Status and Acridine Orange Fluorescence of Mammalian Sperm Nuclei. *J. Androl.* **1992,** *13* (4), 342–348.

39. Dianov, G. L.; Souza-Pinto, N.; Nyaga, S. G.; Thybo, T.; Stevnsner, T.; Bohr, V. A. Base Excision Repair in Nuclear and Mitochondrial DNA. *Prog. Nucleic Acid Res. Mol. Biol.* **2001,** *68,* 285–297.

40. Shamsi, M. B.; Kumar, R.; Bhatt, A.; Bamezai, R.; Kumar, R.; Gupta, N. P.; Das, T.; Dada, R. Mitochondrial DNA Mutations in Etiopathogenesis of Male Infertility. *Indian J. Urol.* **2008,** *24* (2), 150.

41. Schwartz, M.; Vissing, J. Paternal Inheritance of Mitochondrial DNA. *N. Engl. J. Med.* **2002,** *347* (8), 576–580.

42. Dinesh, V.; Shamsi, M.; Dada, R. Supraphysiological free Radical Levels and Their Pathogenesis in Male Infertility. *Reprod. Sys. Sexual Disord.* **2012,** *10* (1), 114.

43. Stuppia, L.; Franzago, M.; Ballerini, P.; Gatta, V.; Antonucci, I. Epigenetics and Male Reproduction: The Consequences of Paternal Lifestyle on Fertility, Embryo Development, and Children Lifetime Health. *Clin. Epigenetics* **2015,** *7* (1), 120.

44. Tremellen, K. Oxidative Stress and Male Infertility—A Clinical Perspective. *Hum. Reprod. Update* **2008,** *14* (3), 243–258.

45. Aitken, R. J.; Baker, M. A. Causes and Consequences of Apoptosis in Spermatozoa; Contributions to Infertility and Impacts on Development. *Int. J. Dev. Biol.* **2013,** *57* (2–4), 265–272.

46. Zini, A.; Libman, J. Sperm DNA Damage: Clinical Significance in the Era of Assisted Reproduction. *Can. Med. Assoc. J.* **2006,** *175* (5), 495–500.

47. Shaha, C.; Tripathi, R.; Mishra, D. P. Male Germ Cell Apoptosis: Regulation and Biology. *Philos. Trans. R. Soc. Lond. B: Biol. Sci.* **2010,** *365* (1546), 1501–1515.

48. Aitken, R. J.; Koppers, A. J. Apoptosis and DNA Damage in Human Spermatozoa. *Asian J. Androl.* **2011,** *13* (1), 36.

49. Aitken, R. J.; Findlay, J. K.; Hutt, K. J.; Kerr, J. B. Apoptosis in the Germ Line. *Reproduction* **2011,** *141* (2), 139–150.

50. Sanocka, D.; Kurpisz, M. Reactive Oxygen Species and Sperm Cells. *Reprod. Biol. Endocrinol.* **2004,** *2* (1), 12.

51. Hosen, M. B.; Islam, M. R.; Begum, F.; Kabir, Y.; Howlader, M. Oxidative Stress Induced Sperm DNA Damage, A Possible Reason for Male Infertility. *Iran. J. Reprod. Med.* **2015,** *13* (9), 525–532.

52. Koppers, A. J.; Garg, M. L.; Aitken, R. J. Stimulation of Mitochondrial Reactive Oxygen Species Production by Unesterified, Unsaturated Fatty Acids in Defective Human Spermatozoa. *Free Radic. Biol. Med.* **2010,** *48* (1), 112–119.

53. Tavilani, H.; Goodarzi, M. T.; Vaisi-Raygani, A.; Salimi, S.; Hassanzadeh, T. Activity of Antioxidant Enzymes in Seminal Plasma and Their Relationship with Lipid Peroxidation of Spermatozoa. *Int. Braz. J. Urol.* **2008,** *34* (4), 485–491.

54. Aitken, R. J.; Curry, B. J. Redox Regulation of Human Sperm Function: From the Physiological Control of Sperm Capacitation to the Etiology of Infertility and DNA Damage in the Germ Line. *Antioxid. Redox Signal.* **2011,** *14* (3), 367–381.

55. Zini, A.; San Gabriel, M.; Baazeem, A. Antioxidants and Sperm DNA Damage: A Clinical Perspective. *J. Assist. Reprod. Genet.* **2009,** *26* (8), 427–432.

56. Mishra, S.; Kranthi, V.; Kumar, R.; Malhotra, N.; Mohanty, K., Oxidative Damage to Sperm DNA: Clinical Implications. *Andrology* **2014,** *3* (116), DOI: 2167-0250.1000116.

57. Wright, C.; Milne, S.; Leeson, H., Sperm DNA Damage Caused by Oxidative Stress: Modifiable Clinical, Lifestyle and Nutritional Factors in Male Infertility. *Reprod. Biomed. Online* **2014,** *28* (6), 684–703.

58. Dada, R.; Kumar, S. B.; Chawla, B.; Bisht, S.; Khan, S. Oxidative Stress Induced Damage to Paternal Genome and Impact of Meditation and Yoga—Can It Reduce Incidence of Childhood Cancer?. *Asian Pac. J. Cancer Prev.* **2016,** *17* (9), 4517–4525.

CHAPTER 3

MANAGEMENT AND PREVENTION OF HYPERTENSION IN THE ELDERLY: A YOGIC APPROACH

SATISH G. PATIL[1*] and SHANKARGOUDA S. PATIL[2]

[1]Department of Physiology, BLDE University's Shri B.M. Patil Medical College, Hospital & Research Centre, Vijayapura 586103, Karnataka, India

[2]Department of Medicine, BLDE University's Shri B.M. Patil Medical College, Hospital & Research Centre, Vijayapura 586103, Karnataka, India

*Corresponding author. E-mail: sathupatil@yahoo.co.in

ABSTRACT

As the life span of human is increasing, the population of elderly individuals is growing rapidly worldwide. Hypertension with vascular aging is one of the major risk factor for cardiovascular (CV) morbidity and mortality in elderly individuals. Apart from a risk factor for CV disease, hypertension is also a significant risk for stroke, chronic kidney disease, cognitive impairment, and dementia. Hypertension in older individuals is often accompanied by multiple comorbidities that not only affect their management tremendously but also their quality of life and longevity. In this chapter, evidence-based comprehensive holistic approach for the management of hypertension in the elderly by yogic life-style modality will be discussed.

3.1   INTRODUCTION

Hypertension with vascular aging is one of the major risk factors for cardiovascular (CV) morbidity and mortality in elderly individuals. It accounts for the third leading cause of global burden of disease. According to the WHO, hypertension is the most common cause of preventable death in both developed and developing countries.[1] As the life span of human is increasing, the population of elderly individuals is growing rapidly world-wide. Globally, the population of elderly is projected to increase from the present 901 million to 2.1 billion by 2050.[2] Projections beyond 2016 made by the United Nation have indicated that India will have about 198 million persons above 60 years of age in 2020 and 326 million in 2050.[3]

Elderly people being at high risk to develop hypertension and their increasing number implies that they represents the largest population of hypertensive subjects in India and worldwide. Apart from a risk factor for CV disease, hypertension is also a significant risk for stroke, chronic kidney disease, cognitive impairment, and dementia.[4,5] Studies have shown that reduction of systolic blood pressure (SBP) by 10 mmHg and diastolic blood pressure (DBP) by 5 mmHg in elderly hypertensive patients is associated with a decrease in myocardial infarction by 25%, stroke by 40%, congestive heart failure by 50%, and overall mortality by 10–20%.[6,7] Management of hypertension in elderly patients is challenging because they are often accompanied by multiple comorbidities. Multiple drug therapy and their side-effects affect the quality of life and longevity. Despite the available literature and evidence showing that lifestyle modalities such as yogic lifestyle can control blood pressure (BP) and improve quality of life, it is often overlooked in the management of hypertension.

3.2   EPIDEMIOLOGY

The prevalence of hypertension in the elderly ranges from 50% to 75%, and it is estimated that two out of three individuals over 75 years of age suffer from hypertension.[6,8] According to the Framingham Heart Study, about 60% of the population by age 60 years develops hypertension. In the same study, it was also estimated that the prevalence of hypertension may increase to about 65% in men and 75% in women by age 70. Also, it has been observed that nearly 85% of the individuals with normal BP up to the age of 55 year were later developed hypertension over 20–25 years (their residual lifetime risk) of follow-up study.[9,10] According to the Seventh Report of the Joint National Committee on Prevention, Detection, Evaluation and Treatment of High Blood Pressure (JNC-7), two-thirds of individuals after 65 years have hypertension.[11] In India, the prevalence of hypertension in the elderly above 60 years ranges from 40% to 60%.[12–14] Hypertension is more prevalent in elderly women than men.[6,14]

3.3   PATHOPHYSIOLOGY

Homeostatic regulation of BP within its normal range to ensure an adequate tissue blood flow to vital organs requires co-ordination of several complex interacting physiological systems. Age-associated changes in this complex regulatory system and vascular tissue results in change in the normal baseline of BP. The pattern of hypertension in the elderly is different from that of young and middle-aged individuals. After the age of 55 years, SBP increases while DBP falls or remains unchanged with age, resulting in isolated systolic hypertension (ISH). The hallmark of hypertension in the elderly is increased vascular resistance.[6] Essential hypertension in the elderly is multifaceted and involves complex mechanism.

Arterial stiffness: The reduction of vascular compliance with age due to stiffening of arteries is the major contributor for the development of hypertension in the elderly. Stiffness and dilatation are two major changes that occur in elastic arteries, particularly in the aorta. Due to aortic stiffening, it fails/decline to expand and recoil during ventricular systole and diastole, respectively. Decline/failure in optimum expansion of aorta leads to elevation in SBP, while failure/decline in recoiling results in lowering of DBP causing widening of pulse pressure (PP) with advancing age. PP is the best marker of arterial stiffness.[15]

Endothelial dysfunction: Endothelial cell structure and functional integrity are important for various vital CV functions including homoeostatic regulation of BP.[16] Vascular endothelium regulates several physiological properties of the blood vessel including vasodilatation, vascular permeability, and antithrombotic properties. One of the key molecules of endothelium that maintains vascular homoeostasis and integrity is nitric oxide (NO). Nitric oxide is a strong vasodilator. Sufficient bioavailability of NO is critical due to normal functioning of endothelium. With advancing age, bioavailability of NO is decreased resulting in endothelial dysfunction. Endothelial dysfunction is characterized by a shift of the normal endothelial function toward reduced vasodilator capacity, a proinflammatory state, and prothrombotic properties.[17] Impaired NO-mediated vasodilatation is a potential contributor for stiffening of arteries and increasing peripheral vascular resistance, a pathognomonic characteristic of hypertension in the elderly.[18,19] Vascular oxidative stress plays an important role in the mechanism of reduction of bioavailability of NO and endothelial dysfunction. Hence, age-associated increase in oxidative stress has been implicated as one of the underlying causes of hypertension.[20–23]

Autonomic dysfunction: An age-related increase in sympathetic nervous system activity has been demonstrated by higher plasma nor-epinephrine levels[24] and muscle sympathetic nerve activity.[6,25] This rise in plasma nor-epinephrine levels with age is thought to be a compensatory mechanism for age-related decrease in beta-adrenergic response.[25] Age-related decline in baroreceptor sensitivity leads to relatively greater activation of sympathetic nervous system (compensatory mechanism) for a given level of BP.[6] Sympathetic overactivity increases vascular tone, vascular stiffness, and, thus, hypertension. Age-related arterial stiffness has been linked with increased sympathetic activity in hypertensive[26] and also in healthy subjects.[27] Increased sympathetic activity is also associated with endothelial dysfunction.[28,29]

Impaired neurohormonal regulation: Age-associated decline in neurohormonal mechanisms such as the renin–angiotensin–aldosterone system contributes to elevation in BP in the elderly. Elderly individuals have 40–60% lower levels of plasma renin activity than younger ones.[30] This decreased plasma renin activity has been attributed to the effect of age-related nephrosclerosis on the juxtaglomerular apparatus.[31] Plasma aldosterone levels also declines with age. Age-related changes in kidney function associated with decreased ability to excrete sodium load may also contribute to an elevation of BP in the elderly.

Molecular mechanisms: Epigenetic studies the interaction of DNA and its expression with the environment. Environmental factors such as diet, stress, obesity, smoking aging, and inactivity or sedentary lifestyle directly affect the incidence of hypertension.[32] A strong link between shorter telomere length and hypertension has been reported. Telomere shortening can be used as predictor for developing hypertension.[32]

3.4   DIAGNOSIS AND CLASSIFICATION OF HYPERTENSION IN THE ELDERLY

3.4.1   DIAGNOSIS OF HYPERTENSION

Since BP is more variable in the elderly individuals, hypertension should never be diagnosed on the basis of a single measurement of BP. A strong association between arterial stiffness and auscultatory gap has been reported, particularly in the elderly.[33] Normally, the measurement of BP depends on measuring on how much force it takes to compress an artery. To compress the stiffened arteries, the sphygmomanometer reading is falsely increased leading to false measurement of BP and misdiagnosis of hypertension. Hence, it has been recommended that the diagnosis of hypertension should be based on the average of a minimum of nine BP readings that have been measured on three separate visits.[6] A diagnostic evaluation for finding the secondary causes of hypertension should be done as per the standard guidelines.[11,34,35]

3.4.2   CLASSIFICATION OF HYPERTENSION

Joint National Committee on Prevention, Detection, Evaluation, and Treatment of High Blood Pressure defined criteria for normal BP and classified hypertension into prehypertension, Stage 1 hypertension, and Stage 2 hypertension. JNC classification of hypertension is shown in Table 3.1. Since isolated diastolic hypertension is so uncommon among older individuals, JNC classified an older patient's hypertension based entirely on the level of their SBP into: Stage-1 hypertension between 140 and 159 mmHg and Stage-2 hypertension, ≥160 mmHg.[11,35]

European Society of Hypertension and European Society of Cardiology[34, 36] classified BP into three categories: optimal, normal, and high normal, while hypertension has been classified into three grades: Grade-1 (mild), Grade-2 (moderate), Grade-3 (severe), and ISH. In the elderly, ISH is more common that can be graded into Grade-1, -2, and -3 on the basis of SBP values as shown in Table 3.2. JNC has omitted ISH in its 7th and 8th guidelines.

TABLE 3.1   Classification of Blood Pressure for Adults According to JNC7 Guidelines.

Classification	SBP (mmHg)	DBP (mmHg)
Normal	≤120	And ≤80
Prehypertension	120–139	or 80–89
Stage 1 hypertension	140–159	or 90–99
Stage 2 hypertension	≥160	or ≥100

TABLE 3.2   Classification of Blood Pressure for Adults According to ESH/ESC 2007 Guidelines.

Classification	SBP (mmHg)	DBP (mmHg)
Optimal	≤120	And ≤80
Normal	120–129	80–84
High normal	130–139	85–89
Hypertension		
Grade-1 (mild)	140–159	90–99
Grade-2 (moderate)	160–179	100–109
Grade-3 (severe)	≥180	≥100
Isolated systolic hypertension	≥140	≤90

3.4.3 TYPES OF HYPERTENSION

- *Essential hypertension:* A rise in BP of unknown cause is termed as essential, primary, or idiopathic hypertension. Essential hypertension is a heterogeneous disorder, with different patients having different causal factors that lead to high BP.[37,38] It accounts for 90–95% of all cases of hypertension.
- *Secondary hypertension:* A rise in BP of known underlying cause is termed as secondary hypertension. The prevalence of secondary hypertension ranges between 5% and 10%.[39] The etiology for secondary hypertension in the elderly are renal artery stenosis, coarctation of aorta, aldosteronism, pheochromocytoma, and hyperthyroidism.[40,41]
- *White-coat hypertension:* It is defined as the presence of an elevated BP (≥140/90 mmHg) in an office/clinic setting or in medical environment, but with normal BP when measured at home or normal day time ambulatory BP. It is more common in the elderly.[42,43]

- *Resistant hypertension*: It is more prevalent in elderly hypertensive patients. It is defined as BP that remains uncontrolled despite the concurrent use of three optimally dosed antihypertensive agents of different classes.[44,45] One of the three antihypertensive agents should be diuretic.[46]

3.5 MANAGEMENT OF HYPERTENSION IN THE ELDERLY

Hypertension in elderly individuals is often accompanied by multiple comorbidities that not only affect their management tremendously but also their quality of life and longevity.[6] Hypertension with multiple comorbidities requires multiple-drug prescription increasing the cost of treatment and economic burden on individuals, family, and country. Lifestyle modalities are strongly recommended in the management of hypertension and prevention of CV disease. It has also been recommended not to start drug therapy soon after the diagnosis of hypertension, if SBP is between 140 and 179 mmHg and not associated with any CV risk factors such as diabetes, cholesterolemia, etc.[34]

3.5.1 *PHARMACOLOGIC APPROACH*

The elderly individuals suffering from ISH are often resistant to pharmacological therapy. An attempt to reduce the SBP aggressively lowers DBP (normally decreased with age) resulting in decreased coronary blood flow.[46] It has been observed that antihypertensive drug can control BP but fails to check/control the progression of arterial stiffness. Furthermore, it has been documented that arterial stiffness increases at faster rate in well-controlled hypertensive patients when compared to individuals with normal BP.[47] Moreover, arterial stiffness is an independent and strong predictor of CV morbidity and mortality in hypertensive patients without any overt CV disease [48,49] as well as in healthy elderly individuals.[50] These information suggests that even after maintaining the BP at optimal level, elderly patients remain at CV risk due to increased arterial stiffness. Currently, pharmacological drugs are not available to reduce arterial stiffness in the elderly.

3.5.2 YOGIC APPROACH

Yoga is a psycho-somatic-spiritual discipline, which includes various mind–body techniques that help to achieve a harmony between our mind, body, and soul.[51] Yoga has been shown beneficial for CV health. It has many established health benefits and is emerging as an important lifestyle modality for prevention and management of CV risk. A meta-analysis of 3168 participants from 44 randomized controlled studies showed clinically important beneficial changes in CV risk factors with yoga.[52]

The goal of yogic management in the elderly with hypertension is (1) to control BP and associated CV risk factors; (2) to reduce number of antihypertensive drugs and their dosage (if patient is on drug therapy); and (3) to improve the quality of life. Yogic lifestyle management includes counseling on lifestyle habits (Yama and Niyama), dietary management (Pratyahara), exercises to improve endurance and flexibility (asana), breathing exercises (pranayama), physical and mental relaxation techniques (Dharana and Dhyana), and various techniques to purify mind and body (kriyas). Figure 3.1 shows the flowchart for yogic management of essential hypertension. Lifestyle changes have been recommended as the first line of intervention for subjects with high normal BP, Grade-1 and -2 hypertension, and as a complementary therapy for Grade-3 hypertensive patients associated with or without CV risk factors.[34] Elderly patients with high-normal BP/prehypertension can be managed by only yogic lifestyle.

Patients with Grade-1 and 2 hypertension should be managed initially by yoga therapy and wait for several months in case of Grade-1 hypertension and for several weeks in case of Grade-2 hypertension, if not associated with any CV risk factors. In cases of Grade-1 and 2 hypertension with 1 or 2 CV risk factors, the yoga therapy can be tried for several weeks. However, if yogic management fails to reduce the BP to the level of recommended target (SBP ≤140 mmHg) then drug (antihypertensive) therapy can be commenced with yoga therapy.[34]

```
                    ┌─────────────────────────────┐
                    │  Diagnostic Evaluation of BP │
                    └─────────────────────────────┘
```

| SBP: 120-139 | SBP: 140-159 | SBP: 160-179 | SBP: ≥180 |
| DBP:80-89 | DBP:≥90 | DBP:≥90 | DBP:≥90 |

| Yogic Management | Yogic Management | Yogic Management | Yogic Management + Drug therapy |

| BP Controlled SBP:≤140 | If BP Uncontrolled after several months of yogic management | BP Controlled SBP: ≤ 140 | If BP Uncontrolled after several weeks of yogic management |

| Maintain Yogic Management | Initiate Drug Therapy + Yogic Management | Maintain Yogic Management | Initiate Drug Therapy + Yogic Management |

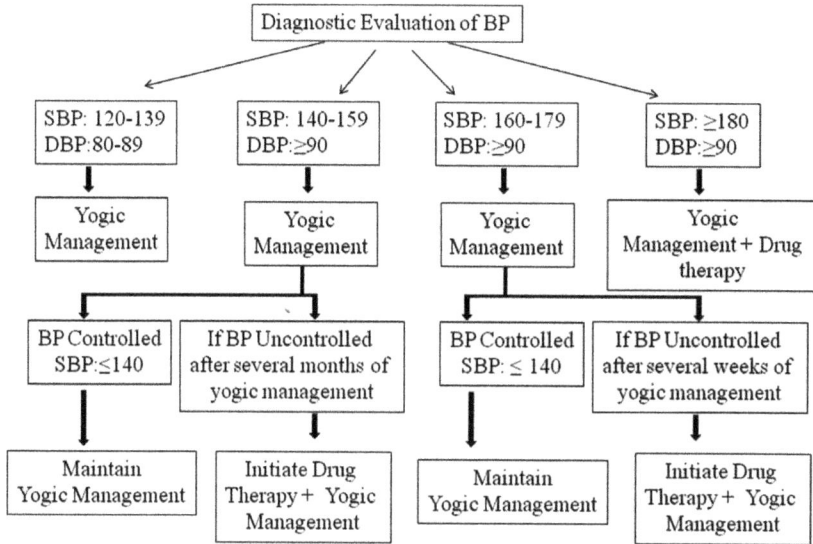

FIGURE 3.1   The flowchart for yogic management of essential hypertension in the elderly.

Control of diet is a primary concern in yogic management, and it plays an important role in health and beneficial modulation of BP in elderly. Purity of food leads to purity of mind. Yoga emphasizes on consumption of sattvik (healthy) food in moderate (Mitahara) quantity. Seasonal foods, fresh fruits, fresh vegetables, nuts, seeds, legumes, whole grains, and dairy products (milk and curd) are sattvik foods. It is advisable to avoid ghee (clarified butter) and butter. Dietary approaches to stop hypertension (DASH) diet with rich fruits, vegetables, low-fat dairy foods, whole grains, and nuts was shown as an effective and beneficial in Stage-1 ISH. In this study, diet rich in fruits and vegetables, DASH diet, and control diet for 8 weeks was given to three groups, respectively. DASH diet lowered SBP by 11.2 mmHg when compared to control group.[53] In another study, a comprehensive approach including walk, yoga, and dietary modifications was more effective than DASH diet on BP control, medication use, and CV risk factors.[54] Patients should also be advised to avoid alcohol, smoking, meat, and reduce salt intake. Satisfactory sleep is very important for a health and to control hypertension. Early to bed and early to rise is good for health. However, time to bed and rise should be gradually modified.

A systematic review (6 studies involving 386 patients) on effect of yoga on essential hypertension has showed yoga as an effective modality for lowering BP. The studies included in this review had a wide variation in the age of subjects from 20 to 75 years and total duration of intervention ranged from 6 to 12 weeks. They reported that yoga has significantly lowered SBP (−2 to −29.17 mmHg) and DBP (−0.74 to −23.67 mmHg) when compared to conventional treatment or no treatment.[55] However, studies demonstrating yoga effects on hypertension in elderly individuals are least available. There are few published studies on yoga effects on hypertension in elderly individuals (Table 3.3).[56-60] Data of these studies suggests that yoga therapy is effective and beneficial in the management of hypertension in the elderly.

The first randomized controlled trial (RCT) of yoga (transcendental meditation (TM)) on mild hypertension in older American-Africans demonstrated a reduction in SBP by 10.7 mmHg and DBP by 6.4 mmHg. This study had included three interventions: (1) TM, (2) passive muscle relaxation (PMR), and (3) lifestyle modification education control (EC) program. TM is yoga-based mental technique, while PMR is a physical-based technique for stress reduction. TM and PMR intervention consisted of 20 min session twice a day for 3 months. TM was twice better than progressive muscle relaxation.[56]

In another RCT, a clinically relevant BP reducing effect with yoga (integrated yoga program) in Indian elderly male subjects with increased PP (high normal BP/Grade-1 hypertension) was reported. This study has given an intervention of integrated yoga program and stretching exercise with walking for two groups of subjects, respectively. Yoga program included loosening practices (sukshama vyama for 10 min), maintaining postures (Asanas: Utkatasana, Padhastasana, Ardhachakrasana, Trikonasana, Bhujangasana, Ardha Salabasana, Ardha Ustrasana, Shashankasana for 15 min), breathing practices (Anuloma Viloma and Brahmari Pranayama for 5 min), and meditation (cyclic meditation for 25 min) for 1 h daily for 6 days in a week. A clinically significant reduction of SBP by 13.23 mmHg was documented.[57]

A complementary yoga therapy (Kundalini yoga) with antihypertensive drugs has been showed more effective in reducing BP and improving quality of life than only pharmacological therapy. Further, it has been shown that individuals who have practiced yoga at home were more benefitted that those who practiced in class.[58]

TABLE 3.3 Impact of Yoga on Hypertension in Elderly Individuals.

Study (year)	Total sample size (yoga/control)	Age (years) mean age ± SD (range)		Design	Duration	Intervention time per session per day/week	Forms of yoga	Control	Baseline blood pressure SBP/DBP (mmHg)	Mean change	
		Yoga	Control							SBP (mmHg)	DBP (mmHg)
Schneider et al. (1995)	127 (Yoga-36/PMR-37, EC-38)	63.7 ±7.0 (55–85)	1. 69.2±7.2 2. 67.4±7.9 (55–85)	RCT	12 weeks	20 min twice daily	TM	1. PMR 2. EC	Yoga—145.4/93.7 PMR—144.3/89.2 EC—150.4/91.7	−10.7	−4.7
Patil et al. (2014)	42 (21/21)	69.42± 5.32 (60–80)	69.52±6.59 (60–80)	RCT	6 weeks	60 min daily for 6 days per week	Asanas, pranayama, meditation	Walking exercise	Y—147.23/74.95 C—147.0/75.52	−4.14	0.38
Wolff et al. (2013)	83 Y1—28 Y2—28 C—27	Y1: 66.2 ±7.7 Y2: 64.0 ±10.3 (20–80)	60.8±11.0 (20–80)	MC	12 weeks	30 min daily	1. Kundalini Yoga 2. Left nostril breathing, spinal flex	Treatment as usual (anti-hypertensives)	Y1—143.8/89.0 Y2—143.6/88.4 C—144.3/89.8	Y1: 2.6 Y2: −4.4	Y1: −0.6 Y2: −5.2
Patil et al. (2015)	60 (30/30)	68.5± 4.85 (60–80)	69.3 ± 5.9 (60–80)	RCT	12 weeks	60 min daily for 6 days per week	Asanas, pranayama, cyclic meditation	Walking exercise	Y—146.07/74.25 C—145.72 /75.5	−13.23	1.0

EC, education control; MC, matched control; PMR, passive muscle relaxation; RCT, randomized controlled trial; TM, transcendental meditation.

3.6   PREVENTION OF HYPERTENSION IN THE ELDERLY

Though there are few data, available evidence suggests that yoga can prevent hypertension in the elderly. As discussed in the pathophysiology above, age-associated changes in the structure (arterial stiffness) and function (endothelial dysfunction) of the artery contributes to the development of hypertension in the elderly. Reduction in arterial stiffness along with BP following yoga intervention for 12 weeks has been documented. The same study has also shown an enhancement in bioavailability of NO suggesting that yoga induce beneficial changes in the endothelial function.[57] A cohort on patients with coronary artery disease has shown an enhancement in the endothelial-dependent vasodilatation in yoga practitioners.[61]

Age-associated oxidative stress is also implicated in the development of hypertension possibly through the development of endothelial dysfunction. Yoga practice for 12 weeks has showed significant reduction in oxidative stress and enhancement in antioxidant capacity in elderly hypertensives.[62]

Sufficient data is available to prove that yoga can induce beneficial modulation in autonomic balance and reduce sympathetic activity.[57,63] A trial of yogic pranayama breathing called Bhastrika on a background of hatha yoga (4 months) on pulmonary function and autonomic function in 76 elderly individuals were studied. In the yoga group, there were significant reduction in sympathetic activity and improvement in the respiratory function.[63]

3.7   CONCLUSION

Yogic management covers all lifestyle modalities such as dietary control, lifestyle counseling, physical exercise with relaxation techniques to improve physical fitness and stability, voluntary regulation of breathing, and mental relaxation techniques to reduce stress and control mind. All these in total help to relax mind and body, reduce stress, and improve the coordination of complex BP regulatory systems and quality of life of the elderly. Data shown represent that a comprehensive approach with yogic diet, sukshama vyama (loosening practices), pranayama (slow breathing practices), and meditation can be prescribed for prevention and management of hypertension in the elderly. The proportion of practice of sukshama vyama, pranayama, and meditation may be 2:1:4. Though there are few data on influence of yoga on hypertension in elderly population, it is recommended for the holistic management of hypertension. No adverse effect of yoga has been reported. However, large and high quality clinical trials on both therapeutic and preventive effects of yogic lifestyle on hypertension in the elderly are needed.

KEYWORDS

- hypertension
- elderly
- yoga
- management
- prevention

REFERENCES

1. Ezzati, M.; Lopez, A. D.; Rodgers, A.; Van der Hoorn, S.; Murray, C. J.; Comparative Risk Assessment Collaborating Group. Selected Major Risk Factors and Global and Regional Burden of Disease. *Lancet* **2002,** *360,* 1347–1360.
2. Department of Economic and Social Affairs, Population Division, United Nations. *World Population Ageing 2015.* 2015. www.un.org/esa/population/publications/worldageing19502050/ (accessed Dec 29, 2016).
3. Kowal, P.; Williams, S.; Jiang, Y.; Fan, W.; Arokiasamy, P.; Chatterji, S. Aging, Health and Chronic Conditions in China and India: Results from the Multinational Study on Global Ageing and Adult Health (SAGE). In *National Research Council. Aging in Asia: Findings From New and Emerging Data Initiatives*; Smith, J. P., Majmundar, Eds. The National Academic Press: Washington, DC, 2012; pp 415–437.
4. Young, A. J. H.; Klag, M. J.; Muntner, P.; Whyte, J. L.; Pahor, M.; Coresh, J. Blood Pressure and Decline in Kidney Function: Findings from the Systolic Hypertension in the Elderly Program (SHEP). *J. Am. Soc. Nephrol.* **2002,** *13,* 2776–2782.
5. Zeiman, S. J.; Melenovsky, V.; Kass, D. A. Mechanisms, Pathophysiology, and Therapy of Arterial Stiffness. *Arterioscler. Thromb. Vasc. Biol.* **2005,** *25,* 932–943.
6. Supiano, M. A. Hypertension. In *Hazard's Geriatric Medicine and Gerontology*; Halter, J. B., Ouslander, J. G., Tinetti, M. E., Studenski, S., High, K. P., Asthana, S., Eds. 6th edn. McGraw Hill Medical Publishers, New Delhi, India,2009; pp 975–982.
7. Law, M.; Wald, N.; Morris, J. Lowering Blood Pressure To Prevent Myocardial Infarction And Stroke: A New Preventive Strategy. *Health Technol. Assess.* **2003,** *7*(31), 1–94.

8. Lloyd-Sherlock, P.; Beard, J.; Minicuci, N.; Ebrahim, S.; Chatterji, S. Hypertension Among Older Adults in Low- and Middle-Income Countries: Prevalence, Awareness and Control. *Int. J. Epidemiol.* **2014,** *43*(1), 116–128.

9. Levy, D.; Larson, M. G.; Vasan, R. S.; Kannel, W. B.; Ho, K. K. The Progression from Hypertension to Congestive Heart Failure. *JAMA* **1996,** *275*(20), 1557–1562.

10. Vokonas, P. S.; Kannel, W. B.; Cupples, L. A. Epidemiology and Risk of Hypertension in the Elderly: The Framingham Study. *J. Hypertens. Suppl.* **1988,** *6*, S3–S9.

11. Chobanian, A. V.; Bakris, G. L.; Black, H. R.; Cushman, W. C.; Green, L. A.; Izzo, J. L. Jr et al. Joint National Committee on Prevention, Detection, Evaluation, and Treatment of High Blood Pressure; National Heart, Lung, and Blood Institute; National High Blood Pressure Education Program Coordinating Committee. Seventh Report of the Joint National Committee on Prevention, Detection, Evaluation, and Treatment of High Blood Pressure. *Hypertension* **2003,** *42*(6), 1206–1252.

12. Radhakrishnan, S.; Balamurugan, S. Prevalence of Diabetes and Hypertension Among Geriatric Population in a Rural Community of Tamilnadu. *Indian J. Med. Sci.* **2013,** *67*, 130–136.

13. Kalavathy, M. C.; Thankappan, K. R.; Sarma, P. S.; Vasan, R. S. Prevalence, Awareness, Treatment and Control of Hypertension in an Elderly Community-Based Sample in Kerala, India. *Natl. Med. J. India* **2000,** *13*(1), 9–15.

14. Chinnakali, P.; Mohan, B.; Upadhyay, R. P.; Singh, A. K.; Srivastava, R.; Yadav, K. Hypertension in the Elderly: Prevalence and Health Seeking Behavior. *N. Am. J. Med. Sci.* **2012,** *4*(11), 558–562.

15. Lee, H. Y.; Oh, B. H. Aging and Arterial Stiffness. *Circ. J.* **2010,** *74*(11), 2257–2262.

16. Stauss, H. M.; Persson, P. B. Role of Nitric Oxide in Buffering Short-Term Blood Pressure Fluctuations. *New Physiol. Sci.* **2000,** *15*, 229–233.

17. Endemann, D. H.; Schiffrin, E. L. Endothelial Dysfunction. *J. Am. Soc. Nephrol.* **2004,** *15*(8), 1983–1992.

18. Wilkinson, I. B.; Qasem, A.; McEniery, C. M.; Webb, D. J.; Avolio, A. P.; Cockroft, J. R. Nitric Oxide Regulates Local Arterial Distensibility In Vivo. *Circulation* **2002,** *105*, 213–217.

19. Fitch, R. M.; Vergona, R.; Sullivan, M. E.; Wang, Y. X. Nitric Oxide Synthase Inhibition Increases Aortic Stiffness Measured by Pulse Wave Velocity in Rats. *Cardiovasc. Res.* **2001,** *51*, 351–358.

20. Ceriello, A. Possible Role of Oxidative Stress in the Pathogenesis of Hypertension. *Diabetes Care* **2008,** *2*, S181–S184.

21. Mateos-Caceres, P. J.; Zamorano-Leon, J. J.; Rodriquez-Sierra, P.; Macaya, C.; Lopez-Farre, A. J. New and Old Mechanism Associated with Hypertension in the Elderly. *Int. J. Hypertens.* **2012,** *2012*, 150107.

22. Briones, A. M.; Touyz, R. M. Oxidative Stress and Hypertension: Current Concepts. *Curr. Hypertens. Rep.* **2010,** *12*(2), 135–142.

23. Grossman, E. Does Increased Oxidative Stress Cause Hypertension? *Diabetes Care* **2008,** *31*, S185–S189.

24. Seals, D. R.; Esler, M. D. Human Ageing and the Sympathoadrenal System. *J. Physiol.* **2000,** *528*, 407–417.

25. Malpas, S. C. Sympathetic Nervous System Overactivity and its Role in the Development of Cardiovascular Disease. *Physiol. Rev.* **2010,** *90*(2), 513–557.

26. Mancia, G.; Grassi, G.; Giannattasio, C.; Seravalle, G. Sympathetic Activation in the Pathogenesis of Hypertension and Progression of Organ Damage. *Hypertension* **1999**, *34*, 724–728.

27. Dinenno, F. A.; Jones, P. P.; Seals, D. R.; Tanaka, H. Age-Associated Arterial Wall Thickening is Related to Elevations in Sympathetic Activity in Healthy Humans. *Am. J. Physiol. Heart Circ. Physiol.* **2000**, *278*, 1205–1210.

28. Hijmering, M. L.; Stroes, E. S.; Olijhock, J.; Hutten, B. A.; Blankestijn, P. J. Sympathetic Activation Markedly Reduces Endothelium-Dependent, Flow-Mediated Vasodilation. *J. Am. Coll. Cardiol.* **2002**, *39*(4), 683–688.

29. Thijssen, D. H. J.; Groot, P. D.; Kooijiman, M.; Smits, P.; Hopman, M. T. E. Sympathetic Nervous System Contributes to the Age-Related Impairment of Flow-Mediated Dilation of the Superficial Femoral Artery. *Am. J. Physiol. Heart Circ. Physiol.* **2006**, *291*, H3122–H3129.

30. Epstein, M. Aging and the Kidney. *J. Am. Soc. Nephrol.* **1996**, *7*(8), 1106–1122.

31. Lionakis, N.; Mendrinos, D.; Sanidas, E.; Favatas, G.; Georgopoulou, M. Hypertension in the Elderly. *World J. Cardiol.* **2012**, *4*(5), 135–147.

32. Mateos-Caceres, P. J.; Zamorano-Leon, J. J.; Rodriquez-Sierra, P.; Macaya, C.; Lopez-Farre, A. J. New and Old Mechanism Associated With Hypertension in the Elderly. *Int. J. Hypertens.* **2012**, *2012*, 150107.

33. Foran, T. G.; Sheahan, N. F.; Cunningham, C.; Feely, J. Pseudo-Hypertension and Arterial Stiffness: A Review. *Physiol. Meas.* **2004**, *25*(2), R21–R33.

34. Mancia, G.; De Backer, G.; Dominiczak, A.; Cifkova, R.; Fagard, R.; Germano, G.; Grassi, G.; Heagerty, A. M.; Kjeldsen, S. E.; Laurent, S.; Narkiewicz, K.; Ruilope, L.; Rynkiewicz, A.; Schmieder, R. E.; Struijker Boudier, H. A.; Zanchetti, A.; Vahanian, A.; Camm, J.; De Caterina, R.; Dean, V.; Dickstein, K.; Filippatos, G.; Funck-Brentano, C.; Hellemans, I.; Kristensen, S. D.; McGregor, K.; Sechtem, U.; Silber, S.; Tendera, M.; Widimsky, P.; Zamorano, J. L.; Kjeldsen, S. E.; Erdine, S.; Narkiewicz, K.; Kiowski, W.; Agabiti-Rosei, E.; Ambrosioni, E.; Cifkova, R.; Dominiczak, A.; Fagard, R.; Heagerty, A. M.; Laurent, S.; Lindholm, L. H.; Mancia, G.; Manolis, A.; Nilsson, P. M.; Redon, J.; Schmieder, R. E.; Struijker-Boudier, H. A.; Viigimaa, M.; Filippatos, G.; Adamopoulos, S.; Agabiti-Rosei, E.; Ambrosioni, E.; Bertomeu, V.; Clement D.; Erdine, S.; Farsang, C.; Gaita, D.; Kiowski, W.; Lip, G.; Mallion, J. M.; Manolis, A. J.; Nilsson, P. M.; O'Brien, E.; Ponikowski, P.; Redon, J.; Ruschitzka, F.; Tamargo, J.; van Zwieten, P.; Viigimaa, M.; Waeber, B.; Williams, B.; Zamorano, J. L. The Task Force for the Management of Arterial Hypertension of the European Society of Hypertension; The Task Force for the Management of Arterial Hypertension of the European Society of Cardiology. 2007 Guidelines for the Management of Arterial Hypertension: The Task Force for the Management of Arterial Hypertension of the European Society of Hypertension (ESH) and of the European Society of Cardiology (ESC). *Eur. Heart J.* **2007**, *28*, 1462–1536..

35. James, P. A.; Oparil, S.; Carter, B. L.; Cushman, W. C.; Dennison-Himmelfarb, C.; Handler, J.; Lackland, D. T.; LeFevre, M. L.; MacKenzie, T. D.; Ogedegbe, O.; Smith, S. C. Jr, Svetkey, L. P.; Taler, S. J.; Townsend, R. R.; Wright, J. T. Jr, Narva, A. S.; Ortiz, E. 2014 Evidence-Based Guideline for the Management of High Blood Pressure in Adults Report From the Panel Members Appointed to the Eighth Joint National Committee (JNC 8). *JAMA* **2014**, *311*(5), 507–520.

36. Mancia, G.; Fagard, R.; Narkiewicz, K.; Redón, J.; Zanchetti, A.; Böhm, M.; Christiaens, T.; Cifkova, R.; De Backer, G.; Dominiczak, A.; Galderisi, M.; Grobbee, D. E.; Jaarsma, T.; Kirchhof, P.; Kjeldsen, S. E.; Laurent, S.; Manolis, A. J.; Nilsson, P. M.; Ruilope, L. M.; Schmieder, R. E.; Sirnes, P. A.; Sleight, P.; Viigimaa, M.; Waeber, B.; Zannad, F.; Task Force Members. 2013 ESH/ESC Guidelines for the Management of Arterial Hypertension: the Task Force for the Management of Arterial Hypertension of the European Society of Hypertension (ESH) and of the European Society of Cardiology (ESC). *J. Hypertens.* **2013**, *31*(7), 1281–1357.

37. Carretero, O. A.; Oparil, S. Essential Hypertension. Part I: Definition and Etiology. *Circulation* **2000**, *101*(3), 329–335.

38. Messerli, F. H.; Williams, B.; Ritz, E. Essential Hypertension. *Lancet* **2007**, *370*(9587), 591–603.

39. Chiong, J. R.; Aronow, W. S.; Khan, I. A.; Nair, C. K.; Vijayraghavan, K.; Dart, R. A.; Behrenbeck, T. R.; Geraci, S. A. Secondary Hypertension: Current Diagnosis and Treatment. *Int. J. Cardiol.* **2008**, *124*(1), 6–21.

40. Viera, A. J.; Neutze, D. M. Diagnosis of Secondary Hypertension: An Age-Based Approach. *Am. Fam. Physician.* **2010**, *82*(12), 1471–1478.

41. Prisant, L. M.; Gujral, J. S.; Mulloy, A. L. Hyperthyroidism: A Secondary Cause of Isolated Systolic Hypertension. *J. Clin. Hypertens. (Greenwich)* **2006**, *8*(8), 596–599.

42. Celis, H.; Fagard, R. H. White-Coat Hypertension: A Clinical Review. *Eur. J. Intern. Med.* **2004**, *15*(6), 348–357.

43. Verdecchia, P.; Staessen, J. A.; White, W. B.; Imai, Y.; O'Brien, E. T. Properly Defining White Coat Hypertension. *Eur. Heart. J.* **2002**, *23*(2), 106–109.

44. Vongpatanasin, W. Resistant Hypertension: A Review of Diagnosis and Management. *JAMA* **2014**, *311*(21), 2216–2224.

45. Calhoun, D. A.; Jones, D.; Textor, S.; Goff, D. C.; Murphy, T. P.; Toto, R. D.; White, A.; Cushman, W. C.; White, W.; Sica, D.; Ferdinand, K.; Giles, T. D.; Falkner, B.; Carey, R. M.; American Heart Association Professional Education Committee. Resistant Hypertension: Diagnosis, Evaluation, and Treatment: A Scientific Statement from the American Heart Association Professional Education Committee of the Council for High Blood Pressure Research. *Circulation* **2008**, *117*(25), e510–e526.

46. Satoshkar, R. S.; Bhandarkar, S. D.; Rege, N. N. *Pharmacology and Pharmacotherapeutics*, 18th ed.; Popular Prakashan Private Limited, India, 2005; pp 421–422.

47. Benetos, A.; Adamopoulos, C.; Burean, J. M. Labat, C.; Bean, K.; Thomas, F .; Pannier, B.; Asmar, R.; Zureik, M.; Safar, M.; Guize, L . Determinants of Accelerated Progression of Arterial Stiffness in Normotensive Subjects and in Treated Hypertensive Subjects Over a 6-Year Period. *Circulation* **2002**, *105*, 1202–1207.

48. Blacher, J.; Asmar, R.; Djane, S. Aortic Pulse Wave Velocity as a Marker of Cardiovascular Risk in Hypertensive Patients. *Hypertension* **1999**, *33*, 1111–1117.

49. Laurent, S.; Boutouyrie, P.; Asmar, R.; Gautier, I.; Laloux, B.; Guize, L.; Ducimetiere, P.; Benetos, A. Aortic Stiffness is an Independent Predictor of All-Cause and Cardiovascular Mortality in Hypertensive Patients. *Hypertension* **2001**, *37*, 1236–1241.

50. Sutton-Tyrrell, K.; Najjar, S. S.; Boudreau, R. M.; Venkitachalam, L.; Kupelian, V.; Simonsick, E. M.; Havlik, R.; Lakatta, E. G.; Spurgeon, H.; Kritchevsky, S.; Pahor,

M.; Bauer, D.; Newman, A. Health ABC Study. Elevated Aortic Pulse Wave Velocity, a Marker of Arterial Stiffness, Predicts Cardiovascular Events in Well-Functioning Older Adults. *Circulation* **2005**, *111*, 3384–3390.

51. Patil, S. G.; Mullur, L.; Khodnapur, J.; Dhanakshirur, G. B.; Aithala, M. R. Effect of Yoga on Short-Term Heart Rate Variability Measure as an Index of Stress in Subjunior Cyclists: A Pilot Study. *Indian J. Physiol. Pharmac.* **2013**, *57,* 81–86.

52. Cramer, H.; Lauche, R.; Haller, H.; Steckhan, N.; Michalsen, A.; Dobos, G. Effects of Yoga on Cardiovascular Disease Risk Factors: A Systematic Review and Meta-Analysis. *Int. J. Cardiol.* **2014**, *173,* 170–183.

53. Moore, T. J.; Conlin, P. R.; Ard, J.; Svetkey, L. P. DASH (Dietary Approaches to Stop Hypertension) Diet Is Effective Treatment for Stage 1 Isolated Systolic Hypertension. *Hypertension* **2001**, *38*(2), 155–158.

54. Ziv, A.; Vogel, O.; Keret, D.; Pintov, S.; Bodenstein, E.; Wolkomir, K.; Doenyas, K.; Mirovski, Y.; Efrati, S. Comprehensive Approach to Lower Blood Pressure (CALM-BP): A Randomized Controlled Trial of a Multifactorial Lifestyle Intervention. *J. Hum. Hypertens.* **2013**, *27*(10), 594–600.

55. Wang, J.; Xiong, X.; Liu, W. Yoga for Essential Hypertension: A Systematic Review. *PLoS One* **2013**, *8*(10), e76357.

56. Schneider, R. H.; Staggers, F.; Alxander, C. N.; et al. A Randomised Controlled Trial of Stress Reduction for Hypertension in Older African Americans. *Hypertension* **1995**, *26*(5), 820–827.

57. Patil, S. G.; Aithala, M. R.; Das, K. K. Effect of Yoga on Arterial Stiffness in Elderly with Increased Pulse Pressure: A Randomized Controlled Study. *Complement. Ther. Med.* **2015**, *23,* 562–569.

58. Wolff, M.; Sundquist, K.; Larsson Lonn, S.; Midlov, P. Impact of Yoga on Blood Pressure and Quality of Life in Patients with Hypertension—A Controlled Trial in Primary Care, Matched for Systolic Blood Pressure. *BMC Cardiovasc. Disord.* **2013**, *13*, 111.

59. Park, H. S.; Kim, Y. J.; Kim, Y. H. The Effect of Yoga Program on Reduced Blood Pressure in Elderly's Essential Hypertension. *J. Korean Acad. Nurs.* **2002**, *32*(5), 633642.

60. Patil, S. G.; Dhanakshirur, G.; Aithala, M. R.; Das, K. K. Comparison of the Effects of Yoga and Lifestyle Modification on Grade-I Hypertension in Elderly Males: A Preliminary Study. *Int. J. Clin. Exp. Physiol.* **2014**, *1,* 68–72.

61. Sivasankaran, S.; Pollard-Quintner, S.; Sachdeva, R.; Pugeda, J.; Hoq, S. M. The Effect of a 6-Week Program of Yoga and Meditation on Brachial Artery Reactivity: Do Psychosocial Interventions Affect Vascular Tone? *Clin. Cardiol.* **2006**, *29,* 393–398.

62. Patil, S. G.; Dhanakshirur, G. B.; Aithala, M. R.; Naregal, G.; Das, K. K. Effect of Yoga on Oxidative Stress in Elderly with Grade-I Hypertension: A Randomized Controlled Study. *J. Clin. Diagn. Res.* **2014**, *8*(7), BC04–BC07.

63. Santaella, D. F.; Devesa, C. R.; Rojo, M. R.; Amato, M. B.; Drager, L. F.; Casali, K. R.; Montano, N.; Lorenzi-Filho, G. Yoga Respiratory Training Improves Respiratory Function and Cardiac Sympathovagal Balance in Elderly Subjects: A Randomised Controlled Trial. *BMJ Open* **2011 May,** *1*(1), e000085.

PART II
Ayurveda, the Holistic Healthcare System

CHAPTER 4

IMPLEMENTATION OF THE THEORY OF EQUALITY BETWEEN THE UNIVERSE AND INDIVIDUAL IN AYURVEDIC TREATMENT

VIBHA SOOD*, K. L. MEENA, and GOVIND PAREEK

Department of Basic Principles, National Institute of Ayurveda, Jaipur, Rajasthan, India

Corresponding author. E-mail: drvibhasood@gmail.com

ABSTRACT

Ayurveda is India's traditional and natural system of medicine. It emphasizes prevention of disease, rejuvenation of our body system, and extension of life span. In Ayurvedic texts, it is mentioned that all the materials and spiritual phenomena of the universe (*Loka*) are present in the individual (*Purusha*). Similarly, all that present in the individual are also contained in the universe. Thus, the individual is an epitome of the universe. Visualization of the identity of the individual with the universe paves the way for salvation. Realization of the identical nature of the universe and the man brings about real knowledge of things as a person equipped with such knowledge considers himself as responsible for every external event and thus gets rid of the bondage of happiness as well as miseries. In *Ayurveda*, a year is divided into six parts called seasons (*Ritu*), according to the movement of sun. In each season, due to its particular characteristics, human body becomes affected and vitiated by different particular pathological factors (*dosha*). When suitable diet and regimen is followed by man as mentioned in *Ayurveda*, his body system remains in normal condition. When this pattern is not followed by him, he gets affected by diseases due to accumulation of *dosha*. Similarly, when characteristics of a particular season are shown in an excessive way, disasters happen in nature. This theory of equality can be applied in various diseases also. For example, in *Prameha* water element accumulates excessively in body. It is resembled as moisture (*kleda*) in nature. It is responsible for vitiation of *kapha dosha*. During treatment of *prameha* while applying various medicines which act on different properties of *kapha*, *kleda* is also tried to reduce. Therefore, the moisture-controlling medicines like *triphala* and *yava* are given to the patient. Thus, the treatment by dissimilar properties is also based on "Theory of Equality between Universe and Individual." The detailed application of theory will be described in this chapter.

4.1 INTRODUCTION

Ayurveda, the science of life and longevity, is the most ancient healthcare system in the world, and it unites the profound thoughts of medicine and philosophy. It emphasizes prevention of disease, rejuvenation of our body system, and extension of life span. In Ayurvedic text *Charaka Samhita*, it is mentioned that the individual living being is a miniature replica of the universe. Therefore, the universe and the individual human being are under the same laws and in fact based on a continuum which undergoes from the realm of the universe to that of the smallest form of creation. Every factor which is present in the universe also present in the individual and vice versa. This concept of similarity is called *loka purusha samya siddhanta*.[1] Cognition of the similarity of the individual with the universe prepares a way for *Moksha*. This concept of equality between individual and universe is also helpful in etiopathogenesis and treatment of a disease. When the changes occur in individual simultaneously with nature in a compatible form, health is maintained but in a reverse order harmony is lost and disease can arise.

4.2 LITERARY REVIEW

Acharya Charak mentioned in *Shareera Sthana* that an individual is an epitome of universe. Microcosm and macrocosm are in a never-ending interaction with each other. When one who looks equally the entire universe within himself, and his own self in the entire universe, acquires the real knowledge.[2] The conveyance of the soul from one body to another is always guided by his own past actions. Once he realizes that his own past actions are only responsible for everything happening to him, he starts detaching himself from all drastic actions and this kind of manner shows the way of his salvation.

An individual has a *Hetu* (cause), *Utpatti* (birth), *Vriddhi* (growth), *Upaplava* (decay), and *Viyoga* (dissolution). *Hetu* is the cause of manifestation, *utpatti* is process of birth, *vriddhi* is growth, *upaplava* is onslaught of miseries, and *viyoga* is the cessation of the elan vital or dissolution or attainment of the natural state. Perception of the thing that the attachment precedes *dukha* and detachment leads to peace *uparam* is the real knowledge, and this is the motive of similarity between *brahmand* and *purusha*.[3]

This concept is mentioned as *Pind Brahmand Nyaya* (*yat pinde tat brahmande*) in *Yajurveda*. *Acharya Atreya* mentioned in *Charak Samhita* that the subdivisions of universe are countless likewise individual's subdivisions are also countless. *Purusha* (individual) is a constitution of six *dhatu*, viz., *Prithvi, Jal, Teja, Vayu, Akash*, and *Avyakta Brahma*. *Prithvi* constitutes the form of man (*murti*), *Jala* moisture (*kleda*), *Tejas* heat (*santap*), vayu elan vital (*Prana*), akash porous portions (sushira), and Avyakt Brahma the internal soul (*Antaratma*).[4] This concept of similarity has been applied everywhere in Ayurvedic texts for the diagnosis and treatment of the diseases. As *Prameha vyadhi* is a *tridoshaja vyadhi*.[5] *Dushya* involved in it are *meda, mansa, kleda, shukra, rakta, vasa, majja, lasika, rasa,* and *oja*.[6] In description of types of *prameha, kaphaja prameha* is described at first due to its same nature with *nidana, dosha,* and *dushya*. Therefore, *kaphaj prameha* has maximum subtypes. Liquidity of *Kapha dosha* increases excessively in *prameha*,[7] which is due to involvement of vitiated *kleda*. In all types of *prameha, kleda* becomes vitiated. *Kleda* factor in *loka* is resembled as *jal mahabhoot* in *purusha*. In *loka, kleda bhava* naturally increases in *Varsha Ritu*, which subsides automatically in *Sharad Ritu* due to sharp rays of sun. Rainy season comes after the ending of *Adan Kala*. So the body and digestion power are too weak at this time. In rainy season, all the *dosha* get vitiated due to environmental changes. But *vata* and *kapha* become vitiated more.[8] If proper *ritucharya* is not followed, then chances are more to get afflicted by the diseases caused by *vata* and *kapha*. To reduce *kleda bhava*, the drugs having properties like diuretic, astringent, hot in potency, *ruksha* and *kashaya, tikta* or *katu* in rasa are applied to body. *Phaltrikadi Kwatha*, combination of *Amla*, *Haridra*, and *Madhu* and *Yava*, has all these properties.[9]

Rainy season is prone to *Gulma Vyadhi* also. In all types of *gulma* vitiation of *vata dosha* is inevitable.[10] *Vata dosha* is composed of *vayu* and *akasha Mahabhoot*. As mentioned earlier, *akash* is similar to porous parts and *vayu* is similar to *prana* in human body. In *gulma* patient, *jatharagni* should be protected all the time because equilibrium and vitiation of *dosha* depends on it[11] and *Jatharagni* depends on balanced *vayu*.[12] So while doing appropriate treatment to correct other *dosha*, *vayu* should be protected all the time like in the beginning, in the middle, and at the end of therapy. In *gulma, vayu* is already aggravated; so *snehana* and *swedana* are performed to remove obstruction of air in the passage. *Shodhana* is applied in mild form with cautions of upholding *vayu* in controlled condition.[13] Administration of *Sneha* is done carefully only to alleviate aggravated form of *vayu* and to balance the *jatharagni*. With all these, balanced combination of herbal compounds is given orally to keep *vayu* in appropriate state.

In *Ritu Chakra*, autumn comes after rainy season. In rainy season where body has adopted itself for rain and cold, sudden exposure to heat of the sun in autumn causes aggravation of pitta.[14] So *pitta*-related disorders are common in this season. *Rakta piita* is one of them. Due to inappropriate lifestyle and eating behaviors, *pitta* and *rakta* both increase in their ratio. Aggravated *pitta* comes into contact of *rakta*, gets it vitiated and acquires the color and smell of *rakta*. Therefore, it is called *raktapitta*. *Pitta dosha* is composed of *agni mahabhoota*. In *purusha agni* or *tejas mahabhoot* is resembled as *abhisamtaap*. So when it becomes excessive, it produces burning sensation all over the body, a sensation like smoke is coming out of the mouth associated with other *pitta*-related symptoms.[15] So the drugs which are cold in potency, having rasa like *madhur, tikta, kashaya*, are given. *Kashaya* rasa due to its astringent property works as a hemostatic also.[16] Drugs like *vasa, chandana, madhooka* have all these properties. To reduce *abhisantaapjanya trishna* cooled water boiled with *sugandhbala, chandan, ushira, musta*, and *parpatak* are given orally. *Rakta pitta* is a *samtarpanjanya vyadhi*, so in the beginning if patient is not weak, *Stambhan Karma* is not performed. Otherwise, it can arise many complications.[17] Thus, this concept is applied everywhere in *Ayurveda* to know etiology and treatment of the diseases.

4.3 DISCUSSION

Loka purusha samya siddhanta is a base of *Chikitsa Karma*. *Bhava* mentioned in *Charaka Samhita* have prime motive to show the path of salvation. They give the way to get a high state of spiritualism. But they point their utility to treatment also. First six phenomena are mentioned to show similarity of basic constitution of *purusha* with *loka*. *Acharya Charak* has told in his *Samhita* that only gross phenomena are explained here. Further, *Acharya Chakrapani* mentioned in his commentary that universe contains particular phenomena like trees, grass, animals, etc., and individual has ligaments, tendons, artery, etc. These all are enormous in number, and they also can be correlated with each other. Some more spiritual phenomena has been mentioned by *Acharya Charak* in *Purusha Vichaya Shareera*,[18] and further, he has told that some more other phenomena which are common in universe and man also can be perceived by inference.[19]

Here is the list of *bhava* which are mentioned in *Charaka Samhita* to show the similarity between *loka* and *purusha*:

Sl. No.	Lokagata Bhava	Purushgata Bhava
1	*Prithvi*	*Murti*
2	*Aap*	*Kleda*
3	*Teja*	*Abhisantaap*
4	*Vayu*	*Prana*
5	*Viyat*	*Sushir*
6	*Brahm*	*Antaratma*
7	*Vibhuti of Brahm*	*Vibhuti of Antaratma*
8	*Vibhuti of Brahm—Prajapati*	*Vibhuti of Brahm—Man*
9	*Indra*	*Ahankar*
10	*Aditya*	*Adan*
11	*Rudra*	*Rosha*
12	*Soma*	*Prasad*
13	*Vasu*	*Sukh*
14	*Ashwini Kumar*	*Kanti*
15	*Marut*	*Utsah*
16	*Vishvedev*	*Indriya and Indriyartha*
17	*Tama*	*Moh*

18	*Jyoti*	*Gyan*
19	*Srishti*	*Garabhadhan*
20	*Krityuga*	*Balyawastha*
21	*Treta*	*Yuvawastha*
22	*Dwapar*	*Vriddhawastha*
23	*Kaliyug*	*Rogi*
24	*Yugant*	*Mrityu*

4.4 CONCLUSION

The area of application of this theory is very vast. It can be helpful to treat *Manasa Vyadhi* also. In today's era, there has been generated a large gap between human and environment by living materialistic life. *Loka purusha samya siddhanta* is helpful to change the view of a man toward nature. When person thinks himself a part of universe, he will treat the environment and its creations in a right way. In Ayurvedic texts, environmental disturbances are described as *Janpadodhwansa*. The characteristics of *Vikrita Vayu, Jal, Desha, Kala,* and lifestyle during that period with some cautions and medication are also mentioned there.[20] According to the concept of "*Samanyam Vriddhikaranam*," *bhava* which have reduced in body are tried to increase by applying the *Aushadh* and *Aahar–Vihar* of same *bhava*. Similarly, when a particular bhava is increased in body, *Viparita* type of *Aushadha–Aahar–Vihar* is given to the patient (*Hrasa Hetuh Visheshashch*).[21] By doing all these measurements, *Samya* of the body is tried to keep maintained. At the same time, samya between *Purusha* and *Brahmanda* is also equally important to uphold. If this *samya* gets disturbed, *Pralaya* befalls in universe. Thus, *Lok Purusha Samya Siddhanta* is very useful to preserve equilibrium in the universe.

KEYWORDS

- **Ayurveda**
- **bhava**
- **loka**
- **purusha**
- **samya**

REFERENCES

1. Agnivesha. Shareera Sthana 4/13. In *Charaka Samhita*; Trikamji Acharya, Y., Ed.; Chaukhamba Surbharati Prakashan: Varanasi, 2013; pp 318.
2. Agnivesha. Shareera Sthana 5/7. In *Charaka Samhita*; Trikamji Acharya, Y., Ed.; Chaukhamba Surbharati Prakashan: Varanasi, 2013; pp 325.
3. Agnivesha. Shareera Sthana 5/8. In *Charaka Samhita*; Trikamji Acharya, Y., Ed.; Chaukhamba Surbharati Prakashan: Varanasi, 2013; pp 326.
4. Agnivesha. Shareera Sthana 5/5. In *Charaka Samhita*; Trikamji Acharya, Y., Ed.; Chaukhamba Surbharati Prakashan: Varanasi, 2013; pp 325.
5. Agnivesha. Nidana Sthana 4/3. In *Charaka Samhita*; Trikamji Acharya, Y., Ed.; Chaukhamba Surbharati Prakashan: Varanasi, 2013; pp 211.
6. Agnivesha. Nidana Sthana 4/7. In *Charaka Samhita*; Trikamji Acharya, Y., Ed.; Chaukhamba Surbharati Prakashan: Varanasi, 2013; pp 212.
7. Agnivesha. Nidana Sthana 4/6. In *Charaka Samhita*; Trikamji Acharya, Y., Ed.; Chaukhamba Surbharati Prakashan: Varanasi, 2013; pp 212.
8. Agnivesha. Sutra Sthana 6/33–34. In *Charaka Samhita*; Trikamji Acharya, Y., Ed.; Chaukhamba Surbharati Prakashan: Varanasi, 2013; pp 47.
9. Agnivesha. Chikitsa Sthana 6/21,26,40. In *Charaka Samhita*; Trikamji Acharya, Y., Ed.; Chaukhamba Surbharati Prakashan: Varanasi, 2013; pp 448.
10. Agnivesha. Nidana Sthana 3/6. In *Charaka Samhita*; Trikamji Acharya, Y., Ed.; Chaukhamba Surbharati Prakashan: Varanasi, 2013; pp 211.
11. Agnivesha. Chikitsa Sthana 5/136. In *Charaka Samhita*; Trikamji Acharya, Y., Ed.; Chaukhamba Surbharati Prakashan: Varanasi, 2013; pp 442.
12. Agnivesha. Chikitsa Sthana 28/8. In *Charaka Samhita*; Trikamji Acharya, Y., Ed.; Chaukhamba Surbharati Prakashan: Varanasi, 2013; pp 616.
13. Agnivesha. Chikitsa Sthana 5/23,28,31. In *Charaka Samhita*; Trikamji Acharya, Y., Ed.; Chaukhamba Surbharati Prakashan: Varanasi, 2013; pp 437.
14. Agnivesha. Sutra Sthana 6/41. In *Charaka Samhita*; Trikamji Acharya, Y., Ed.; Chaukhamba Surbharati Prakashan: Varanasi, 2013; pp 48.
15. Agnivesha. Nidana Sthana 2/4–6. In *Charaka Samhita*; Trikamji Acharya, Y., Ed.; Chaukhamba Surbharati Prakashan: Varanasi, 2013; pp 205–206.
16. Agnivesha. Sutra Sthana 26/43(6). In *Charaka Samhita*; Trikamji Acharya, Y., Ed.; Chaukhamba Surbharati Prakashan: Varanasi, 2013; pp 145.
17. Agnivesha. Chikitsa Sthana 4/25–28,31. In *Charaka Samhita*; Trikamji Acharya, Y., Ed.; Chaukhamba Surbharati Prakashan: Varanasi, 2013; pp 429–430.
18. Agnivesha. Shareera Sthana 5/4–5. In *Charaka Samhita*; Trikamji Acharya, Y., Ed.; Chaukhamba Surbharati Prakashan: Varanasi, 2013; pp 325.
19. Agnivesha. Shareera Sthana 5/5. In *Charaka Samhita*; Trikamji Acharya, Y., Ed.; Chaukhamba Surbharati Prakashan: Varanasi, 2013; pp 325.
20. Agnivesha. Vimana Sthana 3/7,14–18. In *Charaka Samhita*; Trikamji Acharya, Y., Ed.; Chaukhamba Surbharati Prakashan: Varanasi, 2013; pp 241–242.
21. Agnivesha. Sutra Sthana 1/44. In *Charaka Samhita*; Trikamji Acharya, Y., Ed.; Chaukhamba Surbharati Prakashan: Varanasi, 2013; pp 9.

CHAPTER 5

NANOTECHNOLOGY IN ANCIENT INDIAN HOLISTIC HEALTHCARE

SNIGDHA S. BABU[1], E. K. RADHAKRISHNAN[2*], SABU THOMAS[1,3], and NANDAKUMAR KALARIKKAL[1,4]

[1]International and Inter University Centre for Nanoscience and Nanotechnology, Mahatma Gandhi University, Kottayam 686560, Kerala, India

[2]School of Biosciences, Mahatma Gandhi University, Kottayam 686560, Kerala, India

[3]School of Chemical Sciences, Mahatma Gandhi University, Kottayam 686560, Kerala, India

[4]School of Pure and Applied Physics, Mahatma Gandhi University, Kottayam 686560, Kerala, India

*Corresponding author. E-mail: radhakrishnanek@mgu.ac.in

ABSTRACT

Ayurveda is one of the most powerful and sophisticated holistic healthcare systems in world. Records suggest that Ayurveda has been practiced since Vedic period (~1100 BCE). This ancient healthcare system has made use of nanotechnology, which have gained extreme popularity in recent times, to effectively treat maladies. The concept of particle reduction has been discussed in the ayurvedic scripture *Charaka Samhita* (1500 BCE). Bhasmas are unique metallic/mineral preparations, which are purified and treated with herbs and heated to high temperatures to obtain nanosized therapeutics. The recent improvements in visualization and characterization procedures have helped in elucidating the presence of nanoparticles in bhasma preparations. In this chapter, nanotechnology in the preparation and characterization of bhasma, the ayurvedic nanomedicine, is discussed.

5.1 INTRODUCTION

Nanotechnology has developed by leaps and bounds in the past few decades. Nanomaterials are being utilized widely to improve their performance on various levels. These materials possess unique properties mainly due to their extremely small size and large surface area.

5.1.1 NANOMATERIAL CLASSIFICATIONS

Nanomaterials can be vastly classified as naturally occurring and man-made nanomaterials. Materials such as viruses, proteins, nucleic acids, etc., fall under the naturally occurring materials. The materials that are anthropogenic could be produced unintentionally from combustion of hydrocarbons or through a defined synthesis procedure. Nanotechnology basically deals with intentionally produced nanomaterials.[1] Moreover, nanomaterials are also present in nature in the form of various minerals produced by erosions and volcanic eruptions, in the multilayered nano-structures in the butterfly wings and feet of gecko, and the epicuticular wax crystal structures on lotus leaf surface.[1–5]

5.1.2 NANOTECHNOLOGY IN ANCIENT TIMES

Though the development of electron microscopic techniques has been largely responsible for the dynamic growth in this sector, there have been records on the use of nanomaterials from the ancient times. Nanoparticles were primarily used as colorants in tumblers, ornamental glassware, and medieval paintings.[6] The most iconic example of the use of nano-technology in ancient artifact is the *Lycurgus Cup* from around fourth century BCE. Modern day analytical techniques such as X-ray diffraction and transmission electron microscopy reveals that the artifact consists of nanoparticles made up of gold–silver alloy.[7] Damascus steel sabers from the 17th century were found to have carbon nanotubes and cementite nanowires. Palygorskite clay nanoparticles have been found to render the aesthetically pleasing and highly resistant blue color to Mayan pottery.[8] Clays were used in ancient Cyprus for the bleaching of wools and clothes. Kaolin clay was used to prepare ultra-thin pottery in china during the ninth century. Clay has been used as an internal medicine and for cosmetic purposes around the world.[9] Michael Faraday reported first synthesis of gold nanoparticles in solution in 1857.

5.1.3 NANOMATERIALS IN CONTEMPORARY MEDICINE

Various nanomaterials were being used extensively used by humans for several centuries, and they have been found in nature in inanimate as well as in various animals, insects, and plants. These natural nanostructured materials can help us understand their amazing properties and help us in gaining inspiration for design and engineer high-performance materials.[10–11] With the advent of electron microscopy and various synthetic approaches, nanotechnology is finding itself growing at a very fast rate. Highly investigated nanomaterials are being applied in every aspect of human life imaginable. Nanomaterials have proved to be extremely useful in the field of medicine. The various applications of nanomaterials in contemporary medicine are illustrated in Figure 5.1.

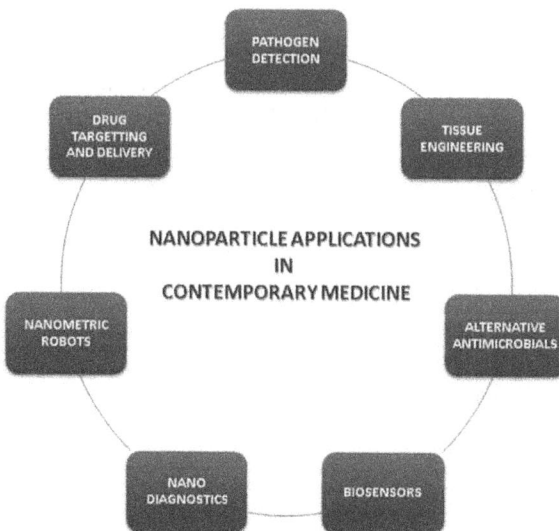

FIGURE 5.1 Nanoparticles used in contemporary medicine.

5.1.4 NANOMATERIALS IN ANCIENT MEDICINE

Though the use of nanomaterials and nanometallic particles is quite recent in contemporary medicine, it has been widely used in an ancient Indian healing system called Ayurveda. This review predominantly deals with Rasa Shastra branch of Ayurveda. Nagarjuna, the eighth century alchemist, is credited with the introduction of metals as medicine. This development saw the advent of a branch of Ayurveda termed "Rasa Shastra," which used herb–metal preparations for treatment of various disorders.

5.2 AYURVEDA

Ayurveda, the science of life, was established and developed over thousands of years ago. Ayurveda works on the principle that mind and body are connected, and it is one of the most sophisticated and powerful holistic healing systems in the world. The ayurvedic records can be traced back to 5000 BCE. It is considered to be an auxiliary knowledge in Vedic tradition. The origin of Ayurveda is said to be found in *Atharvaveda* as well. It is also believed that Sage Agnivesha is the founder of Ayurveda and all his research is compiled in *Agnivesa Samhita*. Charaka, a physician in 300 BC, simplified Agnivesha's compilation and popularized it. Sushruta, an ancient Indian physician, also known as the father of surgery, authored a treatise titled *Susruta Samhita*. *Susruta Samhita* is considered to be the institutional text for Ayurveda.[12–13] Very accurate and detailed surgical accounts have been be found in this epic treatise.[14] Nagarjuna is credited with updating the *Sushruta Samhita*. Atreya Punarvasu, one of the great Hindu sages, was a renowned ayurvedic scholar, and it is believed that the six branches of early Ayurveda are based on his teachings. He is credited as the author of *Bhela Samhita*. The *Charaka Samhita*, the *Sushruta Samhita*, and the *Bhela Samhita* are the three principle early texts on ayurvedic practice. Ayurveda burgeoned during the middle ages in India. The works of Charaka and Sushruta were translated into Chinese and Persian languages. These translational were found to have influenced various European schools of medicine as well.[15–16] Thus, the modern day Ayurveda evolved over the span of a few centuries, and it is currently divided into eight major branches which are illustrated in Figure 5.2.

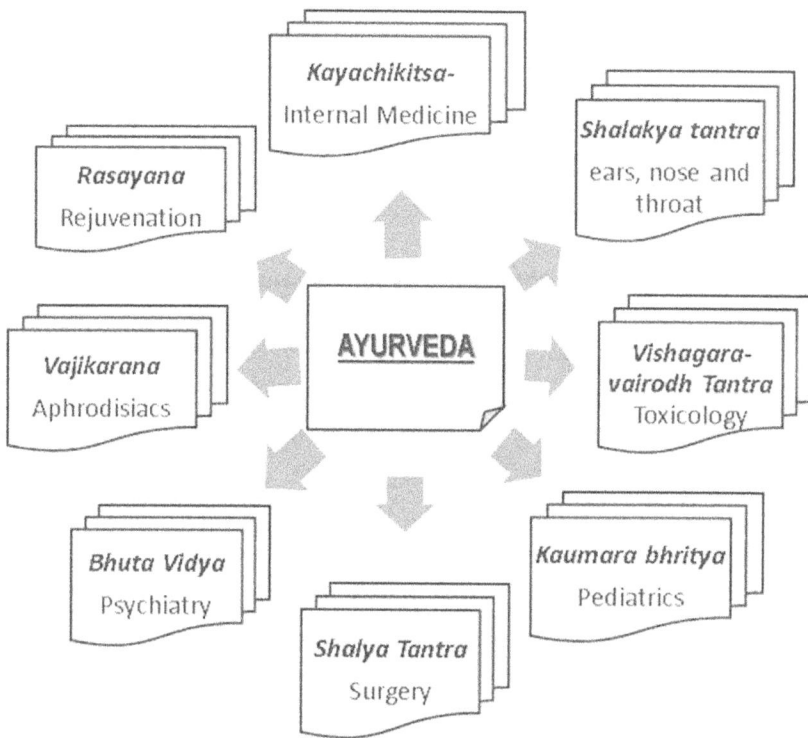

FIGURE 5.2 The eight divisions of Ayurveda.

5.2.1 METALS IN AYURVEDA

Rasa Shastra has been a very important part of Ayurveda since the eighth century.[17] This Shastra usually employs herbo-metallic preparations called bhasmas for curing various maladies. Bhasma roughly translates to residue after incineration. Bhasma is a calcined product in which animal products (horns, shells, feathers), metallic and nonmetallic minerals are converted to ash. The effectiveness of bhasmas in treating various diseases could be attributed to their high level of bio compatibility; moreover, the metallic constituents do not react with the various tissues in the body. These metals are combined with herbs which further enhance the assimilation and delivery of therapeutics. The bhasmas can also be considered to be superior to their herbal counterparts as they have higher stability, longer shelf life, lower dosage, and sustainable availability. These can be broadly classified into metal-based, mineral-based, and herbal bhasmas.

5.2.2 AYURVEDIC NANOMEDICINE

Bhasma preparation involves elaborate, systematic, and time-consuming procedure known as bhasmikarana. The bhasmikarana process converts the bulk metals from their zero-valent state to higher oxidation state, and this conversion of metal to metal oxide could be responsible for the elimination of the toxicity associated with bulk metals. Thus, the bhasmikaran process effectively converts a biologically incompatible substance into a biocompatible one. Some of the commonly used bhasmas are listed in Table 5.1 (adapted from Pal et al.[18]).

TABLE 5.1 Some Commonly Used Bhasmas, Their Starting Material, and Diseases Treated.

Name of bhasma	Raw materials used	Prescribed for
Loha bhasma	Iron, cinnabar	Enlargement of liver, anemia, jaundice
Tamra bhasma	Copper, mercury, sulfur	Anemia, jaundice, digestive disturbance, abdominal disorders
Abhrak bhasma	Calcined purified mica, ash	Respiratory disorders, diabetes, anemia, general weakness
Swarna bhasma	Ash of gold (calcined gold)	Improves body immunity, general weakness, anemia, energetic
Rajat bhasma	Silver ash (calcined silver)	Irritable bowel syndrome, acidity, pitta disorders
Heerak bhasma	Diamond	Severe respiratory tract infection, marrow depression, ovarian cysts, uterine fibroids
Swarnmakshik bhasma	Copper pyrite (calcined), mercury, sulfur	Anemia, jaundice, stomatitis, chronic fever
Vaikrant bhasma	Manganese, sulfur (tourmaline)	Diabetes, can be used in place of diamond ash in case of poor patients

5.2.3 BHASMA PREPARATION

Bhasma preparation involves three basic steps (Fig. 5.3), which are modified according the nature of the raw material used for preparation. The three basic steps are sodhana, marana, and lohitikarana/amritikarana. Sodhana is the purification step in which the external and internal impurities of the raw material is removed. Modification or elimination of undesirable traits in the raw material is carried out. The therapeutic potential is enhanced or modified to suit the end application. The marana step involves the burning or the calcination process. In this process, the purified raw material (metal) is ground in a mortar and pestle with herbal extract and sometimes with trace amounts of other metals. The marana process differs based on the materials used. The organic substances like herbs/animal products are burnt in open air, whereas inorganic substances such as metals are burnt in closed containers. The marana process yields the bhasma, which is usually purified further to make it a suitable therapeutic. Amritikarana translates to "conversion into nectar/ambrosia." The amritikarana process is very crucial in removing the residual toxins (shista dosha) from the bhasma obtained after the marana process. The detoxification step is primarily used for bhasmas of copper, iron, gold, and mica.

5.2.4 QUALITY CONTROL OF BHASMA

The prepared bhasmas are then tested for their purity and integrity using various chemical and physical parameters. This process of testing is called Bhasma Pariksha (Table 5.2). The bhasma is considered consumable only if it passes the prescribed tests. The bhasmas thus produced, after passing all the tests are marketed for various diseases. The bhasmas are administered in very small doses, orally to achieve overall well-being of the affected individuals.

TABLE 5.2   Tests for Checking the Quality of Prepared Bhasma.

Physical properties		Chemical properties	
Varna	Color is dependent on the parent material	Gatarasatva	The bhasma should not taste like the parent metal
Varitara	Floatation in stagnant waters	Nirdhuma	There shouldn't be any fumes
Rekhapurna	Bhasma should be fine enough to fill the furrows of finger tips	Apunarbhava	Inability to regain original metallic form
Unama	A grain of rice should float on a layer of bhasma dispersed in stagnant water	Nirutha	Inability to regain metallic form
Anjana Sannibha	Bhasma should be smooth and irritation free	Amal Pariksha	When mixed with acidic fruit extract, the discoloration of the extract shouldn't occur
Nishchandra	Lusterless when observed under sunlight	Aksharatva	The bhasma should lack alkaline taste
Sukshmatva	Fineness, the particles should be like the pollen of *Pondanus odoratissimus* flower		

5.2.5   CONTEMPORARY INVESTIGATIONS OF BHASMA

Various scientific reports characterizing various bhasmas have been published. State-of-the-art characterization techniques have established without doubt that the ayurvedic bhasmas contain nanosized particles. Some of the sophisticated instruments that have been used for analyzing the bhasma composition include the scanning electron microscope, transmission electron microscope (TEM), energy dispersive X-ray analysis (EDAX), inductively coupled plasma spectroscopy (ICPS), atomic absorption spectroscopy (AAS), X-ray induced photo electron spectroscopy (XPS), etc. The various bhasmas have been investigated using the various sophisticated instruments to determine the nature, crystallinity, composition, biocompatibility, and crystal defects of the materials present in the bhasmas. Swarna bhasma preparations have been found to have gold particles of 56–57 nm dimensions.[19] Ras sindoor (a mercury preparation) was found to contain crystalline mercury sulfide around 25–50 nm.[20] TEM analysis of Yashada bhasma revealed that it contained ZnO particles ranging from 10 to 25 nm.[21] TEM micrographs of lead sulfide, containing naga bhasma, revealed nanosized PbS particles which agglomerated into submicron clusters.[22] Another study revealed that silver nanoparticles ranging from 10 to 60 nm were found in rajatha bhasma.[23]

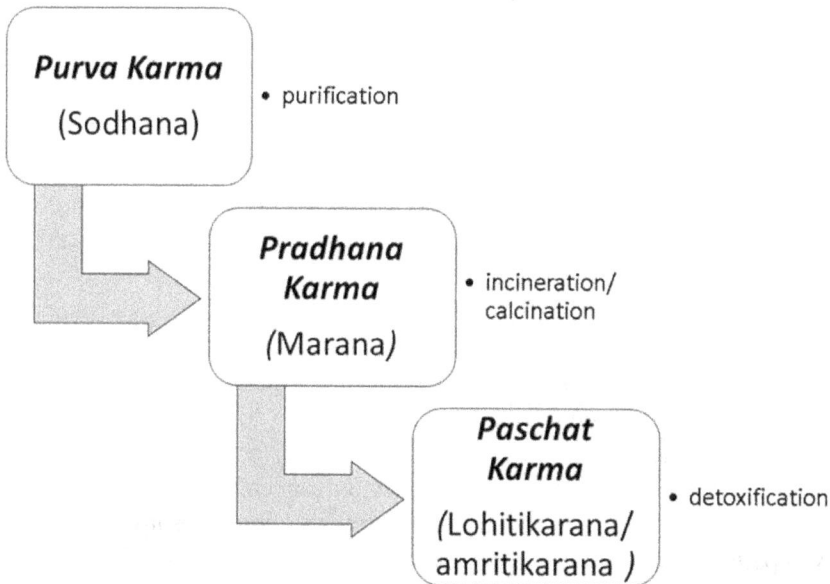

FIGURE 5.3 The basic steps in bhasmikarana process for preparing the ayurvedic bhasmas.

5.2.6 BHASMA COMPOSITION

Various studies have indicated that most bhasmas contain trace amounts of minerals in addition to the primary metal used in the preparation.[21–22, 24] It was also found that some preparations such as swarna bhasma did not have any other metal traces in them.[19] Kumar et al. investigated bhasmas made of calcium, iron, zinc, mercury, silver, copper, tin, and gemstones. They found that in addition to the main constituents, other elements such as essential elements such as sodium, potassium, magnesium, vanadium, calcium, manganese, iron, copper, and zinc were found in microgram per gram of the bhasma. Gold and cobalt were also found in nanograms per gram of the material. These traces elements were found to be chelated with the organic moieties of the herbal extract used in the preparation of the bhasma.[24] The trace elements could also be from the herbs used in the production of bhasma.[22]

5.2.7 BHASMA TOXICITY

Even though bhasmas have been extensively used in the Indian subcontinent for centuries, a lot of controversies are surrounding bhasmas due to the detection of toxic heavy metals in some formulations. Many ayurvedic schools are facing numerous problems in standardizing proper bhasma preparation techniques due to inferior quality raw materials, improper identification of raw materials, the lack of standards, and improper quality control.

From the above studies, the presence of metal nanoparticles or nanoclusters is evident and their size has been found to enhance the bioavailability and therapeutic potential of this age old nanomedicine from ancient India. A large number of patents are being applied for various Ayurveda related products and technologies. Numerous research articles are also being published which makes use of the recent advancements in technology to provide in-depth answers to the mechanisms and processes involved in the therapeutic potential of the bhasma. However, the question of toxicity in these ayurvedic preparations due to improper manufacturing needs to be settled. The increasing demand for ayurvedic medications calls for using stringent processing and testing parameters in order to deliver consistent and excellent quality product to customers.

5.3 CONCLUSIONS

As with all schools of medicine, the ayurvedic methods also need to be updated from time to time. This can be evidenced from how Ayurveda has evolved from its pre-Vedic form to the modern day form. The bhasmas are very useful and potent ayurvedic medicine, which can greatly benefit from the rapid development of nanotechnology and the allied fields. The highly efficient visualization and other characterization techniques used in nanotechnology can be utilized to maintain the quality of the bhasmas. The details of the production process can be monitored in each step of bhasma synthesis. The detailed mechanism of action of the bhasmas can also be investigated. These biosynthesized, nanometric therapeutics can be of great significance in curing diseases with minimal or no side effects.

KEYWORDS

- **nanomedicine**
- **bhasma**
- **Ayurveda**
- **holistic medicine**
- **metallic/mineral preparation**

REFERENCES

1. Schaming, D.; Remita, H. Nanotechnology: From the Ancient Time to Nowadays. *Found. Chem.* **2015,** *17* (3), 187–205.
2. Gao, L.; McCarthy, T. J. The "Lotus Effect" Explained: Two Reasons Why Two Length Scales of Topography Are Important. *Langmuir* **2006,** *22* (7), 2966–2967.
3. Garg, P.; Ghatmale, P.; Tarwadi, K.; Chavan, S. Influence of Nanotechnology and the Role of Nanostructures in Biomimetic Studies and Their Potential Applications. *Biomimetics* **2017,** *2* (2), 7.
4. Nowack, B.; Bucheli, T. D. Occurrence, Behavior and Effects of Nanoparticles in the Environment. *Environ. Pollut.* **2007,** *150* (1), 5–22.
5. Michielsen, K.; Stavenga, D. G. Gyroid Cuticular Structures in Butterfly Wing Scales: Biological Photonic Crystals. *J. R. Soc. Interface* **2008,** *5* (18), 85–94.
6. Brill, R. H. *The Chemistry of the Lycurgus Cup; Proc. 7th Internat. Cong. Glass* **1965,** *223,* 1–13.
7. Barber, D.; Freestone, I. C. An Investigation of the Origin of the Colour of the Lycurgus Cup by Analytical Transmission Electron Microscopy. *Archaeometry* **1990,** *32* (1), 33–45.
8. José-Yacamán, M.; Rendón, L.; Arenas, J.; Puche, M. C. S. Maya Blue Paint: An Ancient Nanostructured Material. *Science* **1996,** *273* (5272), 223.
9. Rytwo, G. Clay Minerals as an Ancient Nanotechnology: Historical Uses of Clay Organic Interactions, and Future Possible Perspectives. *Macla* **2008,** *9,* 15–17.
10. Lynge, M. E.; van der Westen, R.; Postma, A.; Städler, B. Polydopamine—A Nature-Inspired Polymer Coating for Biomedical Science. *Nanoscale* **2011,** *3* (12), 4916–4928.

11. Liu, N.; Lu, Z.; Zhao, J.; McDowell, M. T.; Lee, H.-W.; Zhao, W.; Cui, Y. A Pomegranate-Inspired Nanoscale Design for Large-Volume-Change Lithium Battery Anodes. *Nat. Nanotechnol.* **2014,** *9* (3), 187–192.

12. Bhishagratna, K. L. *An English Translation of the Sushruta Samhita Based on Original Sanskrit text*; Wilkin's Press, Calcutta, India, 1907; Vol. 1.

13. Wujastyk, D. *The Roots of Ayurveda: Selections from Sanskrit Medical Writings*; Penguin, New Delhi, India, 2003.

14. Mukhopādhyāya, G. *The Surgical Instruments of the Hindus: With a Comparative Study of the Surgical Instruments of the Greek, Roman, Arab, and the Modern European Surgeons*; RK Naahar, New Delhi, India, 1977.

15. Chattopadhyaya, D. *History of Science and Technology in Ancient India: Formation of the Theoretical Fundamentals of Natural Science*; Firma KLM Private Limited, Kolkata, India, 1991.

16. Mangathayaru, K. *Pharmacognosy: An Indian Perspective*; Pearson Education, India, 2013.

17. Jha, C. B. *Ayurveda Rasa Shastra*; Choukhambha Surabharati Prakashan: Varanasi, India, 2000, pp 325.

18. Pal, D.; Sahu, C. K.; Haldar, A. Bhasma: The Ancient Indian Nanomedicine. *J. Adv. Pharm. Technol. Res.* **2014,** *5* (1), 4.

19. Rastogi, S. Building Bridges Between Ayurveda and Modern Science. *Int. J. Ayurveda Res.* **2010,** *1* (1), 41.

20. Singh, S. K.; Chaudhary, A.; Rai, D.; Rai, S. *Preparation and Characterization of a Mercury Based Indian Traditional Drug—Ras-Sindoor*; NISCAIR Online Periodicals Repository 2009, *8* (3), *346–351.*

21. Bhowmick, T. K.; Suresh, A. K.; Kane, S. G.; Joshi, A. C.; Bellare, J. R. Physicochemical Characterization of an Indian Traditional Medicine, Jasada Bhasma: Detection of Nanoparticles Containing Non-Stoichiometric Zinc Oxide. *J. Nanopart. Res.* **2009,** *11* (3), 655–664.

22. Singh, S.; Gautam, D.; Kumar, M.; Rai, S. Synthesis, Characterization and Histopathological Study of a Lead-Based Indian Traditional Drug: Naga Bhasma. *Indian J. Pharm. Sci.* **2010,** *72* (1), 24.

23. Sharma, R.; Bhatt, A.; Thakur, M. Physicochemical Characterization and Antibacterial Activity of Rajata Bhasma and Silver Nanoparticle. *AYU* **2016,** *37* (1), 71.

24. Kumar, A.; Nair, A.; Reddy, A.; Garg, A. Unique Ayurvedic Metallic-Herbal Preparations, Chemical Characterization. *Biol. Trace Elem. Res.* **2006,** *109* (3), 231–254.

CHAPTER 6

ENGINEERING ASPECTS OF AYURVEDA: THE MECHANICS AND THERMODYNAMICS OF HUMAN PHYSIOLOGY

G. KUMARAVEL*

Vikram Sarabhai Space Centre, Thiruvananthapuram 695024, India

*E-mail: gnanakumaravel@gmail.com

ABSTRACT

Ayurveda is a science of life, developed and practiced in India for several thousands of years. Even though modern engineering principles are developed during the last few centuries, many of the engineering principles were used in the theory and practice of Ayurveda. In this chapter, the engineering principles embedded in Ayurveda are investigated and an engineering model of Ayurveda is presented. In Ayurveda, the human body, mind, and spirit are considered as a single "system," and the rest of the universe is considered as "surroundings." Both the system and surroundings are made of five elements or panchabhutas. The state of health of the system is governed by the equilibrium and stability characteristics of the system within the system and with respect to the surroundings. The treatment procedure plays the role of control. The conservation laws are applicable as there exist heat and mass transfer between the system and surroundings. The formation of diseases, maintaining health and treatment procedures are modeled in an engineering approach. The engineering approach provides confident that practically every disease is curable. This model can be extended to investigate cause and cure of many diseases.

6.1 INTRODUCTION

The complete knowledge about the existence of universe and the human life is given in four Vedas: Rig, Yajur, Sama, and Atharva. Though Ayurvedic concepts are explained in all the Vedas, Ayurveda is considered as an Upaveda of Atharva Veda.[1] Ayurveda is a classical biological and medical science with well-established principles, developed and practiced in India for several thousand years.[2] The foundation of present day Ayurveda is based on the original texts such as Sushruta Samhita, Charaka Samhita, Astanga Hirudaya, etc., which were written thousands of years before.

According to Vedas, Brahman, which is absoluteness, nonmaterialistic, and superconsciousness, joins with Maya or illusion to form Prakriti or nature, which forms elemental matter.[3] From Prakriti, the three gunas or divine qualities, namely, Satwa—pure and subtleness, Rajas—activeness, and Tamas—inertia, arise, and they interweave to create panchabhutas— the five material elements, namely, Prithvi—Earth, Jala—water, Agni— fire, Vayu—air, and Akash—space.[2] The entire universe is made up of only panchabhutas. Different matters are evolved out of panchabhutas, through different combination and proportion. The Ayurveda considers the human body, mind, and spirit as a single system, and it is made up of the same matter that made this universe. This implies that whatever happens in the universe or surroundings have an influence on the system. The reverse is also true, however smaller it may be. These panchabhutas, Kala (time), direction, soul, and mind are called Dravyas in which Karma (action) and Gunas (qualities) exist in inherent state. Three doshas are formed out of the five elements—Earth and water join to form Kapha Dosha, fire forms Pitta Dosha, and air and space join to form Vata Dosha. The building block of tridoshas from the primordial elements is shown in Figure 6.1.

There are seven types of body–mind–sprit constitutions according to the predominant doshas, namely, Pitta, Vata, Kapha, Pitta–Vata, Kapha– Pitta, Kapha–Vata, and Pitta–Vata–Kapha. At the time of birth, the child acquires any one of the above seven types of constitution. The three doshas are in definite proportion, and they are in balance with each other. This proportion is called "Prakriti" of the person, and it does not change with space and time. But the entire universe is also made up of same five elements associated with the three doshas. Therefore, the food, lifestyle, surroundings, etc., of the person continuously influence on the person's Prakriti. Because of this, the proportion between the doshas may change, and this will cause a deviation in Prakriti of the person. This deviation is called "Vikriti," which is responsible for diseases. The Ayurvedic treatment procedures involve in finding out the Prakriti and Vikriti of the person and treat him accordingly to bring back the deviation to original condition.

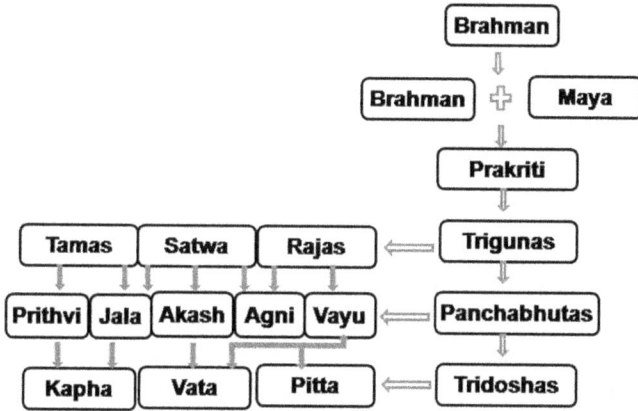

FIGURE 6.1   Building block of tridoshas.

In Ayurveda, food is classified according to tastes, potency (hot or cold), etc. There are six tastes, namely, Madhura (sweet), Amla (sour), Lavana (salt), Katu (pungent), Tikta (bitter), and Kasaya (astringent), based on the combination of panchabhutas in food. Because each dosha is formed out of the five elements and each taste is also made up of the same five elements, the food has its influence on the doshas through taste. Therefore, it is obvious that the food intake of a person should be based on his Prakriti to maintain health. The details are given in Table 6.1.

TABLE 6.1   Six Tastes and Their Constituent Elements.

Sl. No.	Taste	Elements	Influence on doshas
1	Sweet	Earth and water	Increases Kapha; decreases Pitta and Vata
2	Sour	Fire and Earth	Increases Kapha and Pitta; decreases Vata
3	Salt	Water and fire	Increases Kapha and Pitta; decreases Vata
4	Bitter	Air and space	Increases Vata; decreases Pitta and Kapha
5	Pungent	Air and fire	Increases Pitta and Vata; decreases Kapha
6	Astringent	Air and Earth	Increases Kapha and Vata; decreases Pitta

The food consumed is digested by Agni (digestive fire) or the power of transformation, which is a manifestation of fire element. Agni is present everywhere in the body. The Jatharagni, which is present in the stomach, is primarily responsible for digestion. The digested food is transformed into various dhatus or structural components of the body. There are seven dhatus in the body, namely, Rasa (plasma), Rakta (blood), Mamsa (muscle), Medhas (fat), Asthi (bone and cartilage), Majja (bone marrow), and Shukra (reproductive fluids). For each dhatu and each element, there is an Agni, together called Dhatwagni and Bhutagni, respectively. Therefore, including Jatharagni, there are 13 Agnis in the human body, which control digestion, metabolism, etc. Impairment of Agni causes improper digestion and transformation. The improperly digested food is called ama, which is responsible for all diseases, because it out-balances the doshas. In the conversion of digested food to dhatus, waste materials called malas are removed at every stage of conversion. While waste materials are removed from the body by the system, ama is not removed completely by the system. Various Ayurvedic treatments are primarily concerned with removal of ama from the body, thereby balancing the doshas. According to Ayurveda, Arogya (good health) of the system is given by the balanced condition of doshas, dhatus, and malas. The circulation of doshas and dhatus to various parts of the body and the elimination of malas out of the body are carried out through strotas or channels. There are 13 such channels in male and 15 in female bodies. The aggravated doshas can disturb the movement of dhatus in these channels and thereby causing diseases.

In summary, the theory of Ayurveda deals the various combinations and interactions of 3 gunas, panchabhutas, 3 doshas, 6 tastes, 7 dhatus, 13 Agnis, 13 or 15 strotas, malas, ama, etc. It also deals with the interaction of human body with the surroundings, equilibrium with the season, climate, locality, etc. The practice of Ayurveda in treatment of diseases is primarily involved in investigating the system for the disturbed doshas, find out the cause which made it, eliminate the aggravated doshas, and rejuvenate the body for immunity. Because of the systematic, scientific, and methodical approach of Ayurveda, it survived for many thousands of years despite discouragement and ban on it during foreign invasions in India.

The scientific foundations of Ayurveda are brought out by many scholars.[4,5] In the present work, the mechanics and thermodynamic principles embedded in Ayurveda are discussed. Thermodynamics is an engineering science that deals with the interaction between a system and surroundings due to energy transformation involving work, heat, and the properties of matter.[6] The equilibrium, stability, and control of the system are studied in mechanics. In the next section, the principles of Ayurveda are compared to engineering principles. In the third section, the mechanics of human body equilibrium, stability, and control are discussed. The fourth section deals with the thermodynamic aspects. In the fifth section, how the tridoshas act as systems is described. In the sixth, the demand/supply chain of dhatus in the human body is presented. A brief note application of this engineering model in investigating the diseases is given in the seventh section, followed by conclusions.

6.2   ENGINEERING MODEL OF AYURVEDA

At zero absolute temperature and pressure, the three states of matter—solid, liquid, and gases—do not exist, and there is no heat or space within it. They are in frozen state. This can be compared to the Brahman. The frozen material acquires some form of cosmic energy and this creates some movement within the system. This is comparable to Maya. The system consists of three basic things—the mass (m), energy (E), and velocity (v). They are comparable to Tamas, Satwa, and Rajas Gunas, respectively. In other words, Maya joins with Brahman and creates the three gunas. They are comparable to the equation: $E = mc^2$. The mass, energy, and velocity interweave themselves to create three different states of matter—solid, liquid, and vapor. There exist heat and space within the states of matter. The three states of matter—solid, liquid, and vapor—heat, and space are comparable to the panchabhutas—Prithvi, Jala, Vayu, Agni, and Akash, respectively. These five elements form the entire universe. Different matters are evolved from these five elements and human is one such matter. The equilibrium within the human body, mind, and spirit is maintained by three major subsystems—Thermal (Pitta), Mechanical (Vata), and Physical (Kapha) systems. The dominant fluid properties of Pitta, Vata, and Kapha are temperature, pressure, and weight density, respectively. The summary of the above description is given in Table 6.2 and also in Figure 6.2.

TABLE 6.2   Engineering Description of Ayurvedic Principles.

Sl. no.	Ayurveda	Engineering
1.	Brahman	Frozen state of matter (absolute zero temperature and zero pressure)
2.	Maya	Some form of cosmic energy
3.	Trigunas (Maya + Brahman)	Comparable to $E = mc^2$
4.	Satva, Rajas, and Tamas	Energy (E), velocity (v), and mass (m)
5.	Panchabhutas: five elements: Prithvi, Jala, Vayu, Agni, and Akash	States of matter: solid, liquid, and vapor and heat and space
6.	Tridoshas: (Pitta, Vata, Kapha) properties of substance	Dominant material properties: temperature, pressure, and weight density
7.	Tridoshas: (Pitta, Vata, Kapha) functions in human body	Subsystems in human body: thermal, mechanical, and physical systems

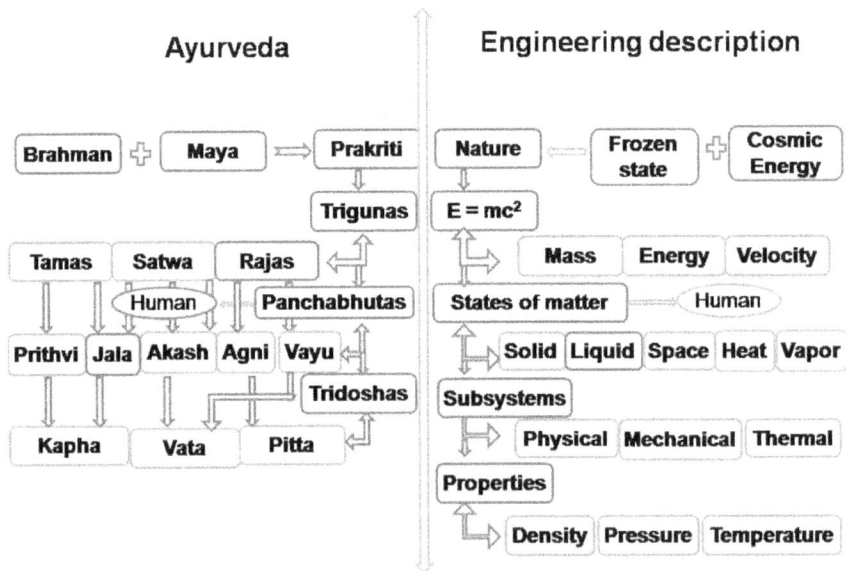

FIGURE 6.2   Engineering description of Ayurvedic principles.

6.3   EQUILIBRIUM, STABILITY, AND CONTROL OF THE SYSTEM

6.3.1   EQUILIBRIUM WITH THE SOLAR SYSTEM

Even though every material is made up of five elements, in each material, one or more of the elements will dominate. For example, Sun is the source of heat energy to Earth through electromagnetic radiation, and therefore, Sun can be considered as element of fire or Agni. Similarly, the planet Earth can be considered as the element of solid, the surface of Earth which contains sea, rivers, and inland water resources as the element of water or Jala and the atmosphere which surrounds the Earth as the element of air or Vayu. The space above atmosphere can be considered as space or Akash.

The human system is an integral part of the universe and both have the same elements in common, any changes in the universe is reflected on the human. Therefore, in order to maintain equilibrium with the universe, Ayurveda recommends the periodical changes in the food and lifestyle according to daily changes and seasonal changes.

The day and night changes are due to rotation of Earth (Dhin) and the Ayurveda divides one day into three equal sessions from sunrise to sunset and one night into three equal sessions from sunset to sunrise. The first session is dominated with Kapha, the middle with Pitta, and the third session with Vata. The change between one session to another session is gradual. Ayurveda recommends "Dinacharya," the food and lifestyle to be followed in each session so as to maintain equilibrium with the changes outside.

The seasonal changes (Ritu) are due revolution of Earth around the Sun, and the Ayurveda recommends "Ritucharya," the food and lifestyle, to be adopted due to seasonal changes. Ayurveda divides 1 year into six seasons, namely, Sisira (late winter), Vasanta (spring), Grisma (summer), Varsa (rainy), Sarad (autumn), and Hemanta (early winter). The first three are categorized as Uttarayana or dry season and the last three are categorized as Daksinayana or wet seasons. Each Dosha accumulates, aggravates, and becomes normal in different seasons. Vata accumulates in summer, aggravates in rainy season, and normalizes in autumn. Pitta accumulates in rainy season, aggravates in autumn, and normalizes in early winter. Similarly, Kapha accumulates in late winter, aggravates in spring, and normalizes in summer. Therefore, the best time to eliminate the aggravated doshas is during the season it gets aggravated. Vata, Pitta, and Kapha are eliminated during rainy, autumn, and spring seasons, respectively. By this process, the conservation of doshas is maintained.

6.3.2 EQUILIBRIUM WITH TIME

The change in Kala or time is called Parinaman. Unlike space, where one can travel to and fro, time is unidirectional. In Ayurveda, the time is considered as one of the Dravyas and the unidirectionality and irreversibility of the time are accounted in treatment of diseases. Even though Prakriti of a person does not change with time, it adopts itself with time through age of the person. The age of person is very important in treatment. Two of the branches of Ayurveda, namely, Bala Chikitsa and Jana Chikitsa deal with childhood and old age diseases, respectively. During childhood and young age, the Prakriti is dominated by Kapha, middle age is dominated by Pitta, and old age is dominated by Vata. This explains why children and youth enjoy playing in hot Sun, whereas middle-aged persons suffer with sunstrokes. Also, as a result of Vata domination, old age people like to travel, talk more, take lead in family functions, get involved in social activities, etc.

There is another factor with respect to time—the time taken to cure a disease. Ayurveda does not support instant cure of any disease because the process of cure is nothing but bringing the doshas to equilibrium, the treatment duration (chikitsa kala) depends on the history of the disease—the time taken for the disease to grow to the present stage. Ideally, the treatment process is a reverse process of disease formation. But, the treatment process need not take the same time duration as that of disease formation. The treatment time for each of the diseases is mentioned in Ayurveda according to strength of the disease (Rogha Bala), strength of the patient (Rogi Bala), age, etc.

6.3.3 EQUILIBRIUM WITH SPACE

The seasonal changes vary from place to place. Therefore, if a person travels from one place to another person, he has to accommodate to the local environment and seasons and change his food and lifestyle accordingly. This way, equilibrium with space is maintained.

6.3.4 STABILITY OF THE SYSTEM

When the internal equilibrium of doshas is disturbed, the system attempts to bring back the doshas to its normal state. Dinacharya and Ritucharya help the system to maintain stability. No treatment is necessary if the system is successful in eliminating the aggravated doshas from the system to the surroundings by itself, and it is possible in healthy system for small disturbances. However, if ama is formed because of the aggravated doshas, then elimination process is difficult. In such cases, treatment—the control process—is to be invoked.

6.3.5 CONTROL OF THE SYSTEM

In Ayurveda, Dosha aggravation is investigated by finding the Prakriti and Vikriti of the person by an astasthana pariksa or eight-fold investigation process. The aggravated, accumulated, or alleviated doshas in dhatus, strotas, etc. and their locations, and the impairment of Agnis are investigated by studying the respective malas for the presence of ama. The aggravated doshas are eliminated through various treatment procedures such as Vamana (vomiting), Virechana (purgation), and Vasti (enema). These procedures eliminate aggravated Kapha, Pitta, and Vata, respectively. The equilibrium, stability, and control of the human body as a system are depicted in Figure 6.3.

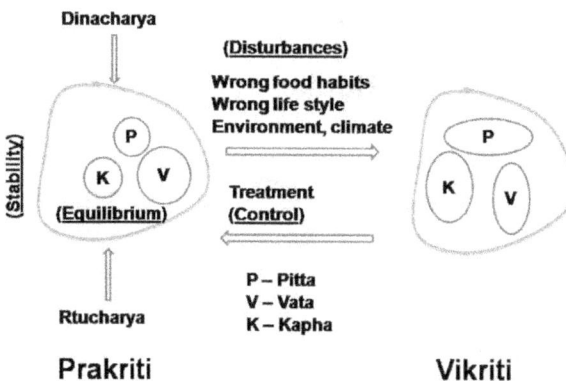

FIGURE 6.3 Description of equilibrium, stability, and control of the system.

6.4   HUMAN BODY AS A THERMODYNAMIC SYSTEM

The surface temperature of a healthy human body remains at 98.4°F irrespective of the surrounding temperature, seasons, climate, and food and lifestyle. Therefore, the human body can be modeled as an isothermal system, operated at a constant surface temperature (T_1), higher than that of the surroundings (T_2), as depicted in Figure 6.4. As a result, there is continuous heat dissipation from system to surroundings, and the system requires a continuous supply of heat energy to maintain external equilibrium with the surroundings. The food, lifestyle, etc. disturb the internal equilibrium of the system. Also, the changes within the surroundings due to change of day and night, wind, climate, seasons, etc. disturb the external equilibrium of the system. These internal and external disturbances shift the equilibrium proportion of doshas away from Prakriti to a perturbed state, or Vikriti, which causes diseases in the system. The Ayurvedic procedures such as Dinacharya and Ritucharya help to maintain equilibrium of the system and treatments play the role of control to maintain stability of the system (Fig. 6.3).

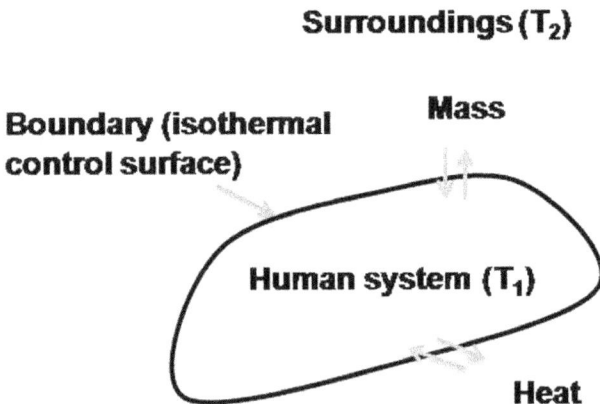

Surroundings (T₂)

**Boundary (isothermal   Mass
control surface)**

Human system (T₁)

Heat

FIGURE 6.4   Human body as a thermodynamic system with its surroundings $(T_1 > T_2)$.

According to Ayurveda, the strength of human body varies with seasons—strongest in winter and weakest in summer.[1,7] In thermodynamics, the maximum efficiency of a heat engine is given by Carnot efficiency $\eta = (T_1 - T_2)/T_1$, where T_1 and T_2 are the temperature of the system (human body) and surroundings, respectively. While T_1 remains constant throughout the year, the average temperature T_2 in a day changes with seasons—highest in summer and lowest in winter. Therefore, strength of the human body can be represented as a function of Carnot efficiency. In modern biology, this phenomenon is linked to metabolism.[8,9]

6.5   TRIDOSHAS AS SYSTEMS

Each of the tridoshas is divided into five types. Vata is divided into Prana, Udana, Vyana, Samana, and Apana. Pitta is divided into Pachaka, Ranjaka, Sadhaka, Alochaka, and Brajaka. Kapha is divided into Avalambaka, Kledaka, Bodhaka, Tarpaka, and Slesaka. Each subsystem has a leader. Prana controls other Vayus, Pachaka controls other Pittas, and Avalambaka controls other Kaphas. Their locations and primary functions are given in Table 6.3.

It can be observed from the table that each of the subsystem carries specific functions; some of them stay together and work together. For example, Samana Vayu and Pachaka Pitta work together for separation of waste and nutrients. Each subsystem, at the end of its function, transfers control to another subsystem. Sequential, selective, and repetitive actions are carried out by these subsystems, as if they are controlled by a software program.

TABLE 6.3   The Subdivisions, Functions, and Locations of Tridoshas.

Dosha	Subdivision	Location	Major function
Vata	Prana	Brain	Moves to respiratory tract; controls respiration, swallowing, belching, sneezing, etc.
	Udana	Chest	Moves to throat, nose, and lungs; controls speech, memory, etc.; responsible for courage, etc.
	Vyana	Heart	Moves all over the body; separation of waste products from the system; nourishment to tissues
	Samana	Stomach	Food absorption; digestion; separation of waste and nutrients

TABLE 6.3   *(Continued)*

Dosha	Subdivision	Location	Major function
	Apana	Lumbosacral	Reproduction and excretory activities; responsible for expulsion of fetus
Pitta	Pacaka	Small intestine	Digestion and assimilation of food; separation of nutrients and waste products
	Ranjaka	Stomach, liver, and spleen	Responsible for intelligence, pride, enthusiasm, etc.
	Alocaka	Eyes	Controls vision
	Bhrajaka	Skin	Controls color and complexion of skin
Kapha	Avalambaka	Chest, shoulder, and sacrum	Water balance; supports body fluid system
	Kledaka	Stomach	Moistens the food
	Bodhaka	Tongue	Controls taste perception
	Tarpaka	Head	Nourishes sense organs
	Slesaka	Joints	Lubricates joints

6.6   DHATUS AND DEMAND/SUPPLY CHAIN

The formation of seven dhatus happens sequentially. Rasa is the essence of properly digested food. From Rasa, Rakta is formed; from Rakta, Mamsa is formed, and so on. The digested food and all dhatus release mala or wastes upon conversion and these malas are removed by Vayu from the body. As seen earlier, improperly digested food creates ama, which is not fully excreted in normal conditions. The presence of ama causes disturbance in the equilibrium of tridoshas. Ama accumulates under the skin. Ama has to be removed from the body through Ayurvedic treatment. While conversion from one dhatu to another, a portion of ama also travels in the chain. Shukra dhatu is at the end of the chain, and there is no mala at the end of the chain. However, the presence of ama in the Shukra indicates impurity. Therefore, the system instructs to eject the Shukra and the command invokes a sexual desire in order to execute ejection. Therefore, a person who has a habit of taking impure food like improperly cooked food, food not compatible with his body constitution, etc. lives with lustful thoughts and higher sexual desires. According to Sushruta, it takes nearly 1 month for the digested food to convert to Shukra. Therefore, Sushruta insists that those couples who plan for a child, should stay away from each other for a month and follow proper food and lifestyle to enable the formation of pure Shukra. On the other hand, children born out of impure Shukra dhatu take birth with unbalanced Prakriti and therefore lead a life with diseases, like plants grown out of poor quality seeds.

In the supply chain from digested food to Shukra, the unutilized Shukra is said to be converted into Ojhas which promotes health of body, mind, and spirit. The Ojhas converts into Tejas finally, which promotes spiritual growth. Therefore, in order to carry a spiritual life, proper food and lifestyle, positive thoughts, and serene environment are advised for the formation of pure Shukra dhatu.

If Shukra dhatu is ejected, it demands a supply from the left neighbor, majja dhatu and after supplying for Shukra dhatu, majja dhatu in turn demands a supply from Asthi and this chain goes on until it reaches Rakta dhatu. The Rakta dhatu has to wait for the arrival of Rasa which in turn comes from digested food. This demand chain is quicker as compared to the supply chain. Therefore, a person involved in sexual activity becomes tired because of the internal mechanisms within the body due to the demand chain and not solely due to the physical activity carried out by him. Also, because of loss of Shukra, which is Kapha in nature, the person feels thirsty. The supply chain and the demand chain of the seven dhatus are depicted in Figure 6.5.

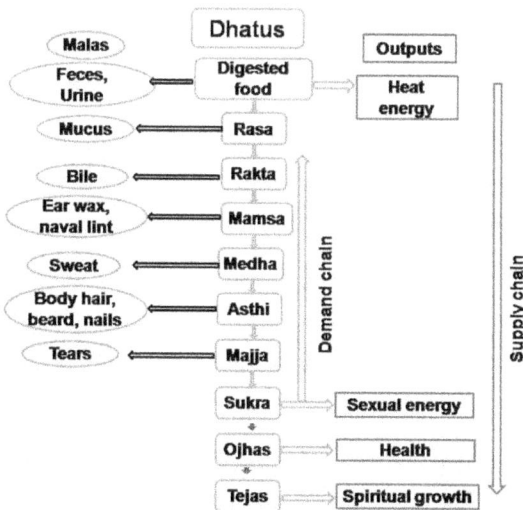

FIGURE 6.5   Seven dhatus—the demand and supply chains.

6.7 INVESTIGATION OF CAUSE AND CURE OF VARIOUS DISEASES

The thermodynamic model of the human system within the framework of Ayurveda can explain the cause of many diseases, and a subject-oriented holistic approach can be useful in treatment of many diseases. Many diseases are classified as due to aggravation of one or more doshas as seen earlier. Some of the examples are discussed here without proof.

When a human body is exposed to sun, heat transfer takes place from the surrounding to the system through solar radiation which directly aggravates Pitta. Therefore, the person is affected by a fever or sunstroke.

Pressure is the driving force for movement of the fluid in a system. In a state of Vikriti due to Vata aggravation, pressure and therefore velocity of the flow within a subsystem is disturbed. Hypertensive heart diseases can be accounted under this category.

Cancer is a disease due to imbalance in all three doshas.[7,10] Any food habit or lifestyle which aggravates all three doshas can destabilize the system, and it may lead to cancer. In smoking, regular application of heated air (Vata and Pitta disturbance) is carried out in Kapha dominated throat region, thus causing tridosha imbalance. This can be interpreted as one of the causes of throat cancer. Investigation of influence of smoking on the subdivisions of tridoshas may throw light on throat and lungs cancers.

Sushruta[7] described about curable and incurable diseases. In a system with curable disease, the disturbed doshas are brought back to its Prakriti state by means of treatment process. But, in a system with incurable diseases, this process is not possible. In thermodynamics, these processes are called reversible and irreversible processes, respectively. By studying Ayurvedic principles in mechanics/thermodynamics perspective, stability criteria for many diseases can be worked out. This will be useful in analyzing cause and cure of many diseases.

It has been explained earlier about the equilibrium of the system (human) with the surroundings. Because both of them are made up of same panchabhutas, the system can maintain equilibrium with the surroundings through mass and energy transfer. Apart from this, there exists a balance between human/animal kingdom and plant kingdom such that for every disease caused by micro-organisms/animals, there exists a plant or combination of plants for its cure. Practically, there is no Ayurvedic preparation without the use of plants. A vast knowledge base is available on the use of various parts of the plants for many diseases. This database has to be modeled to bring out the complementary nature of plants and microorganisms/animals so that new medicines can be prepared for many incurable diseases. For example, Thomas Alva Edison modeled the Rubber plant before he actually discovered it. He brought out the description of a plant with specific qualities and started searching for the plant and discovered it after testing around 17,000 plants. Therefore, a systematic engineering model of Ayurvedic principles will provide confidence that practically every disease is curable, except those governed by time.

6.8 CONCLUSIONS

In the present study, some of the engineering principles embedded in Ayurveda are discussed. The mechanics and thermodynamic model of the human system in the framework of Ayurveda are investigated. This engineering approach can explain the causes of many diseases, and a subject oriented holistic approach can find new treatment procedures for many of the diseases. In further work, the classical texts of Ayurveda will be studied in depth, and the embedded engineering principles will be modeled. These principles will be applied to medical physiology to investigate the cause and cure of many diseases in a unified approach.

ACKNOWLEDGMENTS

My sincere acknowledgments to International Sivananda Yoga Vedanta Centre, Neyyar Dam, Kerala, India for initiating me into Ayurveda and special thanks to Dr. Vishnu, for teaching me this subject.

KEYWORDS

- **Brahman**
- **Maya**
- **trigunas**
- **panchabhutas**
- **tridoshas cosmic energy**
- **mechanics**
- **thermodynamics**

REFERENCES

1. Devanathan, R.; Gopinath, V.; Brindha, P. Ayurvedic Concepts in Vedas. *Health Sci. Int. J.* **2011,** *1*(1), 5–8.
2. Maha Devan, L. *Ayurveda for Beginners,* 5th ed.; Sri Sarada Ayurvedic Hospital: Kanyakumari, India, 2012.
3. Devananda, S. V. *Mediation and Mantras,* 3rd ed.; Om Lotus Publications: New Delhi, 1995.
4. Mishra, L. C. Health Care and Disease Management. In *Scientific Basis for Ayurvedic Therapies*; Mishra, L. C., Ed.; CRC Press: New York, 2004; Chapter 2, pp 15.
5. Shiva Ayyadurai, V. S. The Control Systems Engineering Foundation of Traditional Indian Medicine: The Rosetta Stone for Siddha and Ayurveda. *Int. J. Syst. Syst. Eng.* **2014,** *5*(2), 125–149.
6. Rathakrishnan, E. *Fundamentals of Engineering Thermodynamics*; Prentice-Hall of India: New Delhi, 2005.
7. Bhishagratna, K. K. L. *An English Translation of the Sushruta Samhita*; S. L. Bhaduri: Calcutta, 1916.
8. van Ooijena, A. M. J.; van Marken Lichtenbelt, W. D.; van Steenhoven, A. A.; Westerterp, K. R. Seasonal Changes in Metabolic and Temperature Responses to Cold Air in Humans. *Physiol. Behav.* **2004,** *82*, 545–553.
9. Guyton, A. C.; Hall, J. E. *A Text Book on Medical Physiology,* 10th ed.; Elsevier: India, 2001.
10. Balachandran, P.; Govindarajan, R. Cancer—An Ayurvedic Perspective. *Pharmacol. Res.* **2005,** *51*, 19–30.

CHAPTER 7

HOLISTIC MEDICINE: POSSIBILITIES AND CHALLENGES IN HUMAN REPRODUCTION (GARBHSANSKAR)

TEJAL G. JOSHI[1]* and VRAJESHKUMAR G. KHAMBHOLJA[2]

[1]*CEO, Shree Garbhsanskar Centre*

[2]*Managing Director, Shree Garbhsanskar Centre*

Corresponding author. E-mail: drtejalgjoshi@gmail.com; 108sgc@gmail.com

ABSTRACT

To understand the holistic healthcare, we need to understand the factors those affect human body at grassroots level—the content of the human body, how any disease occurs to the human, and what is holistic medicine. On the idea of ancient Indian Hindu scriptures of teaching the fetus, the approach of holistic healthcare in reproduction at different levels has been designed and tested by the authors.

7.1 HUMAN BEING AS A WHOLE

According to the spiritual science, human being is not just physical body, but it also contains (1) the subtle body, (2) the causal body, and (3) the fragment of the God—the Soul. According to Veda, they are known as sookshma sharir, kaaran sharir, and aatman, respectively. At the time of death of any human being, only physical body is left by a soul and the remaining two bodies remain attached until it attains salvation or get enlightened or get stable in its original form, that is, Aatman. A human is incomplete without all three bodies and soul. For instance, if anyone dies, we call it a dead body of that person, and we do not name it. If a person is unconscious, his mental body (or some part of the brain) does not work, even though the soul and the physical body exist. And the soul without the physical body is no more human. It is called the soul embodied into the subtle and causal bodies.

Understanding the mental body in detail, it is the place where our feelings, emotions, and desires stay. It's accumulated from all previous birth and present birth too. It is made up of three parts: the conscious mind—it is the part of our thoughts and feelings that we are aware of, the subconscious mind—it contains all the impressions required to complete our destiny in current lifetime, and the unconscious mind—this is the aspect of our mind that we are completely unaware of. It contains all the impressions that are associated with our accumulated account.

The subtle body is defined as a part of our being or consciousness that leaves our physical body at the time of physical death. This body consists of the mental body as discussed above, the causal body—the intellect, subtle ego, and the soul. The causal body deals with decision-making process and reasoning abilities. The subtle ego is the feeling that we are separate from God. And the soul is the God principle within us and is our true nature.

Thus, for a human, to work at his full potential and to achieve the objective of his life, alignment of all three bodies and soul is required. The Indian ancient Holy Scripture, Srimad Bhagavad Geeta says that physical body is perishable, but not the soul.

7.2   HOW DISEASE OCCURS?

Around us is a pulsating electromagnetic energy field that is described as a rainbow like aura or as a luminous light body. This 'subtle-energy' field interacts with our physical body by flowing through concentrated spirals of energy. This energy interacts with our ductless endocrine glands and lymphatic system by feeding in good energy and disposing of unwanted energy. When this energy is disturbed or interrupted, there arises the situation what is called a disease. It means, disease starts at energy level first and then it manifests into the physical body. For instance, before we feel fever physically, we actually feel lack of energy in some way or other what we call fatigue or even sometime we feel uneasy. It means for any disease to occur at physical level, it starts from energy level. And mental body and part of the subtle body come under the energy level.

7.3 HOLISTIC MEDICINE

Medicine: It is defined as a natural or chemical agent that helps to diagnose, prevent, cure, control, or mitigation of the disease.

Holistic medicine means, the combo of different intervention which can be used to treat physical body, mental body, or the subtle body of a human being. It is a fact that the conventional way of treatment focuses only on physical body and not on the other parts of a human being.

In short, holistic medicine is a form of healing that considers body, mind, spirit, and emotions—in the quest for optimal health and wellness.

Holistic healers believe that the whole person is made up of interdependent parts and if one part is not working properly, all the other parts will be affected. In this way, if people have physical, emotional, or spiritual imbalances, it can negatively affect their overall health.

7.4 HOLISTIC HEALTHCARE IN REPRODUCTION

Holistic healthcare is a system of comprehensive or total health care, which considers the physical, emotional, social, economic, and spiritual needs of the person; his or her response to illness and the effect of the illness on the ability to meet self-care needs. Holistic healthcare is the modern practice of medicine that expresses this philosophy of care.

A holistic practitioner may use combination of various treatment modalities of healthcare. He uses from conventional medication to contemporary medicine and/or alternative or complementary therapies to treat a patient. For example, person suffering from headache pays a visit to a holistic doctor, instead of using only medication; the doctor will likely scrutinize all the factors that may be causing the headache, such as diet and sleep habits, stress and personal problem, and preferred spiritual practices. The treatment protocol may involve drugs to relieve symptoms; however, lifestyle modifications may also be advised to help prevent the headache from reoccurring. Thus, holistic healthcare is one-stop solution to treat patient in holistic way. According to the above understanding, a holistic healthcare consists of a team of doctors who are specialized in different segments to tackle the various diseases. Such as holistic healthcare in reproduction require team of doctors like gynecologist and obstetrician, in vitro fertility (IVF) specialist, embryologist, anesthetic, holistic healer (Garbhsanskar[1] specialist), fetal medicine specialist, dentist, cosmetologist, dietician, physiotherapist, massage therapist, and even a pediatrician.

7.4.1 HOLISTIC HEALTHCARE IN PRECONCEPTION

It is the healthcare that can provide various ways for expectant couple to conceive the healthy baby. When conception happens, that fertilized cell has all physical, mental, and subtle body with an embodied soul. So to attract a certain kind of soul, one has to raise their levels to match the frequency level of the embodied soul at every level. And that is possible through holistic approach only. Like when a crop is cultivated with good care at every level and each stage right from the selection of seeds, choosing the fertile land, proper season of crop, and atmosphere along with proper fertilizer and if needed pesticides too, the result is sure to get high quality of crops. Same way if one wants to have baby that is better at mind body and embodied soul levels, then pre-conception Garbhsanskar with holistic approach can help couple to reach the goal for their dream child. This approach can be started immediately after marriage or at least one year before conception.

7.4.2 HOLISTIC HEALTHCARE DURING PREGNANCY

In the current time, female choose career progress first and then pregnancy, so it has been observed an increased risk during pregnancy after the age

---

[1]Garbhsanskar: "Garbh" means fetus inside the womb; and "sanskar" is the process of making one better at body, mind, and the embodied soul levels. Hence, Garbhsanskar means the process through which the fetus can be better at mind, body, and the embodied soul levels. This process can be performed on expectant parents, pregnant female as well as during postpartum care. Garbhsanskar specialist is a holistic healer who uses customized form of various natural treatment, alternative and complementary medicines and the training to install good virtues as well as to enhance the intelligence of fetus. This practitioner understands the person as a whole and then tailors a treatment protocol. There are more than 100 therapies, out of which few therapies or blend of more than 10 therapies can be utilized in a customized way according the need of the patient. Garbhsanskar specialist decides it after taking holistic history of a patient.

of 30 years. Moreover, due to drastic change in environment, the natural quality of food has changed that has given rise in pregnancy complication and even sometime hormonal imbalances. Hence, holistic approach has become a need of the time for every pregnancy. During pregnancy fetus development is occurring at various stages. In order to keep watch on its growth, and to minimize the pregnancy complication, as well as its effect on fetus, Garbhsanskar is needed. In addition to that, the future of a baby is the future of parents and of course the future of the nation, so every child matters a lot.

During pregnancy, fetus' physical body and mental body are prepared. 75–80% brain development happens during pregnancy itself. Research has shown that the cognitive function is started way before the birth of a baby. And holistic approach during pregnancy can ensure overall growth of baby. In fact, to stop pruning effect in brain in order to maximize its potential it is required. For that, various treatments of holistic medicine are to be given to the pregnant lady. Holistic approach minimizes the risk factors as well as it also brings positive changes in the life of attending couple and of course healthy, beautiful, intelligent, and virtuous baby is the incentive.

7.4.3 HOLISTIC HEALTHCARE—POSTPARTUM

Holistic healthcare during postpartum period is equally important due to some reasons. First of all, infant's health is dependent on mother's health, so healthy mother can raise healthy child. Moreover, during the first year of babyhood, the rest 20–25% of brain development takes place, so it is crucial to implement certain brain building exercise and innercise (neuron exercise), apart from conventional care. To add to that, positive parenting plays an important role in growth of a baby as good human being.

7.5 POSSIBILITIES

There are en numbers of scopes in holistic healthcare in reproduction. The important one is that it can provide opportunity for employment to the various talents. It is future of medical industry. It can address the under-lying cause of the disease and hence better treatment of patients would be possible. It can also help to reduce the chance of genetic disease in generation. Holistic healthcare in reproduction can help to create better society by helping expectant parents to deliver the virtuous, healthy, and intelligent child. It can also help to minimize the global issues, such as reduction in crime rate by better generation that is good in virtues with good moral values. Overall health and healing of the planet would be possible with holistic healthcare. Globally, it can help to spread love, peace and bliss amongst the people irrespective of their cultures and religions to grow one common among all that is humanity.

7.6   CASE DISCUSSION

We have implemented holistic approach in many cases; here, three such cases with clearly significant result are discussed.

Case-1: A 22-year-old young female having history of thyroid disorder conceived naturally. Her marriage life was not harmonious. In the seventh week of pregnancy, her husband and she visited the gynec hospital, with an objective of abortion as there was a hidden thought of divorce in their mind. Gynecologist referred this case to us. We started their intervention with holistic approach, and at the end, they have delivered a 2.7-kg baby boy successfully, and that baby boy has normal thyroid function at birth. In addition to that, now their marriage life has become full of love, peace, and harmony. They live their life at its full potential.

Case-2: A 25-year-old lady conceived with twin pregnancy. Initially, during her first trimester, doctor suggested her to join holistic Garbhsanskar class, she didn't take it seriously. Then, at the beginning of the third trimester, she was diagnosed with pregnancy-induced hypertension (PIH) and retarded fetal growth less than 1 kg each. She was not responding to the antihypertensive pills. Then, she had to join the class. After 10 days, her alleviated blood pressure came to its normal range. And both fetal growths were also significant. And at the full term, she delivered twin baby girls with an approx weight of 2.5 kg each. Today, all three are quite healthy.

Case-3: A 28-year-old young girl conceived. During her subsequent ultrasound at 11th week doctor diagnosed horizontal 12 mm, 800 g fibroid on external surface of the uterus. That was rapidly growing. Doctor advised her termination of pregnancy and surgical removal of fibroid with a risk of removal of uterus too. Then, she landed into Garbhsanskar class at the 12th week, on the 20th week ultrasound was done again to observe the fibroid. And surprisingly, it became stagnant with the size and weight it was recorded before to join the class. In addition to that her emergency room visit has come down to zero. As of now she is in her last trimester (almost 35th week) enjoying the pregnancy like normal pregnancy, and about to deliver a baby.

7.7 CHALLENGES

There are some challenges in the current time for this philosophy to grow. First of all, not all conventional caregivers are convinced on this concept, hardly 10% of the allopathic practitioner in reproduction believes the use of holistic medicines for their patients. Moreover, the awareness is also a key issue. It is a subject of interest of all to care for agricultural industry to maximize the quality and quantity of crops, but it is not so when it comes to next human generations. Most of the pregnancy happens by default and not by designing some plan. In addition to that, one has to pay a quality time in conversation with patients to make them understand about this healthcare, but doctors don't have much time in their busy OPD. Infrastructure for holistic healthcare is not possible for each and every practitioner, because it requires a lot of finance, and not only space but it also demands quality team work amongst practitioners. It demands healer with spiritual intelligence which is rarely seen in the current time.

KEYWORDS

- Garbhsanskar
- complication during pregnancy
- pregnancy class
- pregnancy-induced hypertension
- gestational diabetes mellitus
- parenting
- 16 Sanskar (Vedic rituals based on science)

PART III
Healing Through Mental Well-Being

CHAPTER 8

WORK-RELATED STRESS AMONG EDUCATORS: PRAYER AS A COPING STRATEGY

ROBIN L. LABARBERA*

Department of Special Education, School of Education, Biola University, 13800 Biola Ave., La Mirada, CA 90639, USA

E-mail: robin.l.labarbera@biola.edu

ABSTRACT

This chapter examines how educators who experience work-related stress feel about prayer as a means of coping with that stress. Existing literature shows that teachers experience significant levels of stress as a result of the ever-growing demands and pressures placed upon them. The severe stress that teachers often experience contributes to a loss of idealism and enthusiasm toward the profession. Other literature associates spiritual practices such as prayer with improved mental health and overall well-being. The study reported in this chapter explored the relationship between work-related stress and the practice of prayer in a sample of 916 Christian educators. Specifically, participants were asked to respond to questions about work-related stress, prayer, and job satisfaction to identify whether prayer helped participants cope with perceived stress and contributed to their job satisfaction. Participants in this study who indicated that they prayed frequently also reported greater satisfaction with their job and valued prayer as a necessary component of their overall well-being.

8.1   INTRODUCTION

Research has shown that teachers experience significant work-related stress and as a result may experience a variety of physical and emotional symptoms such as burnout, depression, anxiety,[29] panic, phobias, confused thinking, general irritation, feelings of powerlessness, and overall emotional exhaustion.[7] Teachers who are under prolonged stress may feel emotionally empty and depressed and may feel like "giving up" and "feel powerless to change what is causing them distress" (see Ref. [30], p 307). Nearly 50% of the teachers will leave the profession before they reach their sixth year of teaching as a result of the stressful conditions teachers are under.[17]

In the literature related to spiritual practices, prayer has a positive association with mental health among participants in all walks of life. For example, Ferguson et al.[11] discussed three impactful studies focused on the role of prayer in mental well-being. Oman and Driskill[25] explored meditation and repetition of certain holy names as a therapeutic practice. Eaken[9] also discussed the health implications of contemplative prayer, and Wong[32] analyzed how prayer provided an antidote to a busy life. University students ($n = 111$) in Belding et al.'s[3] research also reported that prayer and positive self-talk lowered their perceived level of stress. Finally, the connection between prayer and reduced stress was demonstrated in Ferguson et al.'s[11] study of 14 adult parishioners.

In studies examining the effect of prayer and overall well-being, the majority of research has concluded that prayer has a positive impact on one's mental health and overall life-satisfaction. Given the positive impacts of prayer demonstrated in a several studies involving participants from all walks of life, we wondered whether the same results could be found in a sample of Christian educators. This study explored the relationship between work-related stress and the practice of prayer in a sample of Christian teachers. Specifically, 916 Christian educators were invited to respond to questions about work-related stress, prayer, and job satisfaction to identify whether prayer helped participants cope with perceived stress and contributed to their job satisfaction despite their stress experiences. Teachers are reported to experience a high degree of work-related stress, and this study investigated whether prayer helped participants cope with that perceived stress.

8.1.1 EFFECTS OF STRESS

Prolonged stress is linked to a number of physical and emotional health impairments. In the research literature, stress has been associated with high blood pressure, elevated cholesterol levels, cardiovascular disease, chronic fatigue, headaches, and exhaustion.[7] Stress is related to body aches, diabetes, ulcers, a compromised immune system, susceptibility to viral illnesses and other diseases and infections, slower recovery from illness or injury, irregular menstrual cycles, and insomnia.[27] Prolonged stress can also affect the size of the hippocampus and the amygdala and has been linked to impulsiveness, poor executive function, and issues with neuroplasticity.[8]

Stress has also been associated with poor mental health outcomes. The psychological effects of prolonged stress can be anxiety, confused thinking, and feelings of inadequacy, panic, phobias, depression, and emotional exhaustion.[7,13,18] Work-related stress can result in burnout, a condition marked by emotional exhaustion and negative or cynical attitudes. Burnout can lead to depression, which, in turn, has been linked to a variety of other health concerns such as heart disease and stroke, obesity and eating disorders, diabetes, and some forms of cancer. Chronic depression also reduces immunity to other types of illnesses and can even contribute to premature death. Work-related stress has serious implications for one's mental and physical health.

8.2 STRESS AND JOB SATISFACTION AMONG EDUCATORS

Studies have shown that educators experience higher levels of stress than do other professional groups.[7,24] In research dating back to 1990, Punch and Tuettmann[28] found levels of psychological distress among teachers to be twice that of the general population. The demands of administrators, colleagues, and parents; work overload; and student behavior and discipline issues contribute to the experience of work-related stress and burnout. Ever-growing demands and pressures placed upon teachers are associated with high rates of absenteeism and turnover. Nearly 50% of the teachers will leave the profession before they reach their sixth year of teaching as a result of the stressful conditions they are under.[17]

Many times, the job demands appear to outweigh available resources for coping, which leads to the teachers' stress responses,[24] which can be physical or psychological in nature. For instance, physical effects include cardiovascular disease, chronic fatigue, and exhaustion, while psychological effects can be anxiety, confused thinking, feeling inadequate, panic, phobias, depression, emotional exhaustion, and burnout.[7] In research dating back to 1990, Punch and Tuettmann[28] found levels of psychological distress among teachers to be twice that of the general population.

The physical and mental effects of prolonged work-related stress among educators are a serious concern. Research has shown that teachers experience significant physical and emotional symptoms such as burnout, depression, anxiety, insomnia, social isolation, panic, phobias, confused thinking, general irritation, feelings of powerlessness, and overall emotional exhaustion as a result of work-related stress.[7,29] A nationwide survey in the United States found that teachers are physically exhausted, feel their enthusiasm toward teaching has plummeted, and have a sense of overwhelming expectations; they suffer from anxiety, frequent headaches, stomach pains, and high blood pressure.[29] In the present study, our concern for such severe negative outcomes among educators led us to examine how teachers perceived their stress related to work and whether their spiritual practices influenced their sense of job satisfaction.

8.2.1 SOURCES OF STRESS FOR EDUCATORS

Numerous studies discuss the work-related stress associated with the field of education. The top three sources of stress for teachers identified in the literature can be categorized as administrative stress, classroom-based stress, and relational challenges. Administrative stressors include high workload, insufficient planning time, and lack of general support from school administrators[2,7,12,19,21,24]. For instance, Hung's[16] research identified an overwhelming teaching load as a source of stress in a sample of 436 Taiwanese primary teachers, and Richards[29] identified overcommitment at work, with too many duties and responsibilities as a significant source of stress for teachers. Dissatisfaction with working conditions, such as teaching assignment, lack of administrative support, and large teaching load were some of the factors reported in McCarthy et al.'s[24] research.

Finally, low salary, insufficient benefits, and dilapidated buildings were cited as organizational stressors in Akpochafo's[2] research.

The most pervasive of the classroom-based stressors involve direct contact with students, according to Forlin.[12] Such issues include teaching students who may lack motivation, as well as challenges with maintaining student discipline[21,29] and large class sizes.[2] In a nationwide survey of US teachers, Richards[29] found that teaching students who seem "needy" (e.g., students with seemingly significant academic, social, emotional, psychological, and behavioral needs) without sufficient support was a source of stress for teachers. Forlin's[12] research attributed teacher stress to difficulties in meeting the needs of an increasingly diverse classroom population. Additionally, the weight of personal responsibility that teachers often feel for a student's well-being, such as their academic, personal, social, and emotional health,[24] may also heavily contribute to teacher stress.

Teachers have also attributed stress to student behaviors.[26] In one investigation, a factor related to teachers' desire to leave the profession was student behavior and discipline challenges.[5] Van der Wolf and Everaert[31] also blamed continued exposure to challenging behavior for depleting teachers' emotional and physical resources, resulting in loss of satisfaction from teaching. Additionally, dealing with students' challenging behaviors was considered a powerful source of teacher stress in Pang's[26] investigation among over 1200 teachers.

Relationship difficulties have also been cited as sources of stress in the literature.[2,12] Issues such as parent/teacher tension, excessive meetings with parents, and the challenge of meeting parent expectations were reported in Forlin's[12] research. Forlin found that 82% of the teachers in their study indicated that they were challenged with meeting the parents' expectations for their children. Sources of stress in Akpochafo's[2] research included relationships with the headmaster or with colleagues as well.

8.2.2   JOB SATISFACTION AMONG EDUCATORS

Evans[10] defined job satisfaction as "a state of mind encompassing all those feelings determined by the extent to which the individual perceives her/his job-related needs to being met" (p 294). Job satisfaction is the degree to which an individual perceives his/her work as satisfactory as inducing a positive feeling. Based on the literature related to job satisfaction and teaching discussed below, throughout this report, we will consider the term "job satisfaction" to mean participants' commitment to remain in the teaching profession. Overall, the literature demonstrates a clear link between job satisfaction and intentions to stay in the teaching field, and we, therefore, treated the two concepts as parallel.

What kinds of teachers are able to remain in a career working under conditions of overwhelming workloads, challenging students, and difficult parental expectations? When the majority of teachers are disheartened, disappointed, and burned out,[6,7,17,24,28,29] why do some teachers remain satisfied with their jobs and stay in the teaching field for the duration of their careers? In a study of 206 teachers, Bullough and Hall-Kenyon[6] surveyed teacher motivation and well-being, examining the individual qualities of individuals who thrive under seemingly adverse teaching conditions. They argued that teachers who experience their jobs as a "sense of calling" to the profession are more likely to maintain job satisfaction.

Bullough and Hall-Kenyon[6] also asserted that teachers who share a sense of hopefulness are able to meet work demands and remain committed to the teaching profession. "It is this belief that keeps teachers pushing to achieve their goals even when there is considerable opposition—including opposition from children, other teachers, parents and administrators" (p 135). Having a sense of calling influences how teachers respond to the various obstacles presented in their jobs, contributing to protective factors that contribute to thriving as opposed to burnout.[6]

Despite stress work conditions, Bullough and Hall-Kenyon[6] argued that a having a sense of calling and hopefulness increases job satisfaction. Kumcagiz et al. (2014) also attributed job satisfaction to hopefulness. Shaw and Newton[30] believed job satisfaction to be related to school leader attributes. Akbaba[1] maintained that as burnout increases, job satisfaction decreases, and abandonment of the teaching profession results. Researchers in the current study considered the role of religious practices such as prayer in influencing job satisfaction in our sample of Christian teachers when they encounter stressful working conditions.

8.3   COPING WITH STRESS: SPIRITUAL PRACTICES

There is evidence that spirituality and spiritual practices are powerful coping mechanisms for stress. In fact, religious coping is arguably one of the most powerful coping mechanisms, and it has the potential to buffer the damaging effects of stress and negative life events on psychological functioning.[18] People who are more religious or spiritual are better able to cope with stress, they heal faster from illness, and they experience increased benefits to their health and well-being.[23] Religious and spiritual beliefs are negatively correlated with depression and stress.[18]

Praying influences one's state of mind, helping to reduce the effects that stress has on various body organs. It helps beat physical stress, reduces the risk of developing depression and anxiety, and helps provide the strength to deal with day-to-day stress.[18] Prayer helps keep away disorders like heart disease, diabetes, hypertension, ulcers, and migraines, which are all considered to be a result of too much stress.[27]

The practice of prayer has been positively associated with mental health and reduced levels of stress, depression, and anxiety among participants in all walks of life in numerous studies.[3,4,11,13,25] In one large study of German pastoral professionals, participants reported that their trust in God, who guides them and helps to face and accept the demands of life, served to buffer the effects of perceived stress and work burdens to restore life satisfaction.[13] In another study, researchers were interested in learning if the implied presence of a supportive entity, God, would reduce acute stress.[3] They found that participants benefitted significantly from prayer and encouraging self-talk.

Prayer has been found to have a significant relationship with mental health in a number of reports. Kleffman,[20] for example, provided a report of how an Army Chaplain found peace amidst the stress of active duty through centering prayer. Gray,[14] a physician, also found prayer to be an effective coping strategy for the stress of working with cancer patients. And Lawson,[22] an Episcopal priest, asserted that the spiritual practice of daily meditative prayer could help clergy and congregations deal with stress. University students in Belding et al.'s[3] research also reported that prayer and positive self-talk lowered their perceived level of stress. The connection between prayer and reduced stress was also demonstrated in Ferguson et al.'s[11] study of 14 adult parishioners.

Bingaman[4] presented evidence from neuroscience that suggested that spiritual practices help build new neural structures. Bingaman[4] said, "the evidence from neuroscience overwhelmingly suggests that if we want to experience life in all its fullness, if we want, for ourselves and those in our care, to live into the abundance of happiness, love, and wisdom and to be less anxious about tomorrow and our own human nature, we will need to make contemplative spiritual practice more central" (p 487).

Spiritual practices are much more than just comforting rituals to religious individuals. They have the ability to have a positive impact on mood and mental health and to enable tangible reductions in levels of stress. Faith generates optimism, enriches interpersonal relationships, creates support systems, and enhances the quality of life. Scientific research is also emerging which demonstrates promising connections between religiousness and improved mental health. An article by Bingaman[4] demonstrated the plasticity and malleability of the human brain to make a case for greater use of contemplative mindfulness. Bingaman[4] contented that prayer, "brings us into the presence of God" by "reducing the obstacles caused by the hyperactivity of our mind and of our lives" (p 481).

Belding et al.[3] also theorized that "the implied presence of a supportive friend may also reduce stress, and one way to invoke the image of a supportive presence is through prayer to God" (p 180). In the current study, we conceptualized spirituality/prayer as a relationship with God in which believers seek guidance, comfort, and support. Prayer is the spiritual exercise that allows people to communicate directly with God. It is an intensely personal endeavor that can provide a great source of stress relief.

8.3.1 THE CURRENT STUDY

In studies examining the effects of prayer on overall well-being, the majority of research has concluded that prayer has a positive impact on one's mental health and overall life-satisfaction. Given the positive impacts of prayer demonstrated in these studies involving participants from all walks of life, we wondered whether the same results could be found in a sample of Christian educators. As part of a larger study on the spiritual lives of teachers,[15] in this study, we looked at a particular spiritual practice—prayer.

This study explored the relationship between work-related stress and the practice of prayer in a sample of Christian educators. Specifically, 916 Christian educators responded to questions about work-related stress, prayer, and job satisfaction to identify whether prayer helped participants cope with perceived stress and contributed to their job satisfaction despite their stress experiences. Overall, the current data analysis was guided by three questions that were explored through qualitative and quantitative data: (1) What types of job-related stress do Christian educators experience? (2) How do Christian educators feel about their jobs in the presence of such stress? What is their sense of job satisfaction? (3) To what extent does the practice of prayer contribute to participants' feelings about their job?

8.4 METHOD

This study used qualitative and quantitative data from a sample of Christian educators from several different countries, including the United States. A mixed methods approach was taken to gain a better understanding of the phenomenon of stress experienced by participants. Qualitative data analysis was conducted to describe participants' perceived sources of work-related stress. Quantitative data analysis was used to determine participants': (1) sense of job satisfaction or intentions to remain in the teaching profession and (2) practice of the spiritual discipline of prayer. A one-way analysis of variance (ANOVA) was used to assess the relationship of prayer and job satisfaction.

This study was a subset of a larger research project examining the spiritual lives of Christian educators from schools associated with the Association of Christian Schools International.[15] As an extension of that investigation, the current study examined teachers' perceptions of stressors and the strategies employed to mitigate such stress. Of the larger study, 916 participants responded to questions related to the independent and dependent variables in the current study. The survey was conducted through the online tool, SurveyMonkey™.

8.4.1 PARTICIPANTS

The initial survey was partially or fully completed by 1509 teachers living in 38 countries (item 9). Seventy-three percent of these teachers were from the United States and 27% resided in 37 other countries (item 7). Seventy-two percent were female and 28% male (item 6). The mean age was 44 with an age range of 21–76 (item 14). The mean number of years teaching was 16 with a range of 1–52 years of experience (item 3). Respondents' primary teaching responsibilities were PreK-16 with the majority of respondents teaching K-12. Most teachers reported they taught at a private school (88%), followed by international schools (13%), mission schools (7%), and public schools (2%). Teachers reported worshipping in dozens of different denominations with nondenominational (33%) and Baptist (31%) being the highest denomination represented in this study (item 10). A total of 916 participants responded to the questions related to key variables in the current study.

8.4.2   MEASURES

This particular study examines three key variables, which were conceptualized as job satisfaction, sources of stress, and the practice of prayer as a spiritual discipline. To measure job satisfaction, participants were asked quantitative questions to rank how they currently feel about their job with the item: "Which of the following statements most accurately describes how you feel right now as a teacher?" Participants were asked to select one of the following responses: (1) "I love the ministry of teaching. I know this is my calling. I plan on being in teaching, as God leads, for my full career." (2) "Most of the time I like teaching. Even though some days are challenging, overall, I like the students and the teaching process." (3) "I feel up and down. Some days are happy teaching; some days are very frustrating. I often think about a change of job." Or (4) "I feel burned out, frustrated, and ready to quit my job." The preceding item was utilized as the dependent variable. Spiritual disciplines were also assessed by asking two questions—"With what frequency do you practice the following disciplines?" and "Identify the first most important spiritual discipline that supports your ministry as a Christian educator." A list of 22 disciplines followed these prompts.

Qualitative data, in the form of open-ended survey questions, were also included for teachers to specify the aspects of their job they felt contributed to or caused them the most stress. Specifically, sources of stress were analyzed by asking respondents the open-ended question: "What causes you the most stress in your educational role?"

8.5 RESULTS

8.5.1 SOURCES OF STRESS

Participants' open-ended responses were analyzed to provide qualitative data in relation to the circumstances or people they believed contributed to their stress, to address Research Question #1. The most reported source of stress was related to administrative work, which was mentioned by 52% of the educators. The second highest source of stress for participants was classroom-based, mentioned by 22% of educators in the sample (i.e., student discipline issues, finding strategies to teach students who do not engage academically, etc.). Challenging relationships with parents emerged as the third highest response, reported by 15% of the participants (i.e., parent complaints, demands on educators, feeling their child can do no wrong). Of the participants, 11% reported difficult relationships with coworkers or with leadership to be a source of stress for them.

8.5.1.1 ADMINISTRATIVE TASKS

Administrative tasks represented the most commonly reported source of stress for educators in our sample. Comments such as the following were grouped into the "administrative work" category, which reveal the difficulties with completing necessary teaching-related tasks: "Deadlines, paperwork, grading—that causes me the most stress" (participant #1533, Cambodia). "The overloading of tasks. There is never enough time to get everything done. It's always the busyness and the meetings that bring the stress," (participant #401, United States) was a similar response. Overall, there were 13 responses that included the word "paperwork" as a source of stress. The comment by participant #235 (United States) provided a concise summary of this topic: "Paperwork, emails, more paperwork, administrative processes, did I say...paperwork?" Another said, "Paperwork!! I spend way more time than I should doing the paperwork and filling in 'all the little boxes' that takes me away from actual creative preparation for a class" (participant #288, Ecuador).

8.5.1.2 CLASSROOM-BASED STRESS

Factors related to the classroom emerged as the second highest source of stress among educators in our sample. One participant mentioned, "when I explain something several times and the students make little or no effort in trying to understand the concepts" (participant #930, United States) as a source of stress. Participant #1467 from Ukraine said, "I don't like it when kids don't pay attention to my words and even though I'm a teacher they sometimes treat me as their peer." Twenty-four respondents used the word "discipline" in their responses to the question about their greatest source of stress. Comments of this nature included, "Students who continually don't listen to me and talk when they should not causes stress" (participant #378, United States) or "I feel the most stress with handling discipline, especially the teenagers. I want to be consistent, but I also want to reach them. I don't think I've had a breakthrough yet" (participant #1221, United States). Another comment related to discipline was from participant #200, teaching in Honduras, who said, "Being consistent with discipline and rules is stressful. It is difficult in our changing world, which over-emphasizes grace and has lost focus that all actions have consequences." Another participant mentioned that the greatest stress comes from "dealing with students who do not do well academically, do not care or try, and consistently are disrespectful in class" (participant #1063, Canada).

8.5.1.3 CHALLENGING RELATIONSHIPS

The third most significant source of stress among participants in our sample was challenging relationships with parents and with coworkers or leaders. One respondent said, "Unfounded and/or unjust parent complaints" (participant #631, United States) was a source of stress. Another participant phrased it this way: "Parents are making greater demands on educators to 'fix' their children's problems" (participant #326, Ecuador). "Dealing with parents who believe their children cannot be wrong" was stressful, according to another teacher (participant #76, United States). Participant #138 (South Korea) said, "When parents are involved in an issue and support the student without knowing the truth – this can be very stressing." Another said, "At time, parents are so controlling, feel their child is right and don't care to listen to me as the teacher. I want the best for their child, just like they do, but I'm unable to show this. It hurts that parents can be this way and make things so difficult at times" (participant #1218, United States).

Concerning relationships with leadership, one teacher commented, "School leadership being unsupportive and not empathetic" (participant #1132, Indonesia) was stressful, and another said that stress comes from, "peers and some of those in leadership who just really don't get what the focus needs to be" (participant #86, Philippines). An independent samples t-test was conducted to compare sources of stress in male and female participants in our sample. There was no significant difference in scores for male ($M = 1.88$, SD = 1.08) and female ($M = 1.83$, SD = 1.03) groups [$t(8) = 0.64$, $p = 0.52$].

8.5.2   JOB SATISFACTION

Participants responded to the individual question, "Which of the following statements most accurately describes how you feel right now as a teacher?" Slightly more than 64% of the Christian educators in this study love the ministry of teaching and plan on being in teaching for their full career, even with the significant sources of stress they experience. Twenty-eight percent of educators in this sample like their jobs most of the time, 6% feel "up and down," and only 1% feel burned out and ready to quit.

8.5.3   SPIRITUAL DISCIPLINES

Participants were asked to "identify the first most important spiritual discipline that supports your ministry as a Christian educator" out of a list of 22 disciplines, such as prayer, fellowship, individual and corporate worship, rest, solitude, etc. Participants reported that the most regularly practiced discipline was prayer (88.05% of the participants reported they regularly practice this discipline), followed by corporate worship (87.85% of the participants reported they regularly practice this discipline), and fellowship (80% of the participants reported they regularly practice this discipline). Given the high percentage of participants who regularly prac-tice prayer, these data were used in subsequent statistical analysis.

8.5.4 PRAYER'S CONTRIBUTION TO JOB SATISFACTION

In order to determine the relationship between job satisfaction and the practice of spiritual disciplines, a one-way ANOVA was calculated. The results revealed a statistically significant relationship between frequency of prayer and loving the ministry of teaching $[F(3, 912) = 5.433, p = 0.001]$. A Tukey post hoc test revealed that participants were statistically more likely to love the ministry of teaching when they prayed more frequently, compared to the group who reported liking their jobs most of the time $(1.18, p = 0.000)$.

8.6 DISCUSSION

This research identified how stressful a teaching job can be for Christian educators. The most stressful issues fell into four categories. The first is that of a teacher's administrative work. The results of the current study are consistent with the findings reported in previous investigations[2,7,12,19,21,24] that attributed a high workload to increased stress.

A significant number of participants in the current study, despite reports of stress, remain fully committed to their teaching role and plan to stay in the profession throughout the remainder of their career. In our sample, well over half (64%) of the participants love the ministry of teaching and are convinced it is their calling. Consistent with our hypothesis that prayer serves to ameliorate stress, participants in our sample reported a significant relationship between the frequency in which they prayed and job satisfaction.

Prayer, in our investigation, was associated with job satisfaction. Participants who prayed frequently reported greater satisfaction with their job. These findings were consistent with numerous other investigations demonstrating the role of prayer in mediating stress, anxiety, and depression.[3,9,11,25,32]

The findings indicate that those who prayed more frequently were more likely to see teaching as a calling and to remain in the profession for their full career. One implication of this finding is apparent: Christian educators who employ their religious practice of prayer in daily life are more likely to maintain their resilience and their commitment to teaching when faced with difficult or stressful circumstances. The types of individuals who thrive under conditions of overwhelming task loads, disrespectful or inattentive students, and problematic relationships with parents or coworkers must find themselves in need of a copying strategy.

Teachers in our sample valued prayer as a necessary component of their well-being. Davidson and McEwen[8] asserted,

> Just as we as a society are learning to take more responsibility for our physical health by engaging in regular physical exercise, we can also take more responsibility for our minds and brains by engaging in certain mental exercises that can induce plastic changes in the brain and that may have enduring beneficial consequences for social and emotional behavior (p 690).

Prayer, as described in this study, might constitute an ideal intervention to provide positive outcomes.

For individuals who experience sometimes overwhelming work challenges, such improvements in levels of stress due to spiritual practices such as prayer should not be underestimated. One can certainly make a convincing argument that contemplative prayer and meditation in the context of Christian faith helps combat the negativity in our brain that "will surely hold us hostage if we let it" (see Ref. [5], p 484).

8.7 CONCLUSION

In summary, the results of this study suggest an association between frequency of prayer and job satisfaction among Christian educators. It should be understood that we make no claims that prayer causes job satisfaction. The findings from this study merely point to a relationship between the two variables, illuminating the continued level of commitment to the teaching profession even though it is perceived as highly stressful. Learning to cope with stress, through prayer, may help improve teachers' sense of well-being.

Suggestions in this study offer a valuable option to coping with the unrelenting stress that teachers report. The present findings highlight the importance of prayer for dealing with stress and increasing job satisfaction. We believe that perseverance and resilience are dependent upon prayer and therefore of central importance to any successful school improvement or professional development efforts. We also recognize that while prayer is seen as a critical component of resilience for Christian educators, it is unlikely that school authorities could mandate such practices on their campus. Nevertheless, based on the findings in this study, it has been suggested that the regular practice of prayer is a key to maintaining a Christian educator's sense of job satisfaction despite stressful working conditions. Any strategy that serves to strengthen a teacher's sense of hopefulness or satisfaction with the profession is likely to be beneficial to teachers and students alike.

It is apparent that this study offers only a beginning to understanding the nature of teacher stress and coping. While we were convinced that teachers in our sample relied on prayer as a strategy for coping with undesirable working conditions, such is not necessarily the case for all teachers. Also, our research did not include teachers who had left the field due to stressful circumstances, and we can therefore say little about conditions that undermine a teacher's job satisfaction or intent to remain in the profession. Nevertheless, understanding the stressful conditions of teaching, combined with potential strategies for dealing with such stress, deserves our consideration.

KEYWORDS

- stress
- prayer
- educators
- job satisfaction
- spiritual practices

REFERENCES

1. Akbaba, S. A Comparison of the Burnout Levels of Teachers with Different Occupational Satisfaction Sources. *Educ. Sci.: Theor. Pract.* **2014,** *144,* 1253–1261.
2. Akpochafo, G. O. Perceived Sources of Occupational Stress among Primary School Teachers in Delta State of Nigeria. *Education* **2012,** *132*(4), 826–833.
3. Belding, J. N.; Howard, M. G.; McGuire, A. M.; Schwartz, A. C.; Wilsin, J. H. Social Buffering by God: Prayer and Measures of Stress. *J. Relig. Health* **2010,** *49,* 179–187.
4. Bingaman, K. A. The Art of Contemplative and Mindfulness Practice: Incorporating the Findings of Neuroscience into Pastoral Care and Counseling. *Pastoral Psychol.* **2011,** *60,* 477–498.

5. Brown, J.; Davis, S.; Johnson, E. *Teachers on Teaching: A Survey of the Teaching Profession*; Market & Opinion Research International: London, 2002.
6. Bullough, R. V.; Hall-Kenyon, K. M. The Call to Teach and Teacher Hopefulness. *Teach. Dev.* **2011,** *15*(2), 127–140.
7. Chaplain, R. P. Stress and Psychological Distress among Trainee Secondary Teachers in England. *Educ. Psychol.: Int. J. Exp. Educ. Psychol.* **2008,** *28*, 195–209.
8. Davidson, R. J.; McEwen, B. W. Social Influences on Neuroplasticity: Stress and Interventions to Promote Well-Being. *Nat. Neurosci.* **2012,** *15*(5), 689–695.
9. Eaken, L. Origins of Contemplative Prayer, the Development of Medical Imagery Meditation, and Their Impact on Spiritual Life and Health. Unpublished Doctoral Dissertation, San Francisco Theological Seminary, San Anselmo, 2003.
10. Evans, L. Delving Deeper into Morale, Job Satisfaction and Motivation among Education Professionals: Re-examining the Leadership Dimension. *Educ. Manage. Adm.* **2001,** *29*(3), 291–306.
11. Ferguson, J. K.; Willemsen, E. W.; Castaneto, M. V. Centering Prayer as a Healing Response to Everyday Stress: A Psychological and Spiritual Process. *Pastoral Psychol.* **2010,** *59*, 305–329.
12. Forlin, C. Inclusion: Identifying Potential Stressors for Regular Class Teacher. *Educ. Res.* **2001,** *43*(3), 235–245.
13. Frick, E.; Bussing, A.; Baumann, K.; Weig, W.; Jacobs, C. Do Self-Efficacy Expectation and Spirituality Provide a Buffer against Stress-Associated Impairment of Health? A Comprehensive Analysis of the German Pastoral Ministry Study. *J. Relig. Health* **2016,** *55*, 448–468.
14. Gray, E. *Discovering the Center: A Surgeon's Spiritual Journey*; Paulist: New York, 2004.
15. Hetzel, J.; Costillo, D. The Spiritual Lives of Teachers. *Christ. Sch. Educ.* **2013/2014,** *17*(1), 30–35.
16. Hung, C. L. Coping Strategies of Primary School Teachers in Taiwan Experiencing Stress Because of Teacher Surplus. *Soc. Behav. Pers.* **2011,** *39*(9), 1161–1174.
17. Ingersoll, R. M.; Smith, T. M. Do Teacher Induction and Mentoring Matter? *NASSP Bull.* **2004,** *88*(638), 28–40.
18. Kidwai, R.; Mancha, B. E.; Brown, Q. L.; Eaton, W. W. The Effect of Spirituality and Religious Attendance on the Relationship between Psychological Distress and Negative Life Events. *Soc. Psychiatry Psychiatr. Epidemiol.* **2014,** *49*, 487–497.
19. Klassen, R. M.; Chiu, M. M. Effects on Teachers' Self-Efficacy and Job Satisfaction: Teacher Gender, Years of Experience, and Job Stress. *J. Educ. Psychol.* **2010,** *102*(3), 741–756.
20. Kleffman, J. A Journey to Centering Prayer. *Mil. Chaplains Rev.* **1987,** *16*(2), 107–114.
21. Kyriacou, C. Teacher Stress: Directions for Future Research. *Educ. Rev.* **2001,** *53*, 27–35.
22. Lawson, D. *Old Wine in New Skins: Centering Prayer and Systems Theory*; Lantern Books: New York, 2004.
23. Lee, R. *The Superstress Solution*; Random House: New York, 2010.

24. McCarthy, C. J.; Lambert, R. G.; Crowe, E. E.; McCarthy, C. J. Coping, Stress, and Job Satisfaction as Predictors of Advanced Placement Statistics Teachers' Intention to Leave the Field. *NASSP Bull.* **2010,** *94*(4), 306–326.

25. Oman, D.; Driskill, J. Holy Name Repetition as a Spiritual Exercise and Therapeutic Technique. *J. Psychol. Christianity* **2003,** *22*(1), 5–19.

26. Pang, I. Teacher Stress in Working with Challenging Students in Hong Kong. *Educ. Res. Policy Pract.* **2012,** *11*, 119–139.

27. Pietrangelo, A.; Watson, S. *The Effects of Stress on the Body*; Healthline Media, 2014. http://www.healthline.com/health/stress/effects-on-body#overlaySources

28. Punch, K. F.; Tuettmann, E. Correlates of Psychological Distress among Secondary Teachers. *Br. Educ. Res. J.* **1990,** *16*, 369–382.

29. Richards, J. Teacher Stress and Coping Strategies: A National Snapshot. *Educ. Forum* **2012,** *76*, 299–316.

30. Shaw, J.; Newton, J. Teacher Retention and Satisfaction with a Servant Leader as Principal. *Education* **2014,** *135*, 101–106.

31. Van der Wolf, K.; Everaert, H. A. Teacher Stress, Challenging Parents and Problems Students. In *School, Family, and Community Partnership in a World of Differences and Changes*; Castelli, S., Mendel, M., Ravn, B., Eds.; University of Gdansk: Gdansk, 2003; pp 135–146.

32. Wong, J. The Jesus Prayer and Inner Stillness. *Relig. East West* **2005,** *5*, 85–97.

CHAPTER 9

AN APPROACH TO PREDICTING PHYSICALLY HEALTHY AND UNHEALTHY PERSONS USING SUPPORT VECTOR MACHINE CLASSIFIERS BASED ON HANDWRITTEN TEXT

SEEMA KEDAR[1*] and D. S. BORMANE[2]

[1]*JSPM's Rajarshi Shahu College of Engineering, Savitribai Phule Pune University, Pune 411033, India*

[2]*AISSMS COE, Savitribai Phule Pune University, Pune 411033, India*

Corresponding author. E-mail: seemaahkeddar@gmail.com

ABSTRACT

Being healthy is of utmost importance in life. An ill person is not able to live life to its fullest extent. Being healthy makes you feel good and allows you to perform more efficiently and effectively. It also makes one more productive and happier. This chapter suggests an approach to predict whether a person is physically healthy or unhealthy using support vector machine classifier based on handwritten text. It extracts geometric features such as total number of left and right diagonal lines, total number of horizontal and vertical lines, total length of vertical and horizontal lines, total length of left and right diagonal lines, area of skeleton, and regional features such as orientation, major axis length, Euler, and extend from handwriting sample to check whether the writer is physically healthy or not. The proposed approach exhibits 75% accuracy.

9.1 INTRODUCTION

Many people underestimate the importance of good health. To carry out daily activities, good health is necessary.[1] To survive in this world, one should be healthy, both emotionally and physically.[2] Physically healthy person's body functions as it should be without pain, discomfort, or lack of capabilities. One can perform his duties more effectively only when he feels well. Physically fit people do not suffer from cardiac and other health problems. Being ill can affect the performance drastically.[2,3] By analyzing the handwriting, we can predict whether the person is healthy or not.

Handwriting analysis, also known as graphology, is used as a tool for detecting health conditions, personality, and emotions as handwriting occurs through the interactions of many structures and circuits in the brain. As per handwriting analysis, all people suffering from same disease have similar writing features. Similarly, all the physically healthy persons have same kind of writing features. These writing features are studied to predict health condition of a person.[4–11] Predicting health conditions through handwriting analysis is an instant, cost-effective approach.

This chapter presents an approach to predict whether a writer is physically healthy or not. The proposed approach analyzes geometric features such as total number of left and right diagonal lines, total number of horizontal and vertical lines, total length of vertical and horizontal lines, total length of left and right diagonal lines, area of skeleton, and regional features such as orientation, major axis length, Euler, and extend to predict physical fitness of the writer.[12] The system uses support vector machine (SVM) classifier to implement the same. The remainder of the chapter is organized as follows: proposed system is described in Section 9.2, Section 9.3 presents experimental results, and the conclusion is discussed in Section 9.4.

9.2 PROPOSED SYSTEM

As shown in Figure 9.1, the proposed system works in three main steps, namely, preprocessing, feature extraction, and classification. It uses training dataset prepared using JPEG images of handwriting samples of physically healthy and unhealthy persons. All these images are preprocessed.

Then the training feature vector with the abovementioned geometric and regional features is prepared using these preprocessed images.

During testing, the JPEG image of unknown handwriting sample is given as input to the system. The input image is then preprocessed. During preprocessing, the input image is processed and converted to 512 rows and 512 columns image. Noise is removed from it. This enhanced image is given as input to feature extraction step. This step extracts abovementioned geometric and regional features from the image. The testing feature vector for unknown handwriting sample is prepared by combining geometric and regional features. This testing feature vector is compared with training feature vector using SVM classifier. The output is prediction about whether the person is physically healthy or unhealthy.

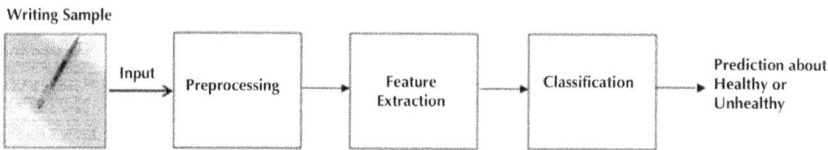

FIGURE 9.1 **(See color insert.)** Block diagram of the proposed system.

9.3 EXPERIMENTAL RESULTS

The data set of 100 handwriting samples of both physically healthy and unhealthy people is used for experimentation. The handwriting samples of both male and female whose age ranges from 20 to 81 are used. Eighty handwriting samples have been used to form training dataset. Out of these, 40 samples are of physically healthy people and remaining 40 are of unhealthy people. The unhealthy handwriting samples include samples of patients suffering from any kind of heart disease, cancer, and diabetes. The testing dataset comprises 20 samples. The proposed approach gives 75% accuracy. The accuracy is calculated using following equation:

$$\text{Accuracy} = \frac{\text{Correctly predicted writing samples}}{\text{Total number of writing samples}} \times 100 \qquad (9.1)$$

$$= \frac{15}{20}$$

$$= 75\%$$

The confusion matrix with predicted class values and actual class values is shown in Table 9.1.

TABLE 9.1   Confusion Matrix.

		Predicted class values		Marginal sum of actual values
		Physically healthy	Unhealthy	
Actual class values	Physically healthy	6	4	10
	Unhealthy	1	9	10
Marginal sum of predicted values		7	13	20

The graph in Figure 9.2 shows the recognition rate of physically healthy and unhealthy class. We obtained 60 and 90% recognition rate for physically healthy and unhealthy classes, respectively.

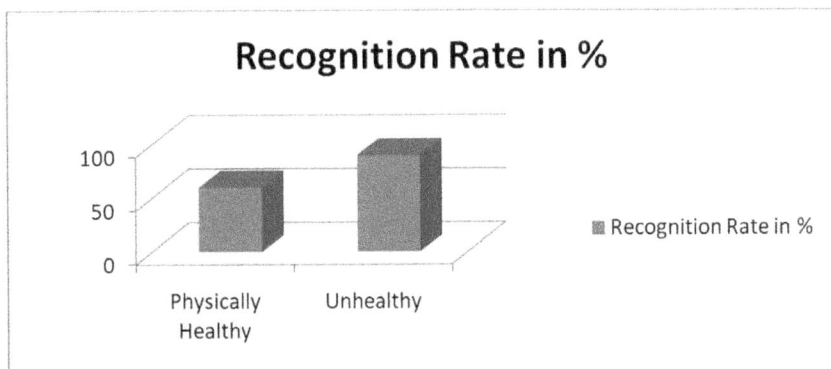

FIGURE 9.2   (**See color insert.**) Recognition rate of physically healthy and unhealthy classes.

9.4   CONCLUSION

The approach for predicting physically healthy and unhealthy person using handwritten text based on graphology is presented here. The training and testing datasets comprises 80 and 20 samples, respectively. 75% accuracy is obtained using SVM classifier. The accuracy can be increased by adding more samples in training dataset of each class.

KEYWORDS

- **physically healthy**
- **unhealthy**
- **support vector machine**
- **handwriting analysis**
- **writing features**

REFERENCES

1. http://www.essaywow.com/health-and-fitness-essays/essay-health-fitness-importance-good-health.html (accessed Feb 2016).
2. Kurtus, R. Importance of Being Healthy. http://www.school-for-champions.com/grades/ importance_of_being_healthy.html (accessed May 24, 2012).
3. The Importance of Physical Fitness https://www.healthstatus.com/health_blog/wellness/the-importance-of-physical-fitness/ (accessed Feb 2016).
4. Thomassen, A. J. W. M; Keuss, P. J. G.; van Galen, G. P. Motor Aspects of Handwriting: Approaches to Movement in Graphic Behavior; North-Holland: Amsterdam, New York, 1983.
5. Plamondon, R.; O'Reilly, C. The Lognormal Handwriter: Learning, Performing and Declining. Front. Psychol. 2013, 4, 945.
6. Kalcheva, E.; Gluhchev, G. In Segmentation and Analysis of Handwritten Scripts from Patients with Neurological Diseases, International Conference on Computer Systems and Technologies, Sofia, Bulgaria, June 19–20, 2003.
7. Greasley, P. Handwriting Analysis and Personality Assessment; Hogrefe Publishing: Boston, 2000; pp 44–51 (Eur. Psychol.).
8. John Antony, D. Personality Profile Through Handwriting Analysis; Anugraha Publications: Tamil Nadu, India, 2008.
9. Backman, R. E. Some Comments Upon the History of Handwriting Analysis, 1964. https://www.ahafhandwriting.org
10. Strang, C. Handwriting in the Early Detection of Disease—A Research Study. The Graphologist (The Journal of the British Institute of Graphologists) 2013, 31 (118).
11. Ünlü, A.; Brause, R.; Krako, K. Handwriting Analysis for Diagnosis and Prognosis of Parkinson's Disease. Proc. Int. Symp. Biol. Med. Data Anal. 2006, 4345, pp 441–450 (Springer Verlag Heidelberg).
12. Kedar, S.; Bormane, D. S. In Heart Disease Prediction Using k-Nearest Neighbor Classifier based on Handwritten Text, Proceedings of the International Conference on CIDM, Dec 5–6, 2015; Vol. 410 (Adv. Intell. Syst. Comput.).

CHAPTER 10

AYURVEDA, YOGA, AND MENTAL HEALTH

ANN HOLADAY*

Anglia Polytechnic, Cambridge University, Cambridge, UK

*E-mail: jivaneesha@gmail.com

ABSTRACT

The causes of mental disturbances are multifaceted and highly complex, but it is clear that the modern medical approach to mental health is limited and largely ineffective judging by the increasing numbers of people suffering from mental disturbances, and the prolific use of psychotropic drugs. There is more violence, suicide, depression, anxiety, addiction than ever before in recent history.

Modern culture, where money is God, is a breeding ground for mental disturbance. Industrialized food available to most people is mass produced, contaminated by chemicals and low in nutritional value, loneliness and isolation is the curse of our time with the dissolution of family and community, to say nothing of toxic media constantly bombarding the mind.

It is known that the prolific use of medications for mental illness causes dependency and adverse side-effects, but no alternative, comprehensive approach has been suggested. It is clear that a new, innovative system is needed. This article looks to Vedic philosophy and the principles of Ayurveda and Yoga for a long-term solution to mental health issues in modern society.

The Vedas recognized mental illness thousands of years ago by understanding the connection between the mind and spirit. Ayurveda and Yoga addresses body, mind, and spirit, gets to the root cause of disease. According to Ayurveda, mental illness is an imbalance of all aspects of being, each one affecting the other. Ayurveda the science of life, with its understanding of the mind through spirituality is very effective and a permanent solution to the mental health issues of today.

10.1   VEDIC PSYCHOLOGY

Mental health issues are probably the most pervasive health issue that modern civilization faces, manifesting in all societies and age groups regardless of race, creed, color, and economic status. Mental illnesses such as schizophrenia and epilepsy have always been recognized, but now there is a syndrome for every mood and disturbance which are treated using counseling and medication. In ancient times, these problems either did not exist or were considered eccentricities and accepted as a normal part of human nature.

Mental disturbances are not created equally, but prevention, early treatment and treating the cause is the best way to address problems. If the cause is not treated, then the problem is masked, will recur and persist. Most psychological disturbances nowadays are the direct result of modern lifestyle and develop because of it; very few are true mental illnesses.

However, modern society forces us to mask symptoms of disturbance because we have to keep working, keep up a standard, keep striving for success, and because we often have no one to depend on, we struggle without support. We have drifted away from our true nature as humans. Families are disintegrating, communities disappearing, and even though we have sophisticated medical systems with numerous psychiatrists, psychologists, counselors, programs, support groups, etc., the problems are only getting worse.

Psychiatry is one of eight specialties in Ayurveda where mental illness is considered to be a spiritual imbalance in which the victim is possessed. Contrary to widespread belief, these were not evil spirits—in fact, Sanskrit does not have a word meaning evil—but were troubled, discontented spirits which embodied themselves in vulnerable people. Psychology, the study of human behavior is not described in the Vedas, but when we study all aspects of body, mind, and spirit as being interconnected, we realize that all diseases have a root cause in the spirit. Therefore, if we connect to our spiritual nature, which has the power to control our mental and physical well-being, mental disturbances can be managed by applying the principles of Ayurveda and Yoga. The law of karma says, "if we have the power to create problems then we have the means to correct them."

Ayurveda is based on the "principle of the five elements" in which the Vedic view of creation is described. Evolution begins with the merging of Purusha (consciousness) and Prakriti (base substance of the universe) into the five elements, earth, water, fire, air, and space.

The five elements are forces of nature and are in every cell of all living things and in all matter. Ayurveda is based on the qualities of these five elements and the principles of "like increases like" and "opposites decrease". Vata is the qualities of air and space which are light, subtle, soft, smooth, cold, rough, dry, and mobile. Pitta is fire which has the qualities of light, dry, subtle, rough, mobile, hot, sharp, and slightly oily. Kapha is water and earth which have the qualities of liquid, oily, cold, heavy, moist, soft, promotes cohesion, wet, stable, tough, and dense.

Vata, Pitta, and Kapha are the "Doshas" which when balanced give good health, and when out of balance cause disease.

10.1.1 COMMON MENTAL DISTURBANCES

- *Stress* is a cause of mental disturbance rather than the disturbance itself. However, many mental health problems are stress related, for example, PTSD (post-traumatic stress disorder). It is impossible to avoid stress in the modern world but Ayurveda and Yoga diet and lifestyle principles can be very effective in managing it.

- *Depression* is a common mental ailment defined as sadness or grief which persists, and is the end result of early signs of mental disturbance. It is important to recognize depression in the early stages. By the time depression is diagnosed, it has already been with the person a long time and maybe deeply rooted. Women are twice as likely to suffer from depression as men indicating hormonal factors. Postnatal (postpartum) depression, PMS (premenstrual syndrome), menopausal depression, and depression during puberty are normal mood fluctuations which must be recognized early. These conditions clearly indicate the mind/body connection.

- *Anxiety* is a feeling of fear, worry, uneasiness, and/or disconnect. It is a normal reaction to demanding situations, which cause stress.

Under normal situations, when the stressor passes so does the anxiety, however in some cases, it becomes a chronic condition.

- *Panic attacks* are a common symptom related to anxiety. They usually happen to the person without warning even when there is no reason to be fearful. However, the perception of danger is very real indeed. A person experiencing a panic attack will often feel as if he or she is about to die or lose consciousness. The fear of a panic attack may lead to phobias.

- *Drug and alcohol addiction* can be defined as the continued use of mood and behavior altering substances despite their adverse consequences. This state creates a condition of tolerance in which the body adapts to the substance and requires increasingly larger amounts to achieve the original effect. Compulsions such as shopping, sex, eating, gambling, exercise, and the computer are also forms of addiction where the person is unable to control their behavior.

- *Pathological grief* is a normal response to loss. The mind has to process in its own time. Each individual grieves in their own way and some people take longer to process grief than others. Pathological grief is when the person becomes totally immersed in their grief and cannot function.

- *Schizophrenia* is a mental disorder characterized by a breakdown of thought processes and emotional response which often manifests as hallucinations, paranoia, and delusion. It is considered to be a genetic disorder which typically begins in young adulthood. No single cause is known. From an Ayurvedic standpoint, it is caused by Vata disturbance in the mind.

- *Attention deficit hyperactivity disorder (ADHD)* is a developmental disorder characterized primarily by attention problems and hyperactivity with symptoms occurring before 7 years of age. It is often associated with learning disabilities.

- *Autism* is a developmental disorder characterized by impaired social interaction, communication, and repetitive behavior with the initial onset of symptoms before 3 years of age.

- *Alzheimer's and dementia* manifest themselves as the same condition, mainly loss of memory and an ability to manage everyday, routine tasks. Alzheimer's is detectable by CT scan and can occur at any age, whereas dementia normally occurs in old age.

- *Suicide* is the result of mental disturbance. It is becoming more and more common in modern society especially amongst young people. It is the result of a total loss of self-worth and the absence of a will do live. Often it is a cry for help.

10.1.2 USE OF PSYCHOTROPIC DRUGS IN MENTAL DISTURBANCE

CCHR (Citizens Commission on Human Rights, www.cchr.org) has gathered alarming statistics on the prolific use of psychotropic drugs in the United States. Almost 25% of the American population is taking psychiatric drugs. The statistics below only shows depression, ADHD, psychosis and anxiety, sleeping pills and tranquilizers are not included. Of particular concern is their use in babies, young children and teens. Giving these types of drugs to the developing mind is not only dangerous, but it creates a lifetime of dependency. The mind, like the body, has a natural tendency to heal itself if managed appropriately, drugs will only block the natural process and mask the problem (Tables 10.1 and 10.2).

TABLE 10.1   CCHR Statistics on the Use of Psychotropic Drugs in the United States.

0–5 years	1,080,168	6–12 years	4,130,340
15–17 years	3,617,593	18–24 years	5,467,615
25–44 years	21,029,136	45–64 years	28,143,196
65+ years	17,404,930	Total number	78,694,222

TABLE 10.2   CCHR Statistics on Psychotropic Drugs by Diagnosis.

	0–5 years	All ages
ADHD	188,899	10,516
Antidepressants	110,516	41,226,394
Antipsychotic	27,343	6,845,303
Antianxiety	727,304	36,472,663

10.1.3   CAUSES, SIGNS, AND SYMPTOMS OF MENTAL DISTURBANCE

Early signs of mental disturbance can be feelings of anxiety, guilt, emptiness, helplessness, hopelessness, pessimism, and worthlessness. Often there is a lack of interest in life and personal appearance, feelings of loneliness and a need to be alone, irritability, restlessness, uncontrollable sorrow, and talk of suicide. Insomnia or excessive sleep and sleeping during the day are all signs of depression. The person may develop digestive problems, over or under eat, have frequent headaches and are often forgetful. Any one of these signs and symptoms can easily be seen as a bad mood or going through a phase and of course they often are. What we tend to do is nothing until it is obvious something is wrong when the problem is chronic, and by then it may be too late.

The causal factors of mental disturbance are as varied as the individuals who suffer from them.

- *Hereditary*: Illnesses such as schizophrenia and epilepsy are considered to be hereditary but at the same time, manifest themselves in puberty which indicates a trigger in the body's physiology affecting the mind. Depression and addictions often run in families but whether this is in fact a genetic trait or because they are behaviors learnt as children is unclear. For example, diabetes is said to be a genetic disorder in modern medicine, but according to Ayurveda, it is the family eating habits.
- *Stressful living*: People in every walk of life are affected by modern living. There are more homicides, suicides, violence, drug and physical abuse, addictions today than ever before in history. These behaviors reflect disturbances of the mind and low mental strength.
- *Lack of family and community*: Modern society is very different from traditional societies, especially since the influence of the women's liberation movement and globalization. Traditionally, women ran the home, managed the children and men were the providers; families and communities remained unchanged for many generations. Now, families are spread out often across continents and the extended family, where all generations live close together, hardly exits. This brings loneliness, isolation and lack of community.

- *Fast-paced living*: Life today is focused on achieving success and striving for a higher standard of living, it seems there is no time to just be and enjoy the simple things in life. Fast-paced living brings with it poor eating habits, eating on the run and not paying attention to the natural rhythms of the body and its connection to nature.
- *Lack of meaningful work*: Corporate takeovers and industrialization have left millions of people without meaningful work. This is clearly evident in India where thousands of farmers are committing suicide because they cannot compete with agri-business and support their families. All over the world small, local family businesses are unable to compete with large corporations who can import mass quantities of goods produced overseas where labor is cheap. There is mass exploitation of workers; companies have no responsibility for or connection to the workers who produce goods for them.
- *Lack of self-sufficiency*: People in general are no longer self-sufficient and depend on the "system" to provide for them. We are losing the ability to make our own clothes, grow our food, and cook for ourselves. We no longer have to build our houses, repair cars, appliances and tools, etc. Without the ability to make a living and to take care of basic needs, there is nothing to do and life has no purpose.
- *Broken homes and single parenting*: There has been a huge increase in the rate of divorce since the Second World War leaving children without a family unit to which they belong. Children need both male and female influences in their upbringing and many children are brought up by single parents without any support. "It takes a village to raise a child."
- *Lack of connection to nature*: Urban areas often don't offer opportunities to commune with nature. Workers are inside, cooped up in office buildings staring at computer screens, in factories, often leave home in the dark and get home after dark. Many are shift-workers whose routine changes from day to day. These are unhealthy lifestyles for humans when there is no connection to nature and a disconnect from the spiritual self.[1]

---

[1] The Vedic view of creation describes the stages of evolution from the merging of Purusha (consciousness) and Prakriti (base substance of the Universe) to the five elements: Earth, water, fire, air, and space. The elements exist in all things meaning that consciousness is in every cell of the mind and body.

10.1.4   CAUSES OF MENTAL DISTURBANCE—AYURVEDIC VIEW

We learn in Ayurveda that mental health and spiritual fulfilment are as important as physical health. If our emotions are disturbed and/or we have no spiritual purpose, we will not be able to heal. Ayurveda treats the cause of disease not just the symptoms and says that the body, mind, and spiritual nature are not only connected but interconnected. For example, if a disease manifests itself in the physical body, the cause of the disease may be a mental disturbance or a spiritual disconnect. In Ayurveda, the body, mind, and spirit must be in harmony for complete healing to take place.

- *Vata in the mind*: Vata is "that which moves" and is the main cause of disturbances in the mind as it creates instability and movement. Too much stimulation and agitation will increase Vata and cause the mind to be disturbed. In everyday living, there are bound to be disturbances—sitting in traffic, rushing to school, pressures at work, financial pressures, etc. If the mind never gets a chance to calm down, rest, and is not nourished properly, it will remain permanently agitated.
- *Vata aggravating diet*: The qualities of Vata are light, dry, and cold. If the intake of foods with the same qualities such as light, dry, cold, stale, canned, processed, junk food, coffee, tea, and alcohol, Vata will be aggravated. Vata being air and space means that aerated foods such as chips, popcorn, carbonated drinks, cookies, crispy, and crunchy foods will increase Vata.
- *Vata aggravating lifestyle*: Multitasking, traveling, fasting, late night work, parties, loud music, and rushing around disturb the mind. Too much time on computers, watching TV and on mobile phones, flickering of screens, and radio waves all aggravate Vata in the mind.
- *Poor quality of mind*: Ayurveda talks about the quality of mind. Sattva is the quality of purity and balance, Rajas is the quality of action and Tamas is the quality of inertia or resistance to action. We must look at the entire picture of ourselves and that of our environment, our diet, lifestyle, and habits. We must change to a Sattvic diet and way of living to attain true happiness which is the key to mental health. If Rajas and Tamas are disturbed by food and drink

such as alcohol, meat, garlic, onions, stale, oily, and spicy foods, the qualities of turbulence and inertia will increase in the mind.

- *Lack of deep, dreamless sleep*: Irregular routines and sleep patterns are common in modern living and since the advent of electricity people stay up late and sleep during the day, all of which disturb Vata and increase Tamas which causes depression.

- *Depravation of Prana*: Prana is the life-force coming into the body through the breath. It is the energy which makes us gasp for air when we hold the breath. Prana supports the mind by allowing the intake of sensory impressions, impulses, feelings, emotions, thoughts, and knowledge. Prana in the mind gives the capacity to communicate and mental adaptability, it allows us to expand our comprehension and arrange our ideas. Prana gives vitality to the mind, the will to live, and to experience life. It is the power of creativity and enthusiasm for life; it is the life-force which enables us to grow and to recover when we get sick. The brain needs serotonin from the sun and Prana from fresh air. If we are not exposed to sunshine, do not have fresh air, and experience the calming effects of nature, Prana will be low and cause depression.

- *Lack of control of sensory material*: The senses are the instruments through which we experience the world and are the bridge between the outside world and the mind (Manas[2]). It is through the five senses that we connect to each of the five elements. The sense of smell connects the mind to the earth element, taste to the water element, touch to the air element, and hearing to the ether element. Thoughts, desires, and emotions arise in the mind and are manifested in an outward direction through the senses. Knowledge comes to the mind through the senses in an inward direction. What comes into the mind through the senses is critical to mental stability; like food it can have either a positive or negative effect. When managing mental health issues, the importance of controlling sensory material must be clearly understood.

---

[2]Manas—The sensate mind. English word "man" comes from this word. It is the semiconscious mind or cognitive intelligence. It is the "outgoing mind" and its job is to get information from the outside world through the senses and to coordinate their activities with the sense organs. Manas is the general capacity for thought and the ability to consider things coming in through the senses. It is an instinctive level of mind, unable to process information only to observe it. It only explores desires such as avoiding pain and seeking pleasure at the level of the senses. As long as we operate at this level, we are merely sensate creatures of habit without values; our energy and thoughts will be directed outward.

- *Misuse of intelligence*: The discriminating mind or intelligence is called the Buddhi in Ayurveda. It acts like the processor of the computer and a filter of information coming into the subconscious— it is the rational mind. It allows understanding, awareness, and the ability to discriminate between truth and falsehood, good and bad. Buddhi gives values and principles and allows us to be objective in our judgment, to question and doubt. It is because of Buddhi that we decide whether something is good for us or not. Anxiety, panic attacks, nervousness, and fear are all symptoms of a weak Buddhi. Addiction is when Buddhi becomes overwhelmed. Prajnaparadha literally means "failure of wisdom". It is the misuse of Buddhi[3]or when we only use its outward function, that is, body and senses for our own selfish desires. Prajnaparadha is considered to be the root cause of all disease. Buddhi is very important to maintaining sanity; it functions properly in Sattva, but in Rajas and Tamas its functions are disturbed.

- *Negative impressions on the subconscious*: The subconscious mind is called Chitta in Ayurveda and can be compared to the hard disk of the computer. It is the bridge between the mind and soul. Chitta is where all life's experiences and images are kept but we are unaware of it constantly taking in and storing our experiences. Deep-seated memories, emotions, habits attachments, and impressions are all stored in the subconscious. Impressions on Chitta are called "Samskaras." The word "scar" comes from this word. Every experience leaves Samskaras on Chitta and not all experiences are positive ones. If a child has a traumatic experience, a deep Samskara is created on Chitta and will lie in wait to raise its ugly head at any time. This is how phobias manifest in the mind when Buddhi is overpowered by Samskaras. There is an automatic reaction and the individual cannot control it, never mind how hard he/she tries. These impressions will affect a person throughout life.

- *Childhood and prenatal trauma*: Mental health begins at conception; if a mother does not want her child, then the child's mental health will be affected throughout life. Buddhi is not developed in

---

[3]Buddhi acts like the processor of the computer and is the rational mind. It allows understanding, awareness, and the ability to discriminate between truth and falsehood, good, and bad. Buddhi gives values and principles and allows us to be objective, in our judgment, to question and to doubt. It is because of buddhi that we decide whether something is good for us or not.

babies and young children leaving Chitta wide open to Samskaras, which is why the early days of development are so important. Everything is recorded even before birth which is why babies, even in the womb, and young children have to be protected from trauma. In Indian culture, babies are not exposed to anyone other than parents and close members of the family for at least 40 days after birth. Birth itself is considered to be a trauma and early days are critical as the baby transitions into the material world.

- *Low Tejas and Ojas*: Ojas is the pure essence of our being and represents our immunity, stamina, feelings of well-being and vitality. In digestion, Ojas is the pure product of reproductive tissue, it is the essence of the tissues and of life. There is said to be eight drops in the heart and death occurs when Ojas are gone. When Ojas are depleted, we are run-down, exhausted, lacking in energy, and depressed. Tejas is a subtle form of Pitta or fire in the mind. It is the fire of perception, inspiration, and awareness. When Tejas is low, the mind is dull and lacking in inspiration.

10.1.5   AYURVEDA AND YOGA TREATMENT STRATEGIES

It takes time for disturbances to manifest themselves and they would not go away overnight or by taking medication to mask the symptoms. It takes a commitment to change by the person, the carers and professionals. All aspects of diet and lifestyle have to change. For example, if we exercise and go to the gym but continue to eat junk food, drink alcohol, and watch violent films we may feel better for a while, but there will not be any permanent change. Everything which goes into the body and mind will have an effect, everything is food and will have either a positive or negative effect.

- *Cleansing diet*: It is commonly known that any type of engine which burns fuel leaves a residue. If these residues are not cleaned periodically the engine would not run properly and if left to build up, will cause the engine to break down. In Ayurveda this residue is called Ama and is defined as a toxic material created in the digestive tract from undigested food. The body cannot absorb it and cannot eliminate it either and a thick slimy material is produced. This is carried by Vata through the system and gets absorbed and trapped in weak areas. The longer Ama stays in the body, the harder and stickier it becomes and eventually is deeply rooted. It adheres to channels and blocks them preventing an efficient flow of blood, lymph urine, etc. It will appear in many forms. It gets into the joints and causes inflammation and arthritis, it is cholesterol blocking the arteries, tumors, stones in the kidneys and gall bladder, and plaques on the brain interrupting nerve impulses.

Causes of Ama accumulation

- *Food* has to be fully digested before additional food is added therefore, snacking is very bad for digestion because food is at different stages of digestion. Hunger is the body's way of telling us that it is ready to receive more food.
- *Overeating*: If the system is overloaded it will clog it up and excessive residue will be created.
- *Weak digestive fire*: If the digestive fire is weak it will not digest food properly. Illness, cold temperatures, cold food and water will reduce the digestive fire.
- *Processed food* contains additives, preservatives, emulsifiers, artificial flavorings, colorings, and chemicals, which the digestive system is not designed to digest and will create Ama. Anything which is foreign to the body will cause disease because it produces Ama.
- *Food preparation*: Microwaving, barbecuing, plastic cookware, aluminum, and nonstick pans add toxins to the food and create Ama.
- *Meat* is very indigestible because the human digestive tract is not designed to digest it. Carnivores have a short digestive tract so after digestion waste is eliminated quickly. Humans have a long digestive tract therefore, meat stays in the tract for a long time and creates toxic material.
- *Ama*: In addition, if farm animals are fed on food which nature does not provide for them and if they are badly treated, the meat will be toxic and produce Ama.
- *Medicines*: Especially antibiotics and supplements in the form of pills will create Ama.

• *Importance of sleep* cannot be overemphasized. Sleep is a function of Buddhi; without proper, deep sleep, Buddhi will not function properly. It is not so much the number of hours of sleep, which can vary from person to person, but the value of deep sleep which leaves us feeling rested and energized. Workers who have irregular hours are more prone to mental and physical problems. Natural sleep follows the circadian rhythms of nature which are described in Ayurveda. The sun goes down during the Kapha time between 6 and 10 p.m. when the energy of the earth is heavy and lethargic. Animals and birds go to sleep at this time. If we stay up past 10 p.m. then we move into Pitta time and get second wind. We must go to bed before 10 p.m. every night and even if we do not sleep, set the alarm for 6 a.m. or before Kapha time begins again. Ayurveda recommends avoiding eating up to 2 h before bed, snacking in the night, and indulging in strenuous mental or physical activity before sleep. A cup of warm milk with some raisins and almonds and a little honey will promote sleep. Calming spices such as nutmeg, cinnamon cardamom, and saffron can be added. Excessive dreaming interferes with deep sleep, it is only in a deep dreamless sleep that we rest in the embodied soul which is when the mind is inactive and the body's functions are involuntary.

* *Simple, easy-to-digest diet* of fresh fruit and vegetables, a variety of whole grains, seeds and legumes (pulses), digestive spices, ([4]cumin, turmeric, fennel, coriander, black pepper, ginger, garlic, mineral salt) ghee, buttermilk, good quality milk, and soft cheese are recommended. Fried, canned, frozen processed food, and complicated food combinations should be avoided.

* *Rules of social and personal behavior*: Yamas[5] and Niyamas[6] help to bring the mind to one-pointedness. They are guidelines for righteous living. Unless we come to terms with ourselves and recognize who we really are, we can never be happy; happiness is the keystone to mental health.

* *Yoga asana* means seat and is the physical practice of stillness to control the body and mind so that pure meditation can occur. In the poses one can relax ones efforts and let the mind slip into infinity.

---

[4]Cumin, turmeric, fennel, coriander, black pepper, ginger, garlic, mineral salt.
[5]YAMAS—Ahimsa: nonviolence towards any living beings. Satya: truthfulness. Achaurya: noncoveting. Brahmacharya: control of sexual energy. Aparigraha: nonstealing.
[6]NIYAMAS—are rules of personal behavior and are lifestyle disciplines for inner development Ishvarapranidhana: surrender to the Divine. Santosha: contentment. Shaucha—purity: Svadhyaya: self-study of mind. Tapas—self-discipline.

Asana practice does not have to be complicated; in fact a simple practice done consistently everyday is more beneficial.

- *Pranayama* is the practice of controlling the breath and is an integral part of asana practice. Prana is often described as the breath, but it is the force which makes us breathe. If we hold the breath and then have to gasp for air, Prana is the energy which makes us gasp. We can increase the life-force through yogic breathing practices and by consuming fresh fruits and vegetables which have Prana, the life force, in them. Prana is in all living things. If we take beans and sprout them, it is the life force in the beans which forces the shoots. If we put a piece of meat in the ground, it will only rot because it has no life force and is dead. It is through Prana that we create higher awareness, it purifies and creates stillness in the mind and allows the development of higher levels of consciousness. When used properly, it will bring the right spiritual direction and will determine inspiration, positivity, and connect us to our inner self. It is through the breath that we consciously connect to subtle sources of energy within us which govern the mind. Prana determines our aspirations and when fully developed allows us to transcend the outer world and promote the evolution of consciousness by surrendering to life and its forces. Pranayama has a calming and purifying effect on the mind. The breath becomes long and subtle and the mind is then ready for concentration. Regular practice will reduce Rajas and Tamas and cultivate Sattvic qualities of the mind.

  - *Anuloma Viloma, Nadi Shodhana, or alternate nostril breathing*: There is a thin membrane between the base of the brain and the nasal passage. Therefore, Anuloma Viloma is effective in bringing Prana (air) to the brain. The right nostril is heating (sun) brings Prana to the left brain. The left nostril is cooling (moon) brings Prana to the right brain; Anuloma Viloma balances the Nadis (subtle energy channels of the body). The most common practice is to breathe in to a count of four and exhale to a count of six. Twelve rounds are customary.

  - *Bhramari*: In this practice, the thumbs are placed on the Tragus[7] the little fingers at the base of the nose at the side of the nostrils. With the tongue to the top of the mouth, a humming sound is

---

[7]Anatomical point: the triangular, muscular structure anterior to the ear canal.

made which creates a vibration in the head. This technique is very effective for dislodging Ama and stimulating the brain. Over time, there will be an improvement in memory, cognitive powers, clarity of thought and improvement in sleep.

- *Shitali* is when the teeth are clenched together and a deep breath is pulled in through the teeth. Alternatively, the tongue is rolled and air sucked in. This is called a cooling breath and useful to remember when heat rises in the body.
- *Laughter*: Laughter is an important practice to have in maintaining mental health. During laughter, there is no thought and the mind is entirely in the joy of the moment. Deep laughter from the lungs eliminates bad air trapped in the lower part of the lungs.

• *Care of the senses*: Proper care of the sense organs from birth is important, especially the control of sensory material entering the mind through the senses. This is especially important for babies and young children.

   - *Hearing—Ether*: The inner ears should be left alone and only the outer ear cleaned. The ears should be kept warm in cold weather, protected from the wind and not be exposed to excessively loud noise. Hot water in the ears such as immersing the head in bath water should be avoided. A little ghee or oil in the ears protects the eardrums.
   - *Touch—Air*: The sense of touch refers mainly to the skin, especially the hands. The skin is the largest organ of the body and indicates overall health. Chemicals in cleaning products, soaps, cosmetics, hair dyes, etc. will be absorbed through the skin including the scalp. Organic oil is the best way to keep the skin clean and then rinse with water and rarely using pure soap.
   - *Sight—Fire*: The eyes are particularly sensitive and should be exercised and rested regularly. Long hours on the computer and watching television will damage the eyes. Eyes should be flushed with clear water (not chlorinated) every morning and a few drops of castor oil or ghee will keep the eyes nourished.
   - *Taste—Water*: The tongue should be scraped every morning to remove Ama and oil held in the mouth to draw toxins from the oral cavity. Oral hygiene is important for physical and mental health.

- *Smell—Earth*: The sense of smell is critical for the sense of taste and should not be overwhelmed with artificial scents (perfumes) and additives in cleaning products. If a chemical has a foul smell, its use should be avoided. Masking the smell with a scent is overriding the body's natural repugnance to a toxic or bad smell. Flushing the nose with water or using a neti pot with a small amount of mineral salt added, clears the nasal passages and sinuses of phlegm.

- *Pratyahara, withdrawal of the senses* is a daily practice of silence except for the sounds of nature. Listening to the silence within brings inner peace and joy. Withdrawal of the senses can be difficult in today's world where there is "sensory overload." Telephones, short bites of information, an emphasis on the physical and sexual aspects of our being, and a barrage of visual images constantly stimulates the mind.

- *Concentration (Dharana)* brings the mind to one-pointedness. It can be done by gazing intently at a candle flame (tradak), a ghee lamp or something unchanging in nature like the ocean, a river, the sky or a mountain view. Concentration is an important practice to master in our world of "scattered thoughts."

- *Meditation (Dhyana)*: The power of meditation has only recently been recognized by modern medicine as a means to connect body, mind and spiritual self. After controlling the senses and practicing concentration, one is able to bring the mind to a meditative state where there is a continuous flow of pure awareness within. It is a state of conscious sleep where we are not aware of time and space. Meditation cannot be taught only techniques to create a state of mind when meditation happens naturally. It takes practice and perseverance but the benefits to healing are immeasurable.

- *Complete absorption in the inner self (Samadhi)* is where the meditator and the meditated become one, meaning Prakriti and Purusha[8] are absorbed into oneness. It is a state of complete awareness beyond the mind and free from desires therefore obtaining total liberation. This state is very difficult to achieve and requires

---

[8]The Vedic view of creation describes the stages of evolution from the merging of Purusha (consciousness) and Prakriti (base substance of the Universe) to the five elements: Earth, water, fire, air, and space. The elements exist in all things meaning that consciousness is in every cell of the mind and body.

a lifetime of practice and only mentioned here for the purpose of explaining the "Eight Limbs of Yoga" (Ashtanga Yoga) from the Yoga Sutras systematized by Patanjali. Samadhi is not a necessary goal for mental health.

Chanting of Mantra is the continuous chant of a Sanskrit word or phrase. "Ohm" is the primordial sound of creation and a powerful mantra. Ohm is in three phases, "Ahh" in the lower chest, "Uhh" in the upper chest, and "Mmm" in the nasal cavity. The sound lasts through the breath. Sanskrit is the language of mantra and evolved from sounds of the universe and of nature. It may be construed that other languages can be substituted, but they will only appeal to the mind and not to the true self. Mantras are effective because they appeal to our spiritual self.

- *Pancha Karma (PK) literally means five actions* which are enema (Vasthi) for Vata pacification, purgation (Verechena) for Pitta and vomiting (Vamana) for Kapha. Nasya is clearing of the nasal passages and (Raktamoksha) Blood Letting. PK is a long, involved process to be done correctly and is prescribed according to the condition of the patient. Therefore, an Ayurvedic diagnosis is critical. The goal in PK is to detoxify all of the tissues and bring all cells to a balanced state.
  - *Abyangha*: A simple Ayurvedic massage. There are other oil massage treatments used in Ayurveda for specific conditions. Ayurvedic massage must not be confused with that of Western massage, the purpose is quite different.
  - *Svedena*: Steam used in specific cases to induce sweating to release toxins through the skin. This would not be recommended for mental conditions where Pitta is aggravated, as it would only increase heat in the body and mind.
  - *Shirodarah*: Shiro means head and Dhara means continuous flow. In cases of severe mental disturbance either warm (for Vata) or cool (for Pitta) oil is used. Treatment is given at the same time of the day for 7–14 days. The duration is 60 min increasing by 10 min each day to 90 min, then decreasing by 10 min to 60 min. Apart from relieving stress, tension and for insomnia, shirodarah can be used for all diseases of the nervous system, in particular, schizophrenia, facial palsy, paralysis,

and epilepsy. Dramatic results of shirodarah accompanied by Ayurvedic herbal medicine are described in Ayurveda. Treatment must be under the guidance of a professional as precautions are necessary for serious conditions. It is a gentle treatment to calm the nervous system and nourish the brain and senses. It is not a "quick fix" and for successful results a sattvic diet and lifestyle must be followed, sleep patterns managed, and daily practices adhered to. Random shirodarah alone will not work. Shirodarah is often given in spas for relaxation and must not be confused with treatment for mental disturbance where it may not be appropriate.

- *Nasya* is the daily application of prescribed oil into the nasal passages through the nose. It is very effective for clearing Kapha from the sinuses and allowing prana to flow freely.
- *Shiro Vasthi* is a method of saturating the skull in medicated oil daily for a period of time for several days.
- *Herbal preparations*: Ayurveda has very effective herbs for sharpening the mind, for example, brahhi, shanka pushpi, and jatamansi. Cinnamon, nutmeg, cardamom, and saffron are calming spices for the mind and good for promoting sleep. Digestive spices (cumin, hing, mineral salt, coriander, fennel, ginger, turmeric) to clear Ama from the system.
- *Marma therapy* can be compared to acupressure in Chinese medicine except the Marma points differ from meridians. The purpose of Marma is to align subtle energies of body and mind.

10.2   AYURVEDIC VIEW OF HEALING THE MIND

According to Ayurveda and yoga, the ultimate goal in life is to achieve self-realization and the main obstacle in doing so is mind. This is because the mind is directed outward; it goes here and there and is always seeking pleasure and desires. We must control the mind so that we can look within, "see" our real self and become "self-realized."

There is a subtle flow of information between the senses, the semiconscious mind (Manas) and the conscious level of mind (Buddhi) which acts as the gatekeeper. Buddhi digests and interprets experiences and information which is then stored in the subconscious (Chitta). Experiences are external; therefore, they are enjoyed by the ego the self-conscious mind (Ahamkara), the force which gives individuality. The ego is a problem for the mind because it causes a division which brings pain and suffering, both mentally and physically.

Ego has to exist for things to happen and we have to have the feeling that this body belongs to me for it to function. Every individual is different and has their own sense of "I," but we tend to believe we are the only important thing. Ego is what gives us a sense of pride, and when operating at this level, ego causes us to look down on others making us prejudiced and "right." Ego identifies itself with the impressions of the mind and is our self-image. It gives us ownership of our emotions as in "I like this" and "I hate you," our identity as in "I am old" and "I am English" and ownership as in "this is my body" and "this is my car." The ego operates through emotions and always wants to enjoy through sensations, and for that, it needs the mind, intelligence and senses. It is through ego that we can expand our mind and achieve focus. But ego is limited because it is never satisfied and therefore makes us unhappy and agitates the mind.

However, the ego is not who we really are but can be considered a waypoint where we make the choice between an outward and inward directed mind. When directed inward, we live in harmony with our true nature and deeper aspects of life. It is where we make a choice between believing that "I am" this body and mind or that "I am" the inner self, which is the real me. "I am Soul." When we recognize that we are not body and mind, we are able to be objective in viewing ourselves and our behavior and are able to change.

The discriminating mind, Buddhi has an outward and an inward function also. When directed outward, we abuse people and nature for our own enjoyment and satisfaction. We tend to discriminate merely through impressions of the mind such as sense objects, pleasures and desires and delude ourselves into thinking this is where happiness and fulfillment lie. We get caught up in ideas about ourselves and believe that the external is reality. We rationalize emotionally without looking at ourselves objectively and seeing the truth.

When Buddhi is directed inward, we have compassion and awareness and are free to manifest pure consciousness. Directed inward Buddhi functions at a high level and allows us to perceive reality, giving us wisdom. Only then can we say we are intelligent, mature, responsible, and free from delusion.

The practice of mantra has the effect of engraining impressions (Samskaras) on the unconscious mind similar to learning by repeating over and over and memorizing. Mantra will erase the impressions rather like cleaning off a mirror in order to "see." However, if Samskaras are deeply rooted, they may be difficult or even impossible to remove. The Buddhi filters experiences and protects the Chitta, but if it is fearful or weak, it will not function properly and Samskaras will be created. Insults, hatred, and emotional hurt create very deep Samskaras and cause disturbances in the mind.

Using Vedic psychology to manage mental health is to go beyond all aspects of the mind through meditation and spiritual practice (Sadhana). It is through Chitta that we connect to cosmic consciousness and Mahat is where pure consciousness appears. In hypnosis and using drugs like LSD we may think that we are having a spiritual experience, but this is only material. Spirituality is beyond Chitta. Ayurvedda gives the wisdom to follow the right diet and lifestyle so that we are healthy physically.

Love is the glue which holds all living beings together. There is a lot of talk about love these days. There are images everywhere in advertising and films of people of all ages about to "make love" which of course means sex. Do we really know what love means anymore? All living beings look for love the moment they are born, babies search for the nipple and the mother not only gives nourishment but nurtures her baby with love. This love is essential for the well-being of all living creatures, human and otherwise. It is unconditional and comes from instinct.

Modern society seems to do everything to bypass love. Farm animals are taken away from their mothers and never allowed to feed naturally so they never feel loved. Therefore, when we eat meat of these animals there won't be the essential ingredient of love, all we have is fear, bewilderment, anxiety, loneliness, and depression; the same problems of the "modern" human.

Everything we put into our body is food, we are what we eat and our food has to contain love in order for love to become part of us. Children brought up on fast food where they eat meat from factory farms, processed and genetically modified food, sprayed fruits, and vegetables served by a person who has no connection to them, will not receive love. When pure food is prepared by a person who loves us, love comes into us and has value far beyond nutrition. It is only by being loved that we learn how to love, not only others but also ourselves and the world in which we live.

There are three kinds of love. Romantic love and infatuation which is captivating and obsessive but changes or wears off. If there is no commitment, this love diminishes and brings fear, uncertainty, insecurity, and sadness. Love which comes out of comfort and familiarity grows, but it has no thrill, no enthusiasm, joy, or fire. Divine love supersedes romantic and comfort love and the closer we get to it, the deeper it becomes. Divine love has comfort, enthusiasm familiarity and never knows boredom.

Forgiveness: Mental disturbances can be due to deep-seated memories engrained in the subconscious. These may be from before birth, as a child or even from a past life. Modern psychology will often diagnose the cause of a disturbance, perhaps abuse, abandonment or not being loved, but in Vedic psychology, it isn't important to know the cause, in fact knowing the cause can often bring up problems with relationships in the person's life. A big part of the healing process is to forgive in one's heart, maybe write a letter, include it in meditation or say it aloud. The power of forgiveness is far reaching, but it does not mean that an against us act is condoned. As long as hurt and revenge are held in the heart against someone or something, true healing of mental disturbance will never be achieved.

10.3 CONCLUSION

Western psychology is based on deep and interesting theories about the mind and human behavior of scholars like Viktor Frankl, Freud, and Adler. But they are limited because they only go to the level of mind and use the mind to describe mind. They cannot explain who this person really is and what it is that drives them. When theories of these great scholars are put into practice, they seem to work but they are incomplete because they don't see the whole picture.

The Vedas describe the mind in great detail and recognize the barriers which it presents when reaching spiritual awareness. The Vedas give a clear explanation of the presence of consciousness in every cell in their theory of creation, and of how matter evolves. When Prakriti and Purusha merge, life evolves, meaning Purusha exists in all living things, in fact Purusha is life itself.

To attain spiritual awareness, we must understand the mind, control it and turn it away from all its desires and wanderings. Modern living is much more complicated than in the days of the Vedas but it was recognized in society thousands of years ago; mankind hasn't changed. The principles of Ayurveda and Yoga, diet, lifestyle, pranayama, meditation, treatments coupled with counseling can have a long-standing effect leaving the person in a position to manage their own mental health successfully without the use of medication. In serious mental illness medication is necessary but can be reduced if proper diet and lifestyle practices are followed. This is Vedic Psychology

KEYWORDS

- Ayurveda
- yoga
- Vedic psychology
- mental health
- mental disturbances
- autism
- depression

Writing Sample

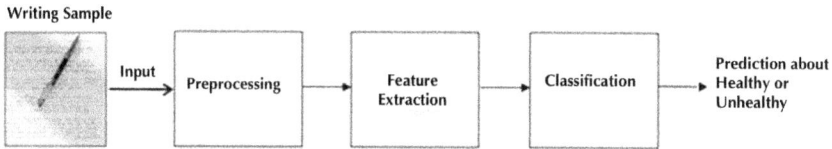

FIGURE 9.1   Block diagram of the proposed system.

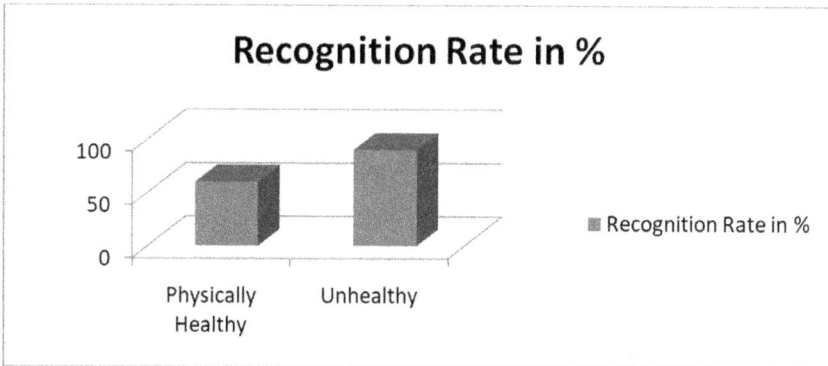

FIGURE 9.2   Recognition rate of physically healthy and unhealthy classes.

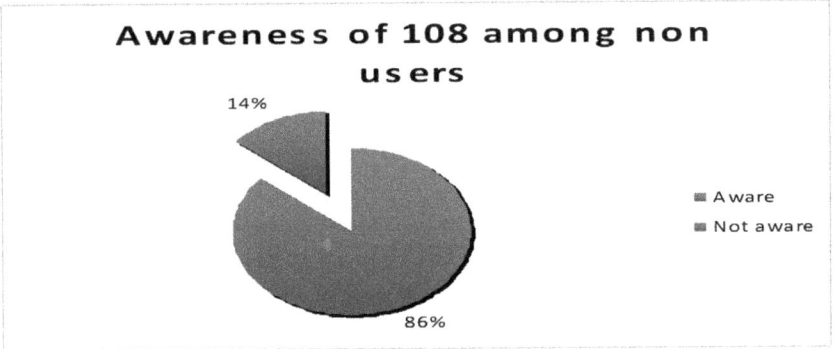

FIGURE 16.1   Awareness of 108 among nonusers.

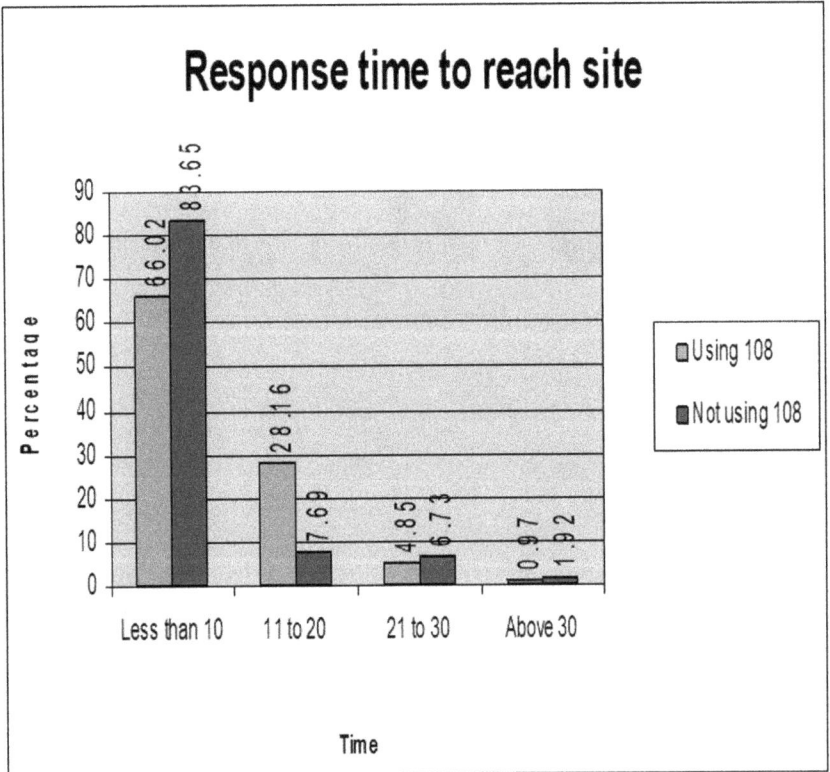

FIGURE 16.2   Time taken by ambulance to reach the emergency site.

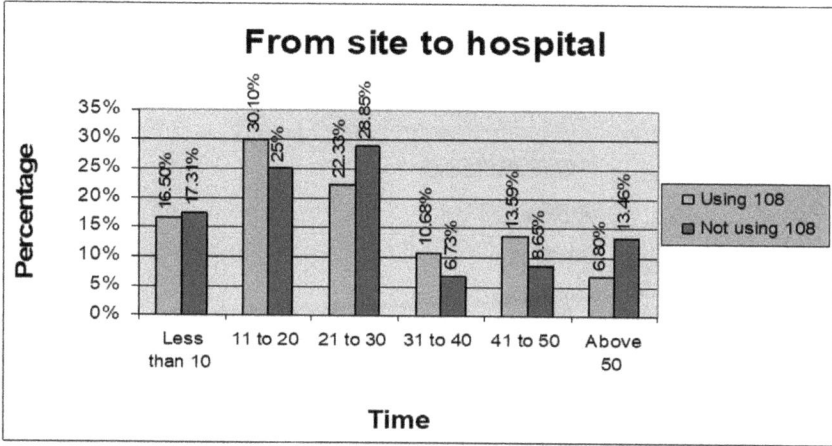

FIGURE 16.3   Time taken for transporting patient from emergency site to hospital.

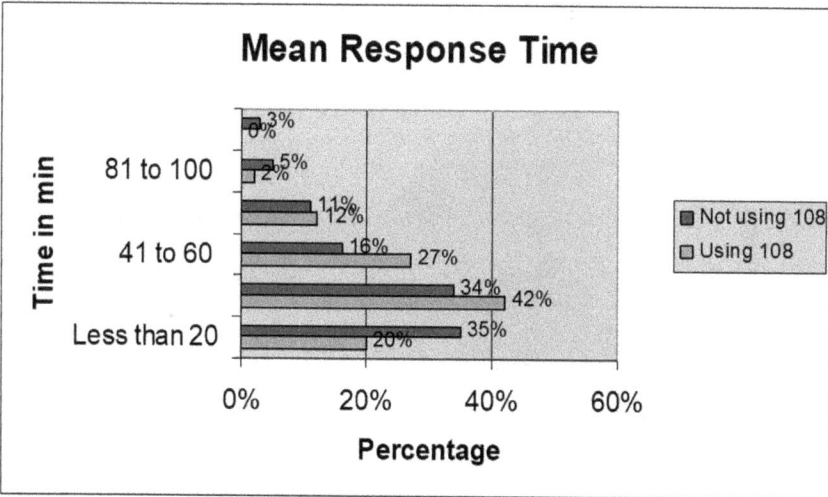

FIGURE 16.4   Mean response time of the vehicle.

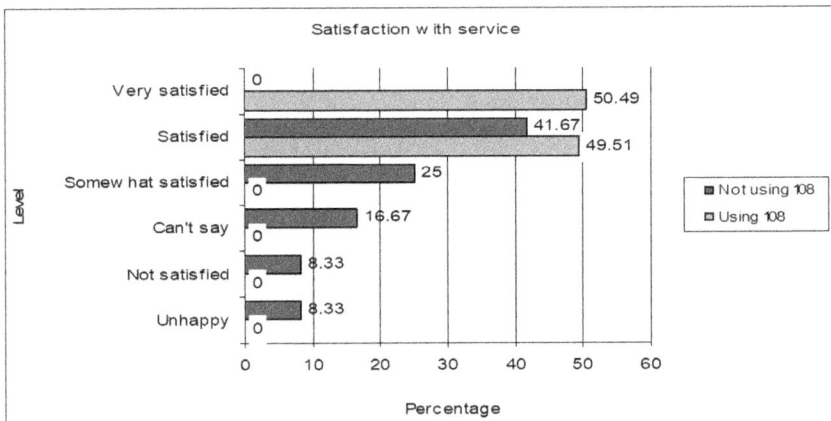

FIGURE 16.5 Satisfaction with the service.

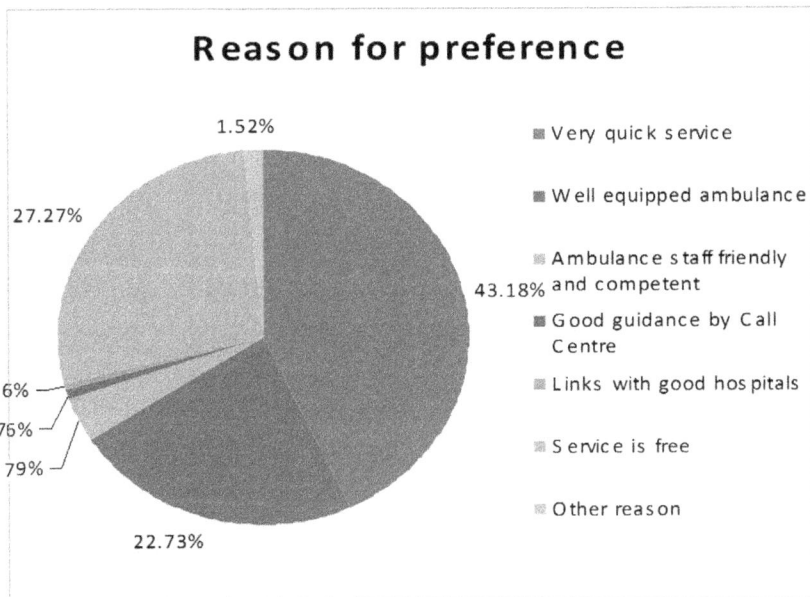

FIGURE 16.6 Reason for preference.

PART IV
Chemicoherbal Treatment Strategies

CHAPTER 11

INTEGRATING HOMEOPATHY IN MAINSTREAM MEDICINE: HOMEOPATHY IN CANCER MANAGEMENT

MANEESHA SOLANKI*

Dhondumama Sathe Homoeopathic Medical College, Pune, Maharashtra, India

*E-mail: dr.maneesha@hotmail.com

ABSTRACT

Today cancer is one of the leading causes of death worldwide, over all socioeconomic classes. The increase in the rate of cancer around the world is over 10 million cancer cases among which 6 million deaths occurring a year globally. Of which 40 lakh new diagnosed cases and 2 lakh reported deaths are in India alone. It is evident that many cancer patients use alternative treatment to the conventional medical care as an adjuvant line of treatment due to the nature and prognosis of the disease.

11.1 INTRODUCTION

Homeopathy as a primary treatment modality for cancer cases is rather uncommon. The philosophical basis of homeopathic treatment encompasses holistic approach and is patient oriented treatment rather than the disease based. Individualization of the patients suffering from the same disease in the treatment is the corner-stone of the homeopathic management. Therefore, not only cell type, location and size of tumor, and extent of disease, but physiologic and psychological status and expressed needs and desires of the patient are the *main factors* that would determine treatment strategy and modality of treatment adopted for a particular individual suffering from cancer.

Hospital is an integral part of the society and patient is the center around which all the efforts of the medical and paramedical staff rotate. A homeopathic hospital setup is no different from a regular hospital, but the time taken to build up the confidence of the patients and society to accept this concept is very challenging.

Treating advanced stage cancer cases in our homeopathic hospital just adds on to our challenges which we face optimistically looking at it as an opportunity that these hopeless cases can become a voice of homeopathy to the society and scientific world and thus justify the system to a level that it is worthy of.

11.2   OBJECTIVES

Our objective while accepting the cases of cancer was to find out whether homeopathic treatment modality, as a primary palliative intervention, either alone or with support of adjuvant treatment, can arrest or control tumor growth, prevent or delay complications normally expected in such cases, maintain normal bodily functions, promote comfort, and provide quality life to these patients or not?

We have carried out this retrospective analysis of in patient department (IPD) admissions for such cases in our hospital for past 3 years. Eighteen patients of advanced stage cancer have opted for the integrated approach and thus were admitted to our hospital.

Diagnosed cases of cancer who were willing to take homeopathic treatment and were admitted to our teaching homeopathic hospital for the period of 3 years, that is, from January 2013 to September 2015 were included in this study.

Out of the 15 cases, 14 were under the conventional cancer treatment, while only 1 was exclusively on homeopathic medicines as per patient's will. All of them received homeopathic medicines based on symptom totality depending on their presenting complaints either acute or chronic constitutional medicine as per the case.

The cases included under our study showed significant effect in relieving the side effects of chemotherapy, radiotherapy, and other associated complaints like restlessness, fear, anxiety, hopelessness, general weakness, etc.

Six cases which were in terminal stage where their relatives had lost hope, we could give them better quality of life in their remaining life span by giving them homeopathic medicines along with a good nursing care, cost effectively.

In all other patients whom we gave homeopathic medicines as an adjuvant therapy, it was observed that the additional economic burden was negligible along with their conventional treatment and nursing care.

Patient who opted for only homeopathic treatment and denied all interventions was very active mentally till the end and could cope up with higher mental abilities like reading and writing on his own till the end.

All these cases came to us as the last ray of hope when the conventional treatment got exhausted.

Cancer being progressive in pathology and heterogeneous in nature possesses a big challenge for its management. Our role while approaching and managing these cases was purely palliative, irrespective of what stage they had come and with what expectations they had.

The plan of treatment we applied to all these cases followed the principles of the system, that is, a thorough homeopathic case taking for individualization and assessing the susceptibility of the patient to ongoing pathology and choosing a most indicated remedy in appropriate potency which either was acute, chronic, constitutional, or antimiasmatic intercurrent remedy as per requirement of the case. Auxiliary treatment is the part and parcel of general nursing care which included acute measures like fluid electrolyte balance, nutritional support, and oxygen therapy as per the need and long-term measures like diet and regimen, bedsore management if any, counseling of patient and their closed ones, and many more intangible things and actions of the hospital personnel involved in the treatment of cases which cannot be measured but have an impact on the overall improvement of the patient.

Herewith, we are giving in brief four such case studies, where homeopathy has played its role as a best palliation.

11.2.1 CASE 1: CANCER OF PYRIFORM SINUS

A detailed history was taken and a thorough physical examination was carried out.

11.2.1.1 CHIEF AND ASSOCIATED COMPLAINTS

Mr. M. K., a 75-year-old male patient, retired 10 years back from the post of manager with very good service record, a diagnosed case of cancer of pyriform sinus. He presented in our hospital outpatient department (OPD) on February 15, 2013, with a painless, hard, localized swelling in the right side of neck; sensation of lump in the throat, and difficulty in swallowing with progressive weight loss, anorexia, and associated complaint of sleeplessness. He was advised to go for immediate excision and reconstructive surgery to be followed by radiation and also chemotherapy. Patient, being extremely frightful of any interventional treatment, opted, therefore, for an alternative treatment, that is, homeopathy.

Since the time he noticed the swelling, he has also noticed gradual weight loss, general weakness, and reduced appetite with difficulty in swallowing, more for liquids than solids and semisolids; sensation as if something is lodged in the throat. Hoarseness of voice aggravated by talking with pain in throat; intermittent dry cough while lying down; increased salivation more at night; and disturbed sleep and great restlessness.

The swelling has remained painless, but gradually increased in size measuring 2.5 cm × 2.5 cm on palpation in the submandibular area on the right side of neck originating beneath the mandible, but not adhering to it. It was hard, with smooth surface and irregular margins, and fixed to the underlying tissue. No other abnormal signs were noted in the neck on examination. Throat: no growth, no displacement of soft palate or uvula noted. Indirect laryngoscopy: irregular mass obliterating the right false vocal cord and adjacent area.

11.2.1.2 PAST HISTORY

No major sickness in the past except low back pain for which he took some homeopathic treatment and had relief from it.

11.2.1.3   FAMILY HISTORY

Two brothers, both have diabetes mellitus (DM); younger brother died of chronic heart disease 2 years ago; grandmother (paternal) died of DM; no history of malignancy in the family.

11.2.1.4   PERSONAL HISTORY

Takes food in gruel form; due to difficulty in swallowing and choking; no regurgitation of food. Cravings: tea^{++}, warm drinks and food^{++}, but now aggravates pain in throat, ice cream^{+}. Thirst: decreased, takes 1–2 glasses of water in a day. Addictions: heavy smoker but stopped for the last 5 years. Perspiration: nothing significant. Urination: 4–5 times during day, 1 or 2 times at night. Stools: daily evacuation, flatulence, occasional constipation. Chilly: needs thick covering and sleeps with head wrapped; intolerance for draught of air. Dreams of dead relatives and colleagues who used to work in his office; fear of operation; anxiety about disease being incurable, and about the family members mainly wife and daughter; fear of disfigurement and disability; fear of injection needles; fear of injuries; fear of after effects of radiation burns; and after effects of chemotherapy.

11.2.1.5   GENERAL EXAMINATION

Tall, average built, fair. Vital data: a febrile; pulse: 82/min, regular; respiratory rate (RR): 20/min.

Blood pressure (BP): 120/70 mmHg. Weight: 40 kg (lost approx. 16 kg in 2 months earlier weighing 56 kg), Pallor^{+}; no other lymphadenopathy; no icterus, cyanosis, clubbing, or peripheral edema noted. All peripheral pulses palpable. Rest nothing abnormal detected (NAD).

11.2.1.6   SYSTEMIC EXAMINATION

Respiratory system (RS): Trachea midline; chest movements bilaterally symmetrical; air entry normal both sides, vesicular breath sounds.

Per abdomen: liver, spleen—not palpable: no free fluid in the peritoneal cavity.

Cardiovascular system (CVS): S_1, S_2 normal, no abnormal findings. Central nervous system (CNS): Higher functions—normal. No neuro-deficit (Tables 11.1 and 11.2).

TABLE 11.1 Following Investigations Were Already Carried Out before Patient Reported to Us.

Date	Investigation	Report
January 30, 2013	Hemogram	Hb—13.9 g%, TLC—6200/cu mm, N—49, L—47, E—02, M—02, B—00; platelets—21,800/cu mm; RBC morphology—NCNC; WBC—reactive lymphocytes+
January 30, 2013	ESR	27 mm at the end of 1 h
January 30, 2013	Chest X-ray	Normal
February 7, 2013	FNAC right submandibular lymph node	Cellular smear showed atypical cells arranged in clumps with pleomorphism and anisokaryosis, hyper chromic nuclei, cells have high N:C ratio. Positive for malignancy? Metastasis from head and neck region
February 7, 2013	USG abdomen and pelvis	Mild grade one fatty change in liver, enlarged prostate–32 g prevoid–199-cc postvoid residue of 4-cc urine
February 7, 2013	Mantoux test	1 mm × 1 mm erythema and induration; TT negative

TABLE 11.2 Investigations Advised after First Visit to Our OPD.

Date	Investigation	Report
February 16, 2013	Hemogram	Hb—14.6 g%, TLC—6000/cu mm, N—51, L—43, E—04, M—02, B—00, platelets—22,200/cu mm, RBC morphology—NCNC
February 16, 2013	BSL	BSL (F)—104 mg/dL, PP—117 mg/dL
February 16, 2013	Lipid profile	Sr. cholesterol—160 mg/dL, HDL—33 mg/dL, Sr. triglycerides—170 mg/dL, VLDL—34 mg/dL, LDL—93 mg/dL, T.Chol/HDChol ratio—4.85(N)

TABLE 11.2   *(Continued)*

Date	Investigation	Report
February 16, 2013	Liver function tests	Sr. bilirubin total—1.46 mg%, direct—0.84 mg%, indirect—0.62 mg%, total proteins—7.2 g/dL, Sr. albumin—4.0 g/dL, Sr. globulin—3.2 g/dL, Sr. alkaline phosphatase—68 IU/L; SGPT—10 IU/L, SGOT—24 IU/L
February 16, 2013	Urine routine	Pus cells—1-2/hpf, Ep cells—occasional, RBC—2-3/hpf
February 16, 2013	RFTs	Sr. urea—29 mg/dL, Sr. creatinine—10 mg/dL
February 16, 2013	CT scan brain CT scan neck	Mild generalized cerebral atrophy-age related. No other abnormality noted. Ill-defined heterogeneous, hypodensity seen involving the root of tongue and tonsillar fossa on right side. Effacement of adjacent fat planes with loss of fat in hyoglossus. Another ill-defined hypodensity seen in region of right pyriform sinus, that is, supraglottic region; finding suggestive of neoplastic etiology. Few discrete, mildly enlarged lymph nodes seen along bilateral IJV level II–IV and submandibular region, largest one measures 2.5 cm × 2.1 cm in size, indenting left submandibular gland and anterior margin of left sternocleidomastoid muscle
February 18, 2013	Sr. PSA	Index value—1 ng/mL (N)
February 18, 2013	2D-Echo	Normal LV dimension, normal LV systolic and diastolic function; LVEF—70%
February 18, 2013	ECG	Sinus rhythm
July 29, 2013	MRI neck	Large lobulated heterogeneously enhancing neoplastic changes involving the epiglottis, right aryepiglottic fold, pyriform sinus, right lateral and posterior oro, and hypopharyngeal walls causing significant compromise of the airway enlarged metastatic lymph nodes along the right upper jugular chain at the level II and submandibular region

TABLE 11.2 *(Continued)*

Date	Investigation	Report
April 12, 2014	2D-Echo	Normal LV dimension, normal LV function and LVEF—60%
April 12, 2014	BSL	F—106 mg/dL, PP—133 mg/dL
April 12, 2014	RFTs	Sr. urea—24 mg/dL and Sr. creatinine—1.2 mg/dL
April 12, 2014	Lipid profile	Sr. cholesterol—145 mg/dL, total cholesterol/HDL ratio—4
April 12, 2014	LFTs	Total bilirubin—0.66 mg%, alkaline phosphatase—300 IU/L, SGPT—28 IU/L, SGOT—30 IU/L, total protein—7.4 g/dL
April 12, 2014	USG abdomen and pelvis	Mild prostatomegaly without significant post urine residue
April 12, 2014	Chest X-ray	Normal

11.2.1.7   HOMEOPATHIC WORKING

Symptoms of the Disease Process: Swelling, pain, difficulty in swallowing, hoarseness, cough, weight loss, sleeplessness, reduced appetite, etc.

Symptoms of the Patient: Chilly, restlessness, awaking around 3 a.m., dreams, cravings, addiction, thirst, salivation, fear, anxiety, sensitive nature, etc.

11.2.1.8   OVERALL GENERAL ASSESSMENT

Advanced irreversible pathology, only palliation is possible. Many individualizing features are still present hence good case for management under homeopathy. May require support in management of the case.

11.2.1.9   PORTRAIT OF DISEASE

Here is a retired, 75-year-old individual who is sensitive and highly anxious, has been a heavy smoker all his life, now developed a chronic irreversible cancerous pathology which is progressing at a moderate speed. Out of fear or dread of after-effects of conventional treatment, he has decided to go for a homeopathic treatment and has come to us. Fortunately for us, in spite of advance pathology and full of common symptoms, he still shows very strong characteristic symptoms on which a constitutional and antimiasmatic remedy could be obtained which if could not cure him, at least shall give him better palliation and a quality life to his remaining life.

11.2.1.10 SYMPTOMS TAKEN INTO CONSIDERATION WHILE PRESCRIBING

1. Anxiety that disease is incurable;
2. Anxiety about his family;
3. Fear of operation;
4. Fear of injection;
5. Mind—sensitive, mental impressions to;
6. Restlessness;
7. Sleeplessness;
8. Dreams of dead people;
9. Chilly;
10. Craving—warm drinks++, ice cream+;
11. Salivation++;
12. Glandular swelling hard painless, submandibular lymph node;
13. Lump swallowing;
14. Pain ears swallowing while cough with constant hawking.

11.2.1.11 TREATMENT

After explaining him and his relatives, the nature and risk of the present illness, the informed written consent was obtained. *Phytolacca 30* dissolved in water in divided doses was prescribed in the OPD and the patient was asked to report after a week (Tables 11.3 and 11.4).

TABLE 11.3 Assessment of the Patient.

Date	Symptoms	Directions
February 2013	–	Phytolacca 30 dissolved in water in divided doses
March 2013	Difficulty in swallowing persisting ↓; swelling neck same; weight 54 kg, vitals stable, anxiety^{++}, mind sensitive^{+}	Silicea 1 M single dose
April 2013	Difficulty in swallowing persisting; pain extending to right ear, salivation^{+++}; night <<; swelling neck same, weight 54 kg vitals stable	Merc. I. F. 30 diluted in water in divided doses
May 2013	Pain swallowing better salivation ↓↓ Wt 54 kg vitals stable, swelling same	Mer. I. F. 200 diluted in water in divided doses
June 2013	Pain swallowing much better; swelling neck same, weight 54 kg, vitals stable	Carcinosin 1 M single dose
July 2013	Pain swallowing much better; swelling neck same, weight 55 kg, vitals stable	SL continued

TABLE 11.3   *(Continued)*

Date	Symptoms	Directions
August 2013	Expectoration stringy; pain swallowing solids morning <<, constant hawking, swelling neck same, Wt 55 kg, vitals stable	Kali bichromicum 200°C diluted in water in divided doses
September 2013	Swelling neck same, marginal improvement; weight 55 kg, vitals stable	SL continued
October 2013	Wt 55 kg, rest same as before	Silicea 1 M single dose
November 2013	General condition much better; neck swelling same; difficulty swallowing >, headache[+++]	Iris V 30 diluted in water in divided doses
December 2013	Same as before, no further deterioration; weight 55 kg, vitals stable, no headache	Carcinosin 1 M single dose
January 2014	Generally over all better, swelling same, wt 56 kg	SL continued

TABLE 11.4 Assessment of the Patient.

February 2014	Same as before, no further deterioration, weight 56 kg, vitals stable, swelling marginally increased, anxiety$^+$, fear^{++}	Silicea 1 M single dose
March 2014	Generally over all better, swelling same, weight 57 kg	SL continued
April 2014	Better, same as above, weight 57 kg	Carcinosin 1 M single dose
May 2014	Better	SL continued
June 2014	Better	SL continued
July 2014	General condition better, difficulty in swallowing$^+$, salvation^{++}, aggravation night, weight 55 kg, vitals stable, anxiety^{++}, fear^{++}, better warm drinks, restlessness$^+$, weakness^{++}	Ars Alb 30 diluted in water in divided doses
August 2014	Same as above intensity ↓↓ weight 53 kg, swelling increased	Ars Alb 30 diluted in water in divided doses
September 2014	Weight 50 kg, swelling increased, difficulty in swallowing^{++}, vitals stable	Carcinosin 1 M single dose
October 2014	Weight 48 kg, swelling increased, anxiety^{++}, fear^{++}, better warm drinks, restlessness$^+$, weakness^{++}	Ars Alb 30 diluted in water in divided doses
November 2014	Weight 46 kg, swelling increased, other symptoms same	Advised hospitalization for nutritional support. Ars Alb 30 diluted in water in divided doses continued
December 2014	Weight 47 kg, swelling same, other symptoms same	Ars Alb 30 diluted in water in divided doses continued

January 2015: Since patient was showing no further improvement, he was advised hospitalization mainly for nutritional support. Nasogastric feeding and or gastrostomy was advised by the surgeon but he refused any intervention. This ultimately resulted into starvation, and on February 2, 2015, he starved to death peacefully. Till his last day of life he continued to do almost everything on his own, he was conscious and oriented, in his last days, he was involved doing the translation of an English novel into Marathi language on his own, till the end of January 2015.

In brief, based on patient's presenting totality, *Phytolacca 30* in repeated doses was administered. Followed by, *Merc. Iod. Flavum 30, Kali bichromicum 30, Iris versicolor 30, and Ars. Alb.30* were given as acute prescriptions from time to time. His chronic constitutional remedy Silicea was repeated as, and when we thought, we got stuck up and disease showed progression. *Carcinosin 1M* was also given at times as an inter-current remedy to boost up the response to indicated remedy during the course of homeopathic intervention from January 2013 to February 2015.

During the course of treatment, the patient showed steady improvement, had less difficulty in swallowing both drinks and food, and had gained weight; his anxiety and fear had resolved. His vital signs were stable, the progression of disease was considerably under control for a long period of almost 2 years, as suggested clinically and corroborated with investigational findings. He was quiet comfortable and stable till the end but succumbed at the end as he did not allow any intervention even as a supportive line of treatment.

11.2.2   CASE 2: A CASE OF HEPATOCELLULAR CARCINOMA (RH-9471/14)

11.2.2.1   PRESENT HISTORY

A 75-year-old male patient, S. B., retired police constable, known case of hepatocellular carcinoma (hepatoma) was admitted in our hospital on May 1, 2014 for homeopathic treatment for his complaints of loose motions, distension of abdomen, marked prostration, loss of appetite, and pedal edema.

He was unable to lift himself, sit, or walk, without the help from his relatives. In March 2014, he was diagnosed as suffering from hepatocellular carcinoma, when his USG abdomen and pelvis showed positive evidence of large hepatic mass which was followed by CT scan showing mass originating in the quadrate lobe, likely due to hepatoma.

He was advised to undergo tapping of ascitic fluid and liver biopsy; he however refused to undergo the same and opted for homeopathy. He and his family members were aware of the nature of his illness and knew that he will not survive more than 3 months, as was communicated to him by the gastroenterologist (Table 11.5).

TABLE 11.5   Laboratory Investigations Carried Out Just Few Days Prior Patient Reported to Us.

Investigation	Report
USG abdomen and pelvis	Evidence of large hepatic mass noted. Size 106 mm × 86 mm in right lobe, advised CT scan for better evaluation
Chest X-ray	NAD
RFTs	BUN 13.4 mg/dL, blood urea 28.8 mg/dL; Sr. creatinine 0.90 mg/dL
HBSAG	Negative
LFT	Bilirubin total: 2.30 mg%; direct: 2.00 mg%; indirect: 0.30 mg%; SGPT: 81.6 IU/L; SGOT: 83.4 IU/L; alkaline phosphates: 116.0 IU/L; total protein 80 g/dL; albumin: 4.0 g/dL; globulin: 4.0 g/dL; A:G ratio: 1.0; prothrombin time: 15 s
BSL (random)	109 mg/dL
Sr. alpha fetoproteins	268.0 IU/mL
Hemogram	Hb: 8.7 g%; RBC: 3.08/cu mm; PCV: 27.1%; WBC: 4400/cu mm; platelets: 250,000/cu mm
CT scan	Mass in quadrate lobe of liver likely due to hepatoma. Measuring 13 cm × 11 cm × 12 cm

Based on his acute presenting totality, *Arsenicum Alb. 30* in water in divided doses was administered. He responded to the drug, and his diarrhea was stopped in less than 8 h. He gradually gained strength and was mobile independently within 10 days and was discharged with advice to attend the OPD. Meanwhile, detailed history was taken and a thorough physical examination was carried out.

11.2.2.2   PAST HISTORY

He gave H/O rickets in childhood; febrile convulsions; hepatitis, twice, once in 1987 and then again in 1997. Prostatectomy in 2000. He also had gastric ulcer in 2003 and with homeopathy he was cured of that.

11.2.2.3 FAMILY HISTORY

Elder brother died of Ca esophagus.

11.2.2.4 PERSONAL HISTORY

Chilly; easily gets tired and fatigue from daily routine. Perspiration presents all over after least exertion. Appetite markedly reduced; thirst reduced; sleep disturbed; dreams of God; Urine—no complaint; lately has become irritable after the onset of illness; God fearing and religious; helpful to others; disciplined and responsible; duty abiding. Mother died when the patient was 9 years old. Looked after by the family. Ill treated by the sister-in-laws and elder brothers but bore it in silence.

11.2.2.5 GENERAL EXAMINATION

Markedly prostrated; pale; grade I dehydrated; pulse: 84/min, regular; RR—24/min; BP—130/68 mmHg; weight: 52 kg; abdominal girth: 97 cm; umbilicus—stretched, presence of free fluid in the abdomen; sacral and pedal edema, pitting; liver enlarged 2 fingers, spleen 1 finger enlarged; no lymphadenopathy.

11.2.2.6 SYSTEMIC EXAMINATION

RS, CVS, and CNS: NAD
Based on his chronic totality Lycopodium 200C single dose weekly was given and Arsenicum album 30°C diluted in water in divided doses was administered. He was advised for a weekly follow-up.

He started regaining his physical strength slowly and progressively. Thereafter, we started him with *Chelidonium majus* mother tincture twice a day, as an organ specific remedy and *Carcinosin 1 M* as an intercurrent medicine. He was under strict clinical supervision with periodic lab investigations to assess the progress of disease (Table 11.6).

TABLE 11.6   Laboratory Investigations.

Date	Investigations done	Reports
July 3, 2014	LFTs	Bilirubin total—1.32 mg%; direct—1.00 mg%; indirect—0.32 mg%; alkaline phosphatase—220 IU/L; SGOT—51 IU/L; SGPT—107 IU/L; total proteins—6.0 g/dL; albumin—2.7 g/dL; globulin—3.30 g/dL
	RFTs	Urea—38 mg/dL; creatinine—1.3 mg/dL
	Hemogram	Hb—8.8 g%; WBC—7000/cu mm; platelet—465,000/cu mm
	AFP	326.78 IU/mL
	ECG	WNL
July 11, 2014	USG abdomen and pelvis	Heterogenous mass in liver as described is more likely s/o neoplastic origin. It is seen to compress upon portal triad causing resultant; proximal IHBRD; splenomegaly—14 cm; gross ascites
July 15, 2014	LFTs	Bilirubin total—1.04 mg%; direct—0.68 mg%; indirect—0.36 mg%; alkaline phosphate—191 IU/L; SGOT—64 IU/L; SGPT—97 IU/L; total proteins—5.4 g/dL; albumin—2.6 g/dL, globulin—2 g/dL
	RFTs	Urea—26 mg/dL; creatinine—1.0 mg/dL
		S. electrolytes: serum Na—118 mEq/L; serum K—4.0 mEq/L; serum Cl—86 mEq/L
	Hemogram	Hb—7.7 g%; WBC—4400/cu mm; platelet—117,000/cu mm
August 2, 2014	LFT	Bilirubin total—0.89 mg%; direct—0.66 mg%; indirect—0.23 mg%; Alk. phosphate—189 IU/L; SGOT—82 IU/L; SGPT—77 IU/L; total proteins—5.6 g/dL; albumin—2.7 g/dL; globulin—2.90 g/dL
	RFTs	Urea—19 mg/dL; creatinine—0.7 mg/dL, S. electrolytes: Na—123 mEq/L; K—4.9 mEq/L; Cl—113 mEq/L
	BT and CT	BT—2 min 10 s; CT—6 min 30 s
	Prothrombin time	18 (control-16) INR—1.12; ISI value—1.0

TABLE 11.6   *(Continued)*

	Hemogram	Hb—7.9 g%; WBC—8200/cu mm; platelet—241,000/cu mm
August 11, 2014	CT scan of abdomen and pelvis	Large, well-defined lobulated moderate heterogeneously enhancing 13 cm × 14 cm × 15 cm (AP, Trans, and craniocaudal) size, soft tissue mass lesion in segment I, III, and VIII of liver. Ill-defined low attenuation nonenhancing areas within the lesion represent of necrotic changes in the central scan. Lesion is compressing of displacing the right and left branches of portal vein with mild compression of left hepatic duct with dilated IHBR in left lobe of the liver. Moderate to gross ascitis
	Hemogram	Hb—7.4 g%; platelet—262,000/cu mm; WBC—4600/cu mm
	RFTs	Sr BUL—57 mg; Sr. creatinine—0.7 mg/dL; Na—119 mEq/L; K—5 mEq/L; Cl—90 mEq/L
	Urine	NAD

He was admitted again on September 19, 2014 for low back pain with a history of fall 2 days back. *Arnica montana 200 tds* was administered on admission. X-ray hip was taken showed # ramus of right pubic bone. Opinion of orthosurgeon was taken who advised him to use lumbar belt. He developed tachypnea and tachycardia. His SpO_2 was 99 at room temperature, he was given *Carbo vegetabilis 30* in repeated deviated doses in water and put on nasal oxygen. His general condition was poor after the fall. He was advised to shift to the ICU for better management which he declined. In 4 days, his vital were stabilized. Again he started gasping on September 28, 2014. Resuscitation was done; cardiopulmonary resuscitation was given and *Carbo vegetabilis 200* once again was administered in deviated doses. He completely recovered from this acute episode and even recovered from the fall.

His stay, thereafter, was uneventful, and he was discharged on October 20, 2014 with advised to come to OPD for follow-up of his treatment of hepatoma, which, he did. We, however, felt that though he recovered from his fall, and though his clinical and lab. data were stable, his vitality has been affected adversely.

In brief, the patient was exclusively on homeopathic treatment till last. On the basis of his presenting complaints, *Ars. Alb. 30* in repeated doses brought back the greatly prostrated, bed-ridden, anorexic patient on his feet. Further, under the stimulation of *Lycopodium 200,* his constitutional remedy, in infrequent doses, *Chelidonium, mother tincture* an organ specific remedy along with *Carcinosin 1 M,* as an intercurrent remedy, has given him the strength of the body and mind to fight back the progressive, irreversible advance pathology of the vital organ, as indicated by his clinical assessment and confirmed by the periodic laboratory findings.

Patient was under strict observation of clinical and lab. parameters with weekly follow-up thereafter.

The last reported information is that he recently sustained another fall and broke his femur neck and died at home during sleep on December 2, 2014 not of cancer but postinjury *pulmonary embolism.*

11.2.3   CASE 3

A 68-year-old female, diagnosed case of ovarian cancer with metastasis and gross ascitis was admitted in the ICU for its management. Patient and the relatives were reluctant and not willing for an invasive as well as aggressive ICU management. Thus, instead of taking her home, they opted for homeopathic treatment and shifted patient to our hospital.

Knowing the grave nature of disease and poor general physical and mental state of patient, after explaining the state of patient to her relatives, we started homeopathic treatment based on the presenting totality of the case and simultaneously started all other auxiliary measures to maintain her nutrition, fluid electrolyte balance, oxygen therapy, as required, along with strict monitoring of her vital signs.

Arsenicum album 30 C potency dissolved in water was given at frequent intervals, and within 48 h of treatment, we could find her mentally more alert and peaceful with stable vital signs. This case was managed in our IPD for about 2 weeks thereafter and patient was discharged in an ambulant state.

Subsequently, she was followed up in our OPD, regularly for about a year. During this period, she needed infrequent IPD admission for her acute ailments and was managed symptomatically. The malignant process remained more or less stagnant without further invasion for a considerable period of time, that is, about 1 year, in this case. The homeopathic treatment offered a complete satisfaction to the patient and her relatives, especially in view of lost hopes and no treatment modalities available in the conventional medicine.

11.2.4 CASE 4

Another case is of a 57-year-old lady diagnosed case of carcinoma of both breasts, who had received radiotherapy and was now advised chemotherapy. After the second cycle of chemotherapy, she started experiencing the adverse effect of chemotherapy; thus, she was admitted in our hospital to overcome the side effects of the chemotherapy. She complained of loss of appetite with nausea and vomiting, hair loss, marked weakness, aphthous ulcers, restlessness, and sleeplessness. Most of these are complaints often found as common adverse effects in a patient receiving chemotherapy. However, for a homeopathic treatment, we had to go beyond this to understand patient as a person, and therefore, a detailed homeopathic history was taken to find out her constitutional remedy as well as her acute remedy which was based on the presenting totality of the case.

Her acute totality comprises of loss of appetite, persistent nausea at the sight and smell of food, and thirstlessness with great retching and weakness. *Ipecacuanha 30 C* was given dissolved in water at frequent intervals as an acute remedy. After the acute complaints were under control, she was administered a single dose of *Lachesis* 200 as a constitutional medicine. This was based on her chronic totality (very religious, weepy cannot bear contradiction, wants to socialize, suspicious, thermally hot, wants fanning, night aggravation and left-sided complaints, etc.). Patient was discharged on the third day of admission and was followed in our OPD regularly.

In this case, her tolerance for further chemo-cycles was less troublesome and well tolerated. Her physical and mental states were stable, irritability was alleviated, her appetite was improved with gradual weight gain.

11.3 CONCLUSION

All these cases were treated and managed on classical method enunciated above. Single medicine, minimum dose, and infrequent repetition of a medicine just to stimulate body's own defense mechanisms were adopted throughout the treatment, following conventional mode for any other disease treated through homeopathy.

The homeopathic intervention in these four cases of cancer with advanced irreversible pathology has given the cost-effective, painless, individualized primary palliative treatment as against the conventional treatment modalities which include surgery, chemotherapy, and radio-therapy. Homeopathic intervention along with supportive care of these patients has successfully arrested/controlled tumor growth, prevented complications, and promoted comfort and good quality of life is possible for a considerable period of time.

The goals usually set in or attempted to achieve, in such primary cancer treatment in conventional cancer management approaches.

"Palliation aims to bring out ease in the last moments of patients life, not just to make patient die peacefully but to make patient live well until he dies."

Although significant progress has been made in cancer treatment and, approximately half of all patients with cancer eventually die of their disease, and one-third of cancer deaths happen within 6 months of diagnosis even when best possible treatment given.

It is a high time for the health-care policy makers to give a thought and build an integrated model for the treatment and management of cancer cases integrating AYUSH therapies as a part of palliative care along with anticancer therapy from the very first time that is beginning from its very diagnosis.

Signs
"+"—intensity of a symptom (mild to severe)
"+"—mild (after probing for long time and then you get the answer)
"++"—moderate (answer that has been obtained after asking leading questions)
"+++"—severe (answer obtained spontaneously on being questioned)

KEYWORDS

- homeopathy
- individualized approach
- integrating cancer management

REFERENCES

1. Hahnemann, S. Organon of Medicine, 6th ed.; B. Jain Publishers: New Delhi, 1990.
2. Kent, J. T. Repertory of the Homoeopathic Materia Medica, 7th ed. (Indian); B. Jain Publishers: New Delhi, 1974.
3. Hering, C. Guiding Symptoms of the Homoeopathic Materia Medica; B. Jain Publishers: New Delhi, 1984.
4. Vokes, E. E.; Golomb, H. M. Oncologic Therapies; Springer-Verlag: Heidelberg, 2002 (Reprint).
5. Grants Atlas of Anatomy, James E Anderson, Reprint 8th Edition 1983.

CHAPTER 12

CHLORPYRIFOS-INDUCED HEPATOTOXICITY AND HEMATOLOGIC CHANGES IN RAT: THE PREVENTIVE ROLE OF *Commiphora mukul*

KANIKA AGGARWAL* and DEVINDER SINGH

Department of Zoology and Environmental Sciences, Punjabi University, Patiala 147002, Punjab, India

Corresponding author. E-mail: kanika_biochem@rediffmail.com

ABSTRACT

Chlorpyrifos (CPF) is a broad-spectrum, chlorinated organophosphate pesticide employed for pest control in various agricultural and animal husbandries. Acute and chronic exposure to CPF can elicit several adverse effects, including oxidative stress. In the present study, we investigated hepatotoxicity and red blood cells (RBC) toxicity of CPF-treated rat and evaluated the antioxidant effect of *Commiphora mukul* (CM) against oxidative stress in the liver tissues and hematological changes of CPF-treated rat. The rats were divided in different groups; group I—control group (vehicle), group II—30 mg/kg CPF, group III—CM 100 mg/kg with 30 mg/kg CPF, group IV—CM 200 mg/kg with 30 mg/kg CPF, group V—CM 400 mg/kg with 30 mg/kg CPF, and group VI—400 mg/kg of CM were administered orally via gavages. The results showed that CM overcame the CPF induced and decreased the levels of superoxide dismutase, catalase, glutathione reductase, lactate dehydrogenase, acid phosphatase, Na^+/K^+-ATPase, and acetyl cholinesterase compared to CPF control. Moreover, CM significantly decreased the lipid peroxidation level induced by CPF as compared to CPF control. The drastic alterations in the shape of the RBC were reverted significantly with the increasing doses concentration of CM. These data suggest that oxidative stress as well as RBC toxicity is involved in CPF-induced toxicity and that CM can protect against the tissue damage as well as RBC toxicity induced by CPF.

12.1   INTRODUCTION

Pesticides are widely used during the production of grains, fruits, and vegetables albeit they can have serious adverse health effects on humans.[1,2] Chemically, it comes under the class organophosphate (OP); moreover, poisoning from OP insecticides from occupational and accidental exposure is the main cause of comorbidity and mortality in the developing countries.[3] The active metabolite of chlorpyrifos (CPF) is an acetylcholinesterase inhibitor.[4] The biotransformation of CPF is done in liver by cytochrome p450 and many other enzymes in microsomal membrane.[5] The toxicity of OP pesticide causes lipid peroxidation (LPO), which consequently can disturb the biochemical as well as physiological functions of liver, kidney, and red blood cells (RBC).[6–8]

Therapeutic uses of *Commiphora mukul* (CM) include nervous diseases, hemiplegia, leprosy, marasmus, muscle spasms, neuralgia, ophthalmia, pyelitis, pyorrhea, scrofula, skin diseases, spongy gums, ulcerative pharyngitis, hypertension, ischemia, hypertension, hemorrhoids, and urinary tract disorders. Research studies showed that CM is effective against several aspects of cardiovascular disease. It reduces the stickiness of platelets and to be an efficacious for hyper lipoproteinemia.[9] It helps to lower cholesterol, to decrease high blood pressure, strengthen the immune system, and eliminate toxins.[10]

CM can improve thyroid functions and of LPO in mice.[11] Extracts of CM were used to manufacture pharmaceutical and cosmetic compositions due to pigmenting and melanocyte agent.[12] Antisebum and antioxidant compositions were made using CM gugulipid components.[14] Cosmetic compounds for skin lightening and antiwrinkle were made from CM species.[13,15] A patent was assigned for a weight control product containing guggul extract.[16] CM is used in other products for control of body weight and cholesterol.[17–19] CM has antihyperglycemic effect in streptozotocin-induced diabetic rats and antifungal effect.[20]   CM has often been used in the roles of inactive pharmaceutical necessities, to make sustained release tablets of other drugs as a sustaining material.[21] It is suitable suspending and emulsifying agent for medicines.[22] CM has been deodorized and sometimes decolorized for inclusion in food like margarine.[23]

12.2   EXPERIMENTAL

12.2.1   CHEMICALS

CPF and CM were procured from Meghmani Organics Limited and Himalaya Drug Company, Bangalore (India), respectively. All other chemicals used in the present study were of analytical grade and were purchased from various chemical suppliers.

12.2.2   ANIMALS AND TREATMENT

Adult male rats of Wistar strain, weighing around 120–180 g were obtained from the central animal house of Panjab University, Chandigarh. All the animals were housed in clean polypropylene cages and were fed standard diet ad libitum (Ashirwad Industries). The animals were allowed to acclimatize to the local vivarium for 7 days. They had free access of water on a 12-h light/dark cycle. The experimental protocols were approved by the Institutional Animal Ethic Committee. The rats were randomly segregated into following six groups with each group having six animals each.

- Group I—Control group (vehicle treated): Animals were administered with corn oil.
- Group II (CPF treated): Animals were administered with 30 mg CPF/kg b. wt., for 28 days.
- Group III (CM + CPF treated): Animals were administered with 100 mg/kg b. wt. along with 30 mg CPF/kg b. wt.
- Group IV (CM + CPF treated): Animals were administered with 200 mg/kg b. wt. along with 30 mg CPF/kg b. wt.
- Group V (CM + CPF treated): Animals were administered with 400 mg/kg b. wt. of CM along with 30 mg CPF/kg b. wt.
- Group VI (CM treated): Animals were administered with 400 mg/kg b. wt. of CM only.

CM was administered as a solution prepared at the 400 mg/5 mL of double distilled water. The dose of CPF used in this study is with reference to the LD_{50} value of CPF and based on doses reported in the literature, which was also standardized in laboratory. CM administration dose concentrations were finalized on the basis of previously published literature assessed pharmacological activities. CPF doses were administered to the animals as reported in the earlier report from this lab.[24,25]

After 28 days of treatment, the animals were fasted overnight and sacrificed by cervical decapitation under light ether anesthesia. Their hepatic tissues were removed, rinsed with ice cold 0.9% (w/v) normal saline, and stored at $-80°C$ for further analysis.

12.2.3 PREPARATION OF HOMOGENATE

A 10% (w/v) tissue homogenate was prepared in 50-mM Tris–HCl (pH 7.4) using Potter-Elvehjem glass homogenizer. Postnuclear supernatant was prepared by centrifuging the homogenate at $1000 \times g$ for 10 min at 4°C, and then, supernatant was again centrifuged at $12,000 \times g$ for 20 min at 4°C to obtain postmitochondrial supernatant (PtMS). Various biochemical assays were performed in the supernatant.

12.2.3.1 LIPID PEROXIDATION

LPO was assayed according to the method reported by Buege and Aust.[26] The molar extinction coefficient for MDA is 1.56×105 M^{-1} cm^{-1}. The results were expressed as nmoles of MDA formed min^{-1} mg^{-1} protein.

12.2.3.2 SUPEROXIDE DISMUTASE

Superoxide dismutase (SOD) activity was assayed in the PtMS according to the method reported by Kono.[27] The results were expressed as units/mg protein, where one unit of enzyme is defined as the amount of enzyme inhibiting the rate of reaction by 50%.

12.2.3.3   CATALASE

Catalase activity was assayed in the PtMS by the method reported by Luck.[28] Results of catalase activity was expressed as µmoles of H_2O_2 decomposed/min/mg protein, using molar extinction coefficient of H_2O_2 (71 M^{-1} cm^{-1}).

12.2.3.4   GLUTATHIONE REDUCTASE

Glutathione reductase (GR) enzyme activity was measured in the PtMS by the method reported by Horn.[29] The results were expressed as nmoles of NADPH oxidized/min/mg protein, using molar extinction coefficient of NADPH (6.22 × 10^6 M^{-1} cm^{-1}).

12.2.3.5   LACTATE DEHYDROGENASE

Lactate dehydrogenase (LDH) activity was assayed spectrophoto-metrically in the PtMS by the method reported by Schatz and Segal.[30] The results were expressed as µmoles of NADH oxidized/min/mg protein. The extinction coefficient (6.3 × 10^3 µmol/L/min) was used to calculate the enzyme activity.

12.2.3.6   ACID PHOSPHATASE

Acid phosphatase activity was assayed in the PtMS by the method reported by Linhart and Walter.[31] The results were expressed as µmoles phenol produced min^{-1} mg^{-1} protein.

12.2.3.7   NA+/K+-ATPASE

Na+/K+-ATPase activity was measured according to the method reported by Quigley and Gotterer.[32] The Na^+-K^+-ATPase activity was computed by subtracting the ouabain insensitive ATPase from the total ATPase. The results were expressed as nmoles of ATP hydrolyzed/min/mg protein.

12.2.3.8   ACETYL CHOLINESTERASE

Acetyl cholinesterase (AChE) activity was determined in the homogenate according to the method reported by Ellman et al.[33] The results were expressed as nmoles of acetylthiocholine iodide hydrolyzed/min/mg protein. The extinction coefficient of 5-thio-2-nitrobenzoic acid (13.6×10^3 M^{-1} cm^{-1}) was used to calculate the enzyme activity.

12.2.3.9   ESTIMATION OF PROTEIN

The protein content was estimated according to the method reported by Lowry et al.[34] using bovine serum albumin as a standard.

12.2.4   SCANNING ELECTRON MICROSCOPY OF BLOOD CELLS

Blood cells were drawn from animals belonging to each of the treatment groups and a drop of blood was immediately fixed in 2.5% glutaraldehyde made in 0.2 M phosphate buffer (pH 7.2). After 1–2 h of fixation, the cells were separated by centrifugation at 1000–1500 rpm. The fixative was discarded and the pellet was resuspended in the phosphate buffer. This process was repeated two times, and the final pellet was suspended in minimum amount of triple distilled water. A drop of sample was smeared on the metallic scanning electron microscope stubs, which were loaded with a conductive silver tape on its top. These stubs were then coated with gold source for 4–5 min to a thickness of 100 Å using sputter ion coater. These specimens were finally observed under electron microscope (JSM-6100, Jeol, Japan) at Regional Sophisticated Instrumentation Center, Panjab University, Chandigarh, India.

12.2.5   STATISTICAL ANALYSIS

All values were expressed as mean ± standard deviation for six observations. The data were analyzed using one-way analysis of variance. Values with $p \leq 0.05$ were considered as statistically significant.

12.3   RESULTS

12.3.1   EFFECT OF CM ON CPF-INDUCED ALTERATIONS IN SOD, CATALASE, AND GR ACTIVITY

In Table 12.1, CPF exposure significantly decreased the SOD activity by 61.46%, catalase activity by 68.13%, and GR activity by 85.79% in group II in comparison to the control group. Further, CM administration decreased the effect of CPF in all the CM + CPF groups by increasing activity of SOD by 41.95%, 107.67%, 158.08%, and 140.41% in groups III, IV, V, and VI, in comparison with the CPF-treated group. Catalase is responsible for the catalytic decomposition of H_2O_2 to oxygen and water.[35] Catalase activity significantly increases in CM along with CPF dose by 68.25%, 155.71%, 196.94%, and 210.03% in groups III, IV, V, and VI when compared to the CPF-treated group. In case of GR, increase in the activity was highly significant by 72.31%, 248.45%, 392.29%, and 578.61% in groups III, IV, V, and VI when compared with the CPF-treated group.

TABLE 12.1   The Effect of In Vivo Administration of CPF, Various Doses of CM + CPF and CM Alone for a Period of 28 Days Daily on the Activities of SOD, Catalase and Glutathione Reductase in the Liver of Male Wistar Rats.

Group	Treatment	SOD activity (IU)	Catalase (µmoles H_2O_2 decomposed/ min/mg protein)	G. reductase (µM NADPH/ min/mg protein)
I	Control	8.72 ± 0.11	34.29 ± 1.38	91.90 ± 0.49
II	30 mg CPF/kg b. wt	$3.36 \pm 0.03^{*\#}$	$10.93 \pm 0.03^{*\#}$	$13.05 \pm 0.06^{*\#}$
III	100 mg CM/kg b. wt + 30 mg CPF/kg b. wt	$4.77 \pm 0.14^{*\$\#}$	$18.39 \pm 0.61^{*\$\#}$	$22.49 \pm 2.09^{*\$\#}$
IV	200 mg CM/kg b. wt +30 mg CPF/kg b. wt	$6.98 \pm 0.12^{*\$\#}$	$27.94 \pm 0.61^{*\$\#}$	$45.48 \pm 2.31^{*\$\#}$
V	400 mg CM/kg b. wt +30 mg CPF/kg b. wt	$8.67 \pm 0.14^{*\$\#}$	$32.45 \pm 1.16^{*\$\#}$	$64.25 \pm 3.58^{*\$\#}$
VI	400 mg CM/kg b. wt	$8.08 \pm 0.13^{*\$}$	$33.88 \pm 0.39^{*\$}$	$88.57 \pm 2.60^{\$}$

CM, Commiphora mukul; CPF, chlorpyrifos; SOD, superoxide dismutase.
Values are mean ± SD of six animals in each group.
$p \leq 0.05$ was considered significant.
Significantly different from control group ($p \leq 0.05$).
$Significantly different from 30 mg CPF/kg b. wt group ($$p \leq 0.05$).
#Significantly different from 400 mg CM/kg b. wt group (#$p \leq 0.05$).

12.3.2 EFFECT OF CM ON CPF-INDUCED ALTERATIONS IN LPO

LPO is the process of oxidative deterioration of polyunsaturated fatty acids due to generation of reactive oxygen species (ROS) under stress conditions.[36] In Table 12.2, CPF exposure significantly increased the LPO by 57.51%, which was significantly decreased by 36.99, 36.11, 39.12, and 60.24% in groups III, IV, V, and VI in comparison with CPF-treated group.

TABLE 12.2 The Effect of In Vivo Administration of CPF, Various Doses of CM + CPF and CM Alone for a Period of 28 Days Daily on Lipid Peroxidation in the Liver of Male Wistar Rat.

Group	Treatment	LPO (nmol MDA/mg protein)
I	Control	3.41 ± 0.27
II	30 mg CPF/kg b. wt	$5.37 \pm 0.08^{*\#}$
III	100 mg CM/kg b. wt +30 mg CPF/kg b. wt	$3.38 \pm 0.22^{\$\#}$
IV	200 mg CM/kg b. wt +30 mg CPF/kg b. wt	$3.43 \pm 0.33^{\$\#}$
V	400 mg CM/kg b. wt +30 mg CPF/kg b. wt	$3.27 \pm 0.29^{*\$\#}$
VI	400 mg CM/kg b. wt	$2.14 \pm 0.13^{*\$}$

CM, Commiphora mukul; CPF, chlorpyrifos.
Values are mean ± SD of six animals in each group.
$p \leq 0.05$ was considered significant.
Significantly different from control group ($p \leq 0.05$).
$Significantly different from 30 mg CPF/kg b. wt group ($$p \leq 0.05$).
#Significantly different from 400 mg CM/kg b. wt group (#$p \leq 0.05$).

12.3.3 EFFECT OF CM ON CPF-INDUCED ALTERATIONS IN LDH, ACP, NA+/K+ ATPASE, AND AChE ACTIVITY

In Table 12.3, CPF reduced the LDH activity by 84.42% in comparison to control group. The highly significant increase in the activity of LDH was 324.00% in group III, 389.62% in group IV, 546.53% in group V, and 495.32% in group VI, when compared to the CPF-treated group. CPF reduced the acid phosphatase (ACP) activity by 46.87%; in comparison to control group, CM decreased the effect of CPF by the increase in the activity of ACP to 42.47, 61.74, 81.78, and 76.16% in groups III, IV, V, and VI, respectively, when compared to the CPF-treated group.

CPF reduced the Na^+/K^+ ATPase activity by 60.11% in comparison to control group. CM treatment along with CPF increases Na^+/K^+ ATPase activity by 103.03, 127.59, 159.74, and 171.19% in groups III, IV, V, and VI, when compared to the CPF-treated group. CPF reduced the AChE activity by 74.14% in comparison to control group. CM resulted in partial recovery of AChE activity by 90.26, 117.54, 135.34, and 168.26% in groups III, IV, V, and VI, when compared to the CPF-treated group.

TABLE 12.3   The Effect of In Vivo Administration of CPF, Various Doses of CM + CPF and CM Alone for a Period of 28 Days Daily on LDH, Acid Phosphatase and Na^+/K^+ ATPase Activity in the Liver of Male Wistar Rats.

Group	Treatment	LDH activity (nmol pyruvate liberated/ min/mg protein)	Acid phosphatase (nmoles/min/ mg protein)	Na^+/K^+ ATPase (nmol of Pi/min/mg protein)	AChE (nmol/ min/mg protein)
I	Control	7.31 ± 1.18	11.85 ± 0.82	66.02 ± 4.10	26.93 ± 0.59
II	30 mg CPF/ kg b. wt	$1.14 \pm 0.01^{*\#}$	$6.29 \pm 0.16^{*\#}$	$26.33 \pm 1.34^{*\#}$	$6.96 \pm 1.01^{*\#}$
III	100 mg CM/ kg b. wt +30 mg CPF/kg b. wt	$4.83 \pm 0.05^{*\$\#}$	$8.97 \pm 0.14^{*\$\#}$	$53.46 \pm 0.41^{*\$\#}$	$13.25 \pm 0.47^{*\$\#}$
IV	200 mg CM/ kg b. wt +30 mg CPF/kg b. wt	$5.58 \pm 0.19^{*\$\#}$	$10.19 \pm 0.22^{*\$\#}$	$59.93 \pm 0.66^{*\$\#}$	$15.15 \pm 0.35^{*\$\#}$
V	400 mg CM/ kg b. wt +30 mg CPF/kg b. wt	$7.37 \pm 0.32^{\$}$	$11.45 \pm 0.14^{\$}$	$68.40 \pm 0.50^{*\$}$	$16.39 \pm 0.55^{*\$\#}$
VI	400 mg CM/ kg b. wt	$6.78 \pm 0.28^{\$}$	$11.09 \pm 0.07^{*\$}$	$71.42 \pm 0.24^{*\$}$	$18.68 \pm 0.29^{*\$}$

CM, Commiphora mukul; CPF, chlorpyrifos; LDH, lactate dehydrogenase.
Values are mean ± SD of six animals in each group.
$p \leq 0.05$ was considered significant.
*Significantly different from control group ($^*p \leq 0.05$).
$^\$$Significantly different from 30 mg CPF/kg b. wt group ($^\$p \leq 0.05$).
$^\#$Significantly different from 400 mg CM/kg b. wt group ($^\#p \leq 0.05$).

12.3.4   MORPHOLOGICAL ALTERATIONS IN ERYTHROCYTES

The alterations in membrane structure and function suggest that CPF exposure might result in morphological changes in erythrocytes, which are critical to its function. Alteration in lipid composition affects the membrane permeability which further leads to the alterations in the cell shape with adverse hematological consequences. Scanning electron micrographs of erythrocytes revealed that administration of CPF resulted in prominent morphological changes in rat erythrocytes. A large number of studies have suggested abnormalities in erythrocyte shape following OP exposure.[37] It is clear from the electron micrographs that the erythrocytes of the control group were perfect discocytes (D), that is, typical biconcave disks as shown in Figure 12.1B. Distortions of normal discocytes to different pathological forms were observed after CPF exposure. Most of the erythrocytes became spherocytes and some prominent changes such as appearance of irregular margins, central and peripheral protuberances, distorted shape were observed after CPF treatment for 28 days (Fig. 12.1C and D). A gradual improvement has seen in groups III and IV. A scanning electron micrograph of erythrocytes of group V (Fig. 12.1G) shows maximum improved erythrocytes topography as compared with CPF-treated group, and group VI (Fig. 12.1A) has almost similar RBC shape as of control group.

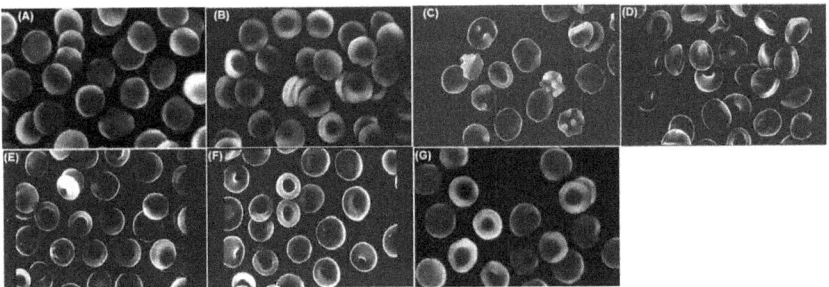

FIGURE 12.1   Scanning electron micrograph of erythrocytes (bar scale = 10 μm) in 400 mg/kg CM group (A), control group (B), 30 mg/kg CPF group (C, D), 100 mg/kg CM + 30 mg/kg CPF group (E), 200 mg/kg CM + 30 mg/kg CPF group (F), and 400 mg/kg CM + 30 mg/kg CPF group (G).

The studies of the morphological feature of cellular elements have great importance for assessing their functional state, vitality, and kinetics.

Observed alterations in the shape of normal RBCs might be due to changes in lipid composition of the membrane. Changes in lipid composition of the membrane were the key reason for such deformities in the shape of RBC's in response to various chemical treatments.[38]

Various experimental studies have shown that oxidative stress in biological systems originates as a result of imbalance between the generation of oxidizing species and cellular antioxidant defenses.[39–46] An inescapable side product of oxidative metabolism is the production of ROS which can damage lipids, nucleic acids, and proteins. In addition, oxidative stress is also a process related to xenobiotic exposure and different levels of environmental contamination.[47] Numerous cellular defense mechanisms exist to prevent the buildup of ROS and collectively help to protect living organisms against oxidative damage. These systems include super oxide dismutase and catalase (which collectively remove superoxide and hydrogen peroxide from the cytoplasm).

12.4   DISCUSSION

In the present study, the tissue considered was liver and blood cells, which have shown more prominent oxidative stress under CPF-induced conditions. The oxidative stress can be marked by LPO, SOD, catalase, and GR levels. Oxidative stress results in increased LPO which affects biochemical enzymes LDH, ACP, Na^+/K^+ ATPase, and AChE. CM might have beneficial effect by preventing oxidative stress. There is a clear need to characterize and relate the CM constituents with their biological activity. Different studies have found that ketonic steroid compounds are the major component of CM.[48,49] Similarly, in our study, the main components in the CM extract were ketonic steroid compounds, such as E- and Z-guggulsterones. Some of the compounds found in the CM extract in the present study possessed antioxidant, antiatherosclerosis, and immunostimulant properties.

12.4.1   SOD AND CATALASE

CM raised the SOD activity, which was reduced by CPF to maximum in group IV, and the studies were corroborate by Verma et al.[50] with different antidotes. Various experimental studies involving CPF administration have shown inhibition in SOD activity in rat liver.[6,840,51–53]

Catalase shows peroxidase activity and catalyzes the oxidation of various hydrogen donors in the presence of relatively lower concentration of H_2O_2.[54] The SOD-catalase system provides the first defense against oxygen toxicity. The concentration of H_2O_2 directly regulates the catalase activity.[55] SOD generates H_2O_2, which is directly removed by catalase and catalase activity is activated only at very high concentration of H_2O_2.[56] CM enhanced the CPF reduced activity of catalase to maximum in group IV. Catalase is a ubiquitous enzyme with primary antioxidant defense component which catalyzes the decomposition of H_2O_2 to H_2O.[57] The present study is confirmed by Verma et al.[50] and Yonar et al.,[58] which showed improvement by different antidotes against CPF on liver of rat and fish, respectively. There are more studies done by various researchers on different organs with similar results.[6–8,59–61]

CM enhances the SOD activity which is supported by different researchers.[11,62–64] CM reduces the toxicity by inhibiting the production of toxic oxygen free radicals.[65] Increase in SOD and catalase activity may be correlated directly to the scavenging of free radicals by CM resulting in protection of SOD, catalase, and GR from ROS such as superoxide anions and hydroxyl radicals.[66] CM treatment resulted in scavenging activity which could exert a beneficial action against alterations caused by the presence of superoxide radicals (O_2 and H_2O_2).[63,68,69] Several studies have reported the modulation of endogenous antioxidants by herbal formulations or plants extracts.[67,70–73]

12.4.2 GLUTATHIONE REDUCTASE

Again in group IV, CM improves the utmost GR activity, decreased due to CPF toxicity. Elsharkawy et al.[74] studied the decrease in GR activity by CPF on rat testicular tissue, which is regained by antidote. GR is responsible for the production of GSH from its oxidized form, GSSG. As GSH is required for the activity of glutathione peroxidase to produce water and oxygen from H_2O_2, GR is an important enzyme required for maintaining high GSH/GSSG ratio.[76] The CPF exposure results in the decrease in GR activity in hepatic tissue in rats.[51,75,77]

Chemically, the heterocyclic ring structure in phytoconstituents of CM has been reported to quench singlet molecular oxygen and exert antioxidant action and protect membrane lipids.[78] The unpaired electron present in the hydroxyl free radical, which is mainly responsible for the CPF-induced damage to the hepatic tissue, might have been trapped and subsequently dismuted by constituents of CM. The protective effect of CM may be associated with the conservation of energy phosphates and substrates, which contributes to an increase in the supply of substrate needed for the synthesis of GSH that protects the cell from reactive metabolites and ROS.[66] The antioxidant property may be related to the antioxidant vitamins, phenolic acids, and micronutrients present in the CM extract.

12.4.3 LIPID PEROXIDATION

Present result of increase in LPO in group IV by CPF is corroborated by Verma et al.[50] who found increase in LPO by CPF. There are several studies done by various researchers on different organs with similar results.[6–8,59–61,79,80] The increased LPO by CPF might be due to free radical mediated membrane damage, and the decreased MDA level in liver following CM treatment might be due to augmentation of endogenous antioxidants. The results support the anti-LPO property of CM in agreement with previous reports.[11,66,82–84] Previous studies have indicated that lipotropes inhibit LPO in cellular membranes as a result of distinct biophysical interactions with membrane lipid bilayer.[81] From this, it can be suggested that CM extract is highly lipotropic and when administered can voluntarily exceed the membrane lipid bilayer just like other lipotropic phytoconstituents. The ability of CM to diffuse into intracellular compartments helps the capabilities of this natural product as an antioxidant.

12.4.4 LACTATE DEHYDROGENASE

In the present study, CPF decreases LDH activity which is supported by Heikal et al.[85] and by OP pesticide in mice liver by El-Shenawy et al.[6] Similar results were found with fishes exposed to OPs.[86–89] Yamano and

Morita[90] observed leakage of LDH in the hepatocytes in incubation medium on pesticide exposure. It suggests the vital role of aerobic metabolism in CPF-induced toxicity, which results in the increased ATP production to meet energy requirement of the cells as energy store got depleted.

The leakage of LDH from hepatic tissue is the diagnostic marker of hepatic toxicity. When hepatic cells are damaged or destroyed due to deficient oxygen supply, production of free radicals and LPO leads to loss of the integrity of cell membranes and renders the membrane more porous and permeable that the membrane may even rupture, resulting in the leakage of this enzyme. In the present study, CM ameliorated LDH activity. The results support the LDH enhancing property of CM in conformity with previous reports by various researchers.[66,71] Treatment with CM prevented depletion of LDH enzyme from hepatic tissue as compared to CPF group, therefore reducing the release of LDH from hepatic tissue into the systemic circulation, which is suggestive of cytoprotective action of CM.

12.4.5 ACID PHOSPHATASE

CM increases ACP, activity decreased due to CPF exposure. Afaf and Hanan[91] found a similar decrease in ACP activity in male albino rats on CPF exposure. Other studies also show similar results, when exposed to OPs.[92,93] Decreased activity may be due to attack of ROS on active sites of enzyme. Bagchi and Stohs[94] supported generation of ROS with lindane, which enhanced LPO and decreased membrane fluidity.

The leakage of ACP from hepatic tissue is due to hepatic toxicity. When hepatic cells are damaged or destroyed due to deficient oxygen supply, production of free radicals and LPO leads to loss of the integrity of cell membranes[66] and renders the membrane more permeable, which results in the leakage of ACP. This accounts for the decreased activities of ACP in hepatic tissue of CPF-challenged rats. In the present study, CM ameliorated the activity of ACP. Treatment with CM prevented depletion of ACP from hepatic tissue as compared to CPF group, therefore reducing the release of ACP from hepatic tissue into the systemic circulation, suggestive of cytoprotective action of CM.

12.4.6   NA⁺/K⁺ ATPase

In the present research, the decreased activity of ATPase by CPF is increased by CM which is supported by Amara et al.[95] in male albino rats on OP exposure. Similar research has been done by several workers showing that the administration of various OPs inhibits Na^+/K^+ ATPase in various other tissues.[96–99]

Experimental results show that Na^+/K^+ ATPase is inactivated by LPO.[100,101] Mishra et al.[102] have shown that LPO decreases the affinity of Na^+/K^+ ATPase for Na^+ and K^+ ions as the active site of enzyme is directly attacked by ROS. Siesms et al.[103] also suggested that oxidative products inhibit Na^+/K^+ ATPase activity. These researchers explained that the active sites of enzyme are directly attacked by ROS. The decline in the activities of antioxidant defense enzymes and enhanced LPO level imply that CPF would have induced the generation of oxygen-free radicals, which peroxidizes the lipid component of hepatic membrane. Bagchi and Stohs[94] supported this with lindane-induced generation of ROS, which enhanced LPO and decreased membrane fluidity. The recovery of Na^+/K^+ ATPase by CM supplementation was probably due to the protective effect of CM against CPF-induced oxidative stress.

12.4.7   ACETYLCHOLINE ESTERASE

AChE is acetylcholine hydrolyzing enzyme which is responsible for cholinergic response termination.[104] In the present research, the decreased activity of AChE by CPF is increased by CM which is supported by Diab et al.[105] and Verma et al.[50] in rat plasma and liver, respectively, and which is regained by different antidotes. Similar inhibition has been reported by various researchers on different organs.[7,8,106]

It was suggested that CPF is metabolically activated by oxidative desulfuration to CPF oxon.[107,108] Due to lipophilic nature of CPF, it inhibits serum and liver AChE and causes delayed toxicity with gradual discharge from the adipose tissues.[106,109,110] The decrease in AChE activity in the present study might be due to phosphorylation of serine at the active site of enzyme. Supplementation of CM improved the CPF-inhibited AChE activity to a limited extent. These results suggest that decrease in AChE activity might be partially due to peroxidation of membrane lipids by CPF and partial protection by CM can be attributed to their antioxidant action.

The mechanism of AChE of CM emerges to be complex and requires further investigation.

In conclusion, these observations showed that CM may prevent toxic effects of CPF on liver and erythrocytes through free radical scavenging activity, upregulation of antioxidant enzymes, membrane stabilizing action, which led to alterations in membrane composition and function, ultimately resulting in altered morphology. Treatment with CM resulted in amelioration in CPF-induced changes, suggesting that CM supplementation would be beneficial. From the discussion held above, it can be concluded that CM works as antidote against CPF. CM is recommended as concomitant supplementation for the protection against severe hepatic damage induced by the CPF as well as other OP pesticides involving oxidative stress-mediated hepatic toxicity.

12.5 SCOPE FOR FURTHER RESEARCH

CM is beneficial but further studies are warranted using different site specific animal models of pesticides in order to judge the effects of these antidotes. Identification of the active ingredients present in the extracts responsible for the observed efficacy of antidotes is also needed. These experiments should be conducted in vitro to know the mechanism of CM protection against CPF toxicity.

KEYWORDS

- *Commiphora mukul*
- chlorpyrifos
- hepatotoxicity
- antioxidant
- electron microscopy

REFERENCES

1. Kaushik, G.; Satya, S.; Naik, S. N. Food Processing a Tool to Pesticide Residue Dissipation a Review. *Food Res. Int.* **2009,** *42,* 26–40.

2. Keikotlhaile, B. M.; Spanoghe, P.; Steurbaut, W. Effects of Food Processing on Pesticide Residues in Fruits and Vegetables: A Meta-Analysis Approach. *Food Chem. Toxicol.* **2010**, *48,* 1–6.

3. Eddleston, M.; Karalliedde, L.; Buckley, N.; Fernando, R.; Hutchinson, G.; Isbister, G. Pesticide Poisoning in the Developing World—A Minimum Pesticides List. *Lancet* **2002**, *360,* 1163–1167.

4. Eyer, F.; Roberts, D. M.; Buckley, N. A.; Eddleston, M.; Thiermann, H.; Worek, F.; Eyer, P. Extreme Variability in the Formation of Chlorpyrifos Oxon (CPO) in Patients Poisoned by Chlorpyrifos (CPF). *Biochem. Pharmacol.* **2009**, *78* (5), 531–537.

5. Foxenberg, R. J.; Mcgarrigle, B. P.; Knaak, J. B.; Ostyniak, P. J.; Olson, J. R. Human Hepatic Cytochrome P450-Specific Metabolism of Parathion and Chlorpyrifos. *Drug Metabol. Dispos.* **2007,** *35*(2), 189–193.

6. El-Shenawy, N. S.; El-Salmy, F.; Al-Eisa, R. A.; El-Ahmary, B. Amelioratory Effect of Vitamin E on Organophosphorus Insecticide Diazinon-Induced Oxidative Stress in Mice Liver. *Pestic. Biochem. Physiol.* **2010**, *96*, 101–107.

7. Mansour, S. A.; Mossa, A. H. Lipid Peroxidation and Oxidative Stress in Rat Erythrocytes Induced by Chlorpyrifos and the Protective Effect of Zinc. *Pestic. Biochem. Physiol.* **2009**, *93*, 34–39.

8. Mansour, S. A.; Mossa, A. H. Oxidative Damage, Biochemical and Histological Alterations in Rats Exposed to Chlorpyrifos and the Antioxidant Role of Zinc. *Pestic. Biochem. Physiol.* **2010**, *96*, 14–23.

9. Ghatak, A.; Asthana, O. P. Recent Trends in Hyper Lipoproteinemias and its Pharmacotherapy. *Indian J. Pharmacol.* **1995**, *27*(1), 14–29.

10. XetaPharm Inc. Gugulon (www.xetapharm.com). 2000.

11. Panda, S.; Kar, A. Gugulu (*Commiphora mukul*) Induces Triiodothyronine Production: Possible Involvement of Lipid Peroxidation. *Life Sci.* **1999**, *65*(12), 137–141.

12. Andre, P.; Lhermite, S.; Pellicier, F. Products Extracted from a Plant of the Genus *Commiphora*, Particularly the *Commiphora mukul* Plant, Extracts Containing Same and Applications Thereof, for example in Cosmetics. U. S. Patent No. 5972341, 1999.

13. Andre, P.; Lhermite, S.; Perllicier, F. Antiwrinkle Cosmetic Compositions Containing Commiphora Extracts. World Patent No. 9710196, 1997.

14. McCook, J. P.; Corey, J. M.; Dorogi, P. L.; Bajor, J. S.; Knaggs, H. E.; Lange, B. A.; Sharpe, E. Antisebum and Antioxidant Compositions Containing Gugulipid and Alcoholic Fraction Thereof. Patent No. 5690948, 1997.

15. Zhang, K. H.; Satpute, P.; Iwata, K.; Tallman, M. T. Cosmetic Compositions for Lightening the Skin Based on Gugulipid and α-Hydroxy Acid, Niacinamide or Phenylalanine. World Patent No. 2001041730, Hindustan Lever Limited of the United Kingdom, 2001.

16. Brink, W. D. Weight Control Product and Method of Treating Hyperlipidemia and Increasing Vigor with Said Product. U. S. Patent No. 6113949, 2000.

17. Ito, N. Health Food Preparation from Commiphora. Japanese Patent No. 08033464, Japan Kokai Tokkyo Koho, 1996.

18. Weisspapir, M.; Schwarz, J. Solid Self-Emulsifying Controlled Release Delivery System for Water-Insoluble Phytosterols in Control of Body Weight and Cholesterol. U.S. Patl Appl Publ, US Patent No. 2002103139, 2002.

19. Gorsek, W. F. Cholesterol Treatment Formulation. U. S. Patent No. 6565896, 2003.
20. Chander, R.; Khanna; A. K.; Pratap, R. Antioxidant Activity of Guggulsterone, the Active Principal of Gugulipid From *Commiphora mukul. J. Med. Arom. Plant Sci.* **2002,** *24,* 370–374.
21. Baveja, S. K.; Rao, K. V.; Arora, J. Examination of Natural Gums and Mucilages as Sustaining Materials in Tablet Dosage Forms. *Ind. J. Pharm. Sci.* **1989,** *51*(4), 115–118.
22. Kakrani, H. K.; Varma, K. C. Suspending and Emulsifying Properties of Guggul Gum. *Indian J. Hosp. Pharm.* **1981,** *18,* 134–138.
23. 23. Beindorf, C.; Husken, H.; Zijp, I. M. (Patent Assignee: Unilever N.V., Netherlands) Deodorization of Guggulipids for Inclusion in Food. European Patent No. 1238590, Eur. Pat. Appl. September 11, 2002. Abstract from CAPLUS 2002:693104.
24. Aggarwal, K.; Singh, D. Toxicological Effects of Chlorpyrifos on Lipid Peroxidation and Inhibition of Some Liver Enzymes in Rat. *Punjab Acad. Sci.* **2011,** *7–8* (1&2), 32–38.
25. Aggarwal, K.; Singh, D.; Singla, S. K. Studies on the Effect of Oxidative Stress Induced by Chlorpyrifos on Antioxidant Hepatic Enzymes in Rat. *World J. Pharm. Pharm. Sci.* **2014,** *3*(11), 523–533.
26. Buege, J. A.; Aust, S. D. Microsomal Lipid Peroxidation. *Methods Enzymol.* **1978,** *52,* 302–310.
27. Kono Y. Generation of Superoxide Radical During Autooxidation of Hydroxylamine and an Assay for Superoxide Dismutase. *Arch. Biochem. Biophys.* **1978,** *186,* 189–195.
28. Luck, H. Catalase. In *Methods of Enzymatic Analysis*; Bergmeyer, H. U., Ed.; Academic Press: New York, 1971; pp 885–894.
29. Horn, H. D. Glutathione Reductase. In *Methods of Enzymatic Analysis*; Bergmeyer, H. V., Ed.; Academic Press: New York, London, 1971; pp 857–881.
30. Schatz, L.; Segal, H. L. Reduction of Alpha—Ketoglutarate by Homogenous Lactic Acid Dehydrogenase—X of Testicular Tissue. *J. Biol. Chem.* **1969,** *244,* 4393–4397.
31. Linhart, K.; Walter, K. Phosphatase (Phosphomono—Esterases). In *Methods of Enzymatic Analysis*; Bergmeyer, H. V., Ed.; Academic Press, New York and London, 1965; pp 944.
32. Quigley, J. P.; Gotterer, G. S. Distribution of (Na$^+$–K$^+$) Stimulated ATPase Activity in Rat Intestinal Mucosa. *Biochem. Biophys. Acta* **1969,** *173,* 456–468.
33. Ellman, G. L.; Courtney, D.; Andres, V.; Featherston, R. M. A New and Rapid Colorimetric Determination of Acetylcholinesterase Activity. *Biochem. Pharmacol.* **1961,** *7,* 88–95.
34. Lowry, O. H.; Rosenbrough, N. J.; Farr, A. I.; Randall, R. J. Protein Measurement with Folin Phenol Reagent. *J. Biol. Chem.* **1951,** *239* (1951), 2370–2385.
35. Chance, B.; Sies, H.; Boveris, A. Hydroperoxide Metabolism in Mammalian Organs. *Physiol. Rev.* **1979,** *59,* 527–605.
36. Niki, F.; Yamamoto, Y.; Takahashi, M.; Yamamoto, K.; Komuro, E.; Miki, M.; Yasuda, H.; Mino, M. Free Radical-Mediated Damage of Blood and Its Inhibition by Antioxidants. *J. Nutr. Sci. Vitaminol.* **1988,** *34,* 507–512.
37. Singh, N. N.; Srivastava, A. K. Haematological Parameters as Bioindicators of Insecticide Exposure in Teleosts. *Ecotoxicology* **2010,** *19,* 838–854.

38. Kumar, V. V. Lipid Molecular Shapes and Membrane Architecture. *Indian J. Biochem. Biophys.* **1993**, *30*, 135–138.
39. Banerjee, B. D.; Seth, V.; Bhattacharya, A.; Pasha, S. T.; Chakrobarty, A. K. Biochemical Effects of Some Pesticides on Lipid Peroxidation and Free-Radical Scavengers. *Toxicol. Lett.* **1999**, *107*, 33–47.
40. Gultekin, F.; Delibas, N.; Yasar, S.; Kilinc, I. In Vivo Changes in Antioxidant Systems and Protective Role of Melatonin and a Combination of Vitamin C and Vitamin E on Oxidative Damage in Erythrocytes Induced by Chlorpyrifos-Ethyl in Rats. *Arch. Toxicol.* **2001**, *75*, 88–96.
41. Oncu, M.; Gultekin, F.; Karaoz, E.; Altuntas, I.; Delibas, N. Nephrotoxicity in Rats Induced by Chlorpyrifos-Ethyl and Ameliorating Effects of Antioxidants. *Hum. Exp. Toxicol.* **2002**, *21*(4), 223–230.
42. Akhgari, M.; Abdollahi, M.; Kebryaeezadeh, A.; Hosseini, R.; Sabzevari, O. Biochemical Evidence for Free Radical-Induced Lipid Peroxidation as a Mechanism for Subchronic Toxicity of Malathion in Blood and Liver of Rats. *Hum. Exp. Toxicol.* **2003**, *22*, 205–211.
43. Abdollahi, M.; Ranjbar, A.; Shadnia, S.; Nikfar, S.; Rezale, A. Pesticide and Oxidative Stress: A Review. *Med. Sci. Monit.* **2004**, *10*(6), 141–147.
44. Sharma, Y.; Bashir, S.; Irshad, M.; Gupta, S. D.; Dogra, T. D. Effects of Acute Dimethoate Administration on Antioxidant Status of Liver and Brain of Experimental Rats. *Toxicology* **2005**, *206*, 49–57.
45. Zama, D.; Meraihi, Z.; Tebibel, S.; Benayssa, W.; Benayache, F.; Benayache, S.; Vlietinck, A. J. Chlorpyrifos-Induced Oxidative Stress and Tissue Damage in the Liver, Kidney, Brain and Fetus in Pregnant Rats. The Protective Role of the Butanolic Extract of *Paronychia argentea* L. *Indian J. Pharmacol.* **2007**, *39*, 145–150.
46. Tuzmen, N.; Canadan, N.; Kaya, E.; Demiryas, N. Biochemical Effects of Chlorpyrifos and Deltamethrin on Altered Antioxidants Defence Mechanisms and Lipid Peroxidation in Rat Liver. *Cell Biochem. Funct.* **2008**, *26*, 119–124.
47. Halliwell, B.; Gutteridge, J. M. C. The Antioxidants of Human Extracellular Fluids. *Arch. Biochem. Biol. Phys.* **1990**, *280*, 1–8.
48. Deng, R. Therapeutic Effects of Guggul and Its Constituent Guggulsterone: Cardiovascular Benefits. *Cardiovasc. Drug Rev.* **2007**, *25*(4), 375–390.
49. Jain, A.; Gupta, V. B. Chemistry and Pharmacological Profile of Guggul: A Review. *Indian J. Trad. Knowl.* **2006**, *5*(4), 478–483.
50. Verma, R. S.; Mehta, A.; Srivastava, N. In Vivo Chlorpyrifos Induced Oxidative Stress: Attenuated by Antioxidant Vitamins. *Pest. Biochem. Physiol.* **2007**, *88*, 191–196.
51. Verma, R. S.; Srivastava, N. Effect of Chlorpyrifos on Thiobarbituric Acid Reactive Substances, Scavenging Enzymes and Glutathione in Rat Tissues. *Indian J. Biochem. Biophys.* **2003**, *40*, 423–428.
52. Ahmed, M. M.; Zaki, N. I. Assessment the Ameliorative Effect of Pomegranate and Rutin on Chlorpyrifos-Ethyl-Induced Oxidative Stress in Rats. *Nat. Sci.* **2009**, *10*(12), 67–77.
53. Khalifa, F. K.; Fatma, A.; Khalil, H. A.; Barakat, M.; Hassan, M. Protective Role of Wheat Germ and Grape Seed Oils in Chlorpyrifos-Induced Oxidative Stress,

Biochemical and Histological Alterations in Liver of Rats. *Aust. J. Basic Appl. Sci.* **2011**, *5*(10), 54–66.

54. Oshimo, N.; Oshimo, R.; Chance, B. The Characteristics of the "Peroxidatic" Reaction of Catalase in Ethanol Oxidation. *Biochem. J.* **1973**, *131*, 555–567.

55. Fornazier, R. F.; Ferreira, R. R.; Vitoria, A. P.; Molina, S. M. G.; Lea, P. J.; Azevedo, R. A. Effects of Cadmium on Anti-Oxidant Enzyme Activities in Sugar Cane. *Biol. Plant.* **2002**, *45*, 91–97.

56. Yu, B. P. Cellular Defenses against Damage from Reactive Oxygen Species. *Physiol. Rev.* **1994**, *1*, 139–162.

57. Cheng, L.; Kellogg, III E. W.; Packer, L. Photoactivation of Catalase. *Photochem. Photobiol.* **1981**, *34*, 125–129.

58. Yonar, M.; Mis, E. S.; Yonar, M.; Ural, S. E.; Silici, S.; Düsükcan, M. Protective Role of Propolis in Chlorpyrifos-Induced Changes in the Haematological Parameters and the Oxidative/Antioxidative Status of *Cyprinus carpio carpio*. *Food Chem. Toxicol.* **2012**, *50*, 2703–2708.

59. Demir, F.; Uzun, F. G.; Durak, D.; Kalender, Y. Subacute Chlorpyrifos-Induced Oxidative Stress in Rat Erythrocytes and the Protective Effects of Catechin and Quercetin. *Pestic. Biochem. Physiol.* **2011**, *99*(1), 77–81.

60. Shittu, M.; Ayo, J. O.; Ambali, S. F.; Fatihu, M. Y.; Onyeanusi, B. I.; Kawu, M. U. Chronic Chlorpyrifos-Induced Oxidative Changes in the Testes and Pituitary Gland of Wistar Rats: Ameliorative Effects of Vitamin C. *Pestic. Biochem. Physiol.* **2012**, *102*, 79–85.

61. Attia, A. A.; ElMazoudy, R. H.; El-Shenawy, N. S. Antioxidant role of Propolis Extract against Oxidative Damage of Testicular Tissue Induced by Insecticide Chlorpyrifos in Rats. *Pestic. Biochem. Physiol.* **2012**, *103*, 87–93.

62. Bellamkonda, R.; Rasineni, K.; Singareddy, S. R.; Kasetti, R.; Pasurla, R.; Chippada, A. Antihyperglycemic and Antioxidant Activities of Alcoholic Extract of *Commiphora mukul* Gum Resin in Streptozotocin-Induced Diabetic Rats. *Pathophysiology* **2011**, *18*, 255–261.

63. Ramesh, B.; Saralakumari, D. Antihyperglycemic, Hypolipidemic and Antioxidant Activities of Ethanolic Extract of *Commiphora mukul* Gum Resin in Fructose-Fed Male Wistar Rats. *J. Physiol. Biochem.* **2012**, *68*(4), 573–582.

64. Sudhakara, G.; Ramesh, B.; Mallaiah, P.; Sreenivasulu, N.; Saralakumari, D. Protective Effect of Ethanolic Extract of *Commiphora mukul* Gum Resin against Oxidative Stress in the Brain of Streptozotocin induced Diabetic Wistar Male Rats. *EXCLI J.* **2012**, *11*, 576–592.

65. Kaul, S.; Kapoor, N. K. Reversal of Changes of Lipid Peroxide, Xanthine Oxidase and Superoxide Dismutase by Cardio-Protective Drugs in Isoproterenol Induced Myocardial Necrosis in Rats. *Indian J. Exp. Biol.* **1989**, *27*, 625–626.

66. Ojha, S.; Bhatia, J.; Arora, S.; Golechha, M.; Kumari, S.; Arya, D. S. Cardioprotective Effects of *Commiphora mukul* against Isoprenaline-Induced Cardiotoxicity: A Biochemical and Histopathological Evaluation. *J. Environ. Biol.* **2011**, *32*, 731–738.

67. Ojha, S. K.; Nandave, M.; Arora, S.; Narang, R.; Dinda, A. K.; Arya, D. S. Chronic Administration of *Tribulus terrestris* Linn Extract Improves Cardiac Function and Attenuates Myocardial Infarction in Rats. *Int. J. Pharmacol.* **2008**, *4*, 1–10.

68. Xu, B.; Moritz, J. T.; Epstein, P. N. Overexpression of Catalase Provides Partial Protection to Transgenic Mouse β-Cells. *Free Radic. Biol. Med.* **1999**, *27*, 830–837.
69. Benhamou, P. Y.; Moriscot, C.; Richard, M. J.; Beatrix, O.; Badet, L.; Pattou, F.; Kerr-Conte, J.; Chroboczek, J.; Lemarchand, P.; Halimi, S. Adenovirus-Mediated Catalase Gene Transfer Reduces Oxidant Stress in Human, Porcine and Rat Pancreatic Islets. *Diabetologia* **1998**, *41*, 1093–1100.
70. Mary, N. K.; Babu, B. H.; Padikkala, J. Antiatherogenic Effect of Caps HT2, A Herbal Ayurvedic Medicine Formulation. *Phytomedicine* **2003**, *10*(6,7), 474–482.
71. Mohanty, I.; Arya, D. S.; Dinda, A.; Talwar, K. K.; Joshi, S.; Gupta, S. K. Mechanisms of Cardioprotective Effect of *Withania somnifera* in Experimentally Induced Myocardial Infarction. *Basic Clin. Pharmacol. Toxicol.* **2004**, *94*, 184–189.
72. Tripathi, Y. B.; Reddy, M. M.; Pandey, R. S.; Subhashini, J.; Tiwari, O. P.; Singh, B. K.; Reddanna, P. Anti-Inflammatory Properties of BHUx, A Polyherbal Formulation to Prevent Atherosclerosis. *Inflammo. Pharmacol.* **2004**, *12*, 131–152.
73. Goyal, S. N.; Arora, S.; Sharma, A. K.; Joshi, S.; Ray, R.; Bhatia, J.; Kumari, S.; Arya, D. S. Preventive Effect of Crocin of *Crocus sativus* on Hemodynamic, Biochemical, Histopathological and Ultrastructural Alterations in Isoproterenol-Induced Cardiotoxicity in Rats. *Phytomedicine* **2010**, *17*, 227–232.
74. Elsharkawy, E. E.; Yahia, D.; El-Nisr, N. A. Chlorpyrifos Induced Testicular Damage in Rats: Ameliorative Effect of Glutathione Antioxidant. *J. Am. Sci.* **2012**, *8*(7), 708–716.
75. Khan, M.; Sobti, R. C.; Kataria, L. Pesticide-Induced Alteration in Mice Hepato-Oxidative Status and Protective Effects of Black Tea Extract. *Clin. Chim. Acta* **2005**, *358*(1–2), 131–138.
76. Carlberg, I.; Mannervik, B. *Glutathione Reductase Methods in Enzymology*; Academic Press: New York, **1985**, Vol. 113, pp 484–490.
77. Wu, H.; Zhang, R.; Liu, J.; Guo, Y.; Ma, E. Effects of Malathion and Chlorpyrifos on Acetylcholinesterase and Antioxidant Defense System in *Oxya chinensis* (Thunberg) (Orthoptera: Acrididae). *Chemosphere* **2011**, *83*(4), 599–604.
78. Zhou, Z.; Yunping, H.; Yunguang, S.; Jia, C. Protective Effect of Clonidine against Toxicity of Organophosphorus Pesticides. *J. Occup. Health* **2001**, *43*, 346–350.
79. Ahmed, N. S.; Mohamed, A. S.; Abdel-Wahhab, M. A. Chlorpyrifos-Induced Oxidative Stress and Histological Changes in Retinas and Kidney in Rats: Protective Role of Ascorbic Acid and Alpha Tocopherol. *Pestic. Biochem. Physiol.* **2010**, *98*, 33–38.
80. Aly, N.; El-Gendy, K.; Mahmoud, F.; El-Sebae, A. K. Protective Effect of Vitamin C against Chlorpyrifos Oxidative Stress in Male Mice. *Pest. Biochem. Physiol.* **2010**, *97*, 7–12.
81. Balkan, J.; Oztezcan, S.; Kucuk, M.; Cevikbas, U.; Kocak-Toker, N.; Uysal, M. The Effect of Betaine Treatment on Triglyceride Levels and Oxidative Stress in the Liver of Ethanol-Treated Guinea Pigs. *Exp. Toxicol. Pathol.* **2004**, *55*, 505–509.
82. Gowrishankar, N. L.; Manavalan, R.; Venkappayya, D.; David, R. C. Hepatoprotective and Antioxidant Effects of *Commiphora berryi* (Arn) Engl Bark Extract against CCl(4)-Induced Oxidative Damage in Rats. *Food Chem. Toxicol.* **2008**, *46*, 3182–3185.

83. Ulbricht, C.; Basch, E.; Szapary, P.; Hammerness, P.; Axentsev, S.; Boon, H.; Kroll, D.; Garraway, L.; Vora, M.; Woods, J. Guggul for Hyperlipidemia: Complement. *Ther. Med.* **2005**, *13*, 279–290.

84. Singh, V.; Kaul, S.; Chander, R.; Kapoor, N. K. Stimulation of Low Density Lipoprotein Receptor Activity in Liver Membrane of Guggulsterone Treated Rats. *Pharmacol. Res.* **1990**, *22*, 37–44.

85. Heikal, T.; Abdel-Tawab, M.; Mossa, H.; Abdel-Rasoul, M. A.; Mare, G. K. The Ameliorating Effects of Green Tea Extract against Cyromazine and Chlorpyrifos Induced Liver Toxicity in Male Rats. *Asian J. Pharm. Clin. Res.* **2013**, *6*(1), 974.

86. Samuel, M.; Sastry, K. V. In Vivo Effect of Monocrotophos on the Carbohydrate Metabolism of the Freshwater Snake Head Fish, *Channa punctatus*. *Pestic. Biochem. Physiol.* **1989**, *34*(1), 1–8.

87. Sastry, K. V.; Siddiqui, A. A. Some Hematological, Biochemical, and Enzymological Parameters of a Fresh-Water Teleost Fish, *Channa punctatus*, Exposed to Sublethal Concentrations of Quinalphos. *Pestic. Biochem. Physiol.* **1984**, *22*(1), 8–13.

88. Ghosh, T. K. Toxic Impact of Three Organophosphate Pesticides on Carbohydrate Metabolism in a Freshwater Fish *Channa punctatus*. *Adv. Biol. Sci.* **1987**, *6*, 20.

89. Goel, A.; Danni, V.; Dhawan, D. K. Protective Effects of Zinc on Lipid Peroxidation, Antioxidant Enzymes and Hepatic Histoarchitecture in Chlorpyrifos-Induced Toxicity. *Chem. Biol. Interact* **2005**, *156*, 131–140.

90. Yamano, T.; Morita, S. Hepatotoxicity of Trichlorfon and Dichlorvos in Isolated Rat Hepatocytes. *Toxicology* **1992**, *76*, 69–77.

91. Afaf, A. E.; Hanan, A. T. E. Chlorpyrifos (from Different Sources): Effect on Testicular Biochemistry of Male Albino Rats. *J. Am. Sci.* **2010**, *6*(7), 252–261.

92. Verma, S. R.; Rani, S.; Dalela, R. C. Pesticide-Induced Physiological Alterations in Certain Tissues of a Fish, *Mystus vittatus*. *Toxicol. Lett.* **1981**, *9*, 327–332.

93. Thenmozhi, C.; Vignesh, V.; Thirumurugan, R.; Arun, S. Impacts of Malathion on Mortality and Biochemical Changes of Fresh Water Fish *Labeo rohita*. *Iran J. Environ. Health Sci. Eng.* **2011**, *8(4)*, 387.

94. Bagchi, M.; Stohs, S. J. In Vitro Induction of Reactive Oxygen Species by 2,3,7,8,-Tetrachlorodibenzo-*p*-Dioxin, Endrin, and Lindane in Rat Peritoneal Macrophages, and Hepatic Mitochondria and Microsomes. *Free Radic. Biol. Med.* **1993**, *14*, 11–18.

95. Amara, I. B.; Soudani, N.; Hakim, A.; Troudi, A.; Zeghal, K. M.; Boudawara, T.; Zeghal, N. Selenium and Vitamin E, Natural Antioxidants, Protect Rat Cerebral Cortex against Dimethoate-Induced Neurotoxicity. *Pestic. Biochem. Physiol.* **2011**, *101*, 165–174.

96. Basha, P. M.; Nayeemunnisa. Effect of Methyl Parathion on Na^+/K^+ and Mg^{2+} Adenosine Triphosphate Activity in Developing Central Nervous System in Rats. *Indian J. Exp. Biol.* **1993**, 31, 785–787.

97. Hazarika, A.; Sarkar, S.N. Effect of Isoproturon Pretreatment on the Biochemical Toxicodynamics of Anilofos in Male Rats. *Toxicology* **2001**, *165(2-3)*, 87–95.

98. Singh, M.; Sandhir, R.; Kiran, R. In Vivo Effects of Organophosphate Pesticides on Rat Erythrocytes. *Indian J. Exp. Biol.* **2004**, *42*, 292–296.

99. Agrahari, S.; Gopal, K. Inhibition of Na^+-K^+-ATPase in Different Tissues of Freshwater Fish *Channa punctatus* (Bloch) Exposed to Monocrotophos. *Pesticide Biochem. Physiol.* **2008,** *92,* 57–60.

100. Sun, A. Y. The Effect of Lipid Peroxidation on Synaptosomal (Na^+, K^+)-ATPase Isolated from the Cerebral Cortex of Squirrel Monkey. *Biochem. Biophys. Acta* **1972,** *266,* 350–360.

101. Hexum, T. D.; Fried, R. Effect of Superoxide Radicals on (Na^+, K^+) Transport Adenosine Triphosphatase and Protection by Superoxide Dismutase. *Neurochem. Res.* **1979,** *4,* 73–92.

102. Mishra, O. P.; Delivoria-Papadpoulos, M.; Cahillane, G.; Wagerle, L. C. Lipid Peroxidation as the Mechanism of Modification of the Affinity of the Na^+, K^+-ATPase Active Sites for ATP, Na^+, K^+ and Strophanthidin In Vitro. *Neurochem. Res.* **1989,** *14,* 845–851.

103. Siesms, W. G.; Sommerburg, C.; John, S.; Van, K.; Frederick, J. G. M. Carotenoid Oxidative Degradation Products inhibit Na^+/K^+-ATPase. *Free Rad. Res.* **2000,** *33,* 427–435.

104. Milatovic, D.; Gupta, R. C.; Aschner, M. Anticholinesterase Toxicity and Oxidative Review Article. *Sci. World J.* **2006,** *6,* 295–310.

105. Diab, A. E. A.; El-Aziz, E. A. A.; Hendawy, A. A.; Zahra, M. H.; Hamza, R. Z. Antioxidant Role of both Propolis and Ginseng against Neurotoxicity of Chlorpyrifos and Profenofos in Male Rats. *Life Sci. J.* **2012,** *9*(3), 987–1008.

106. Murphy, S. D. Toxic Effects of Pesticides. In Casarett and Doull's Toxicology. *Basic Sci. Poisons* **1986,** *3,* 519–581.

107. Sultatos, L. G.; Murphy, S. D. Kinetic Analysis of the Microsomal Biotransformation of the Phosphorothioate Insecticides Chlorpyrifos and Parathion. *Fundam. Appl. Toxicol.* **1983,** *3,* 16–21.

108. Chamber, H. W.; Chamber, J. E. An Investigation of Acetylcholinesterase Inhibition and Ageing, and Choline Acetyltransferase Activity Following a High-Level Acute Exposure to Paraoxon. *Pest. Biochem. Physiol.* **1989,** *33,* 125–131.

109. Chambers, J. E.; Carr, R. L. Inhibition Patterns of Brain Acetylcholinesterase and Hepatic and Plasma Aliesterases following Exposures to Three Phosphorothionate Insecticides and their Oxonsin Rats. *Fundam. Appl. Toxicol.* **1993,** *21,* 111–119.

110. Capodicasa, E.; Scapellato, M. L.; Moretto, A.; Caroldi, S.; Lotti, M. Chlorpyrifos-Induced Delayed Polyneuropathy. *Arch. Toxicol.* **1991,** *65,* 150–155.

CHAPTER 13

ROLE OF HERBS AND THEIR DELIVERY THROUGH NANOFIBERS IN PHARMACOTHERAPY OF DEPRESSION

GINPREET KAUR[1], MIHIR INVALLY[1], HIRAL MISTRY[1], PARNIKA DICHOLKAR[1], and SUKHWINDER BHULLAR[2,3*]

[1]Department of Pharmacology, Shobhaben Pratapbhai Patel School of Pharmacy & Technology Management, SVKM's NMIMS, Vile Parle (West), Mumbai 400056, Maharashtra, India

[2]Department of Mechanical Engineering, Bursa Technical University, Bursa, Turkey

[3]St. Boniface Hospital Albrechtsen Research Centre, Winnipeg, Manitoba, Canada

*Corresponding author. E-mail: sbhullar@sbrc.ca

ABSTRACT

Depression is a type of mood disorder in which a person feels sad, anxious, restless, irritable, helpless, or guilty, resulting in loss of interest in daily activities. Depression is however related to neurodegeneration of nerve cells which causes neurodegenerative diseases such as Alzheimer's and Parkinson's. These synthetic drugs which are used for the treatment of depression include selective serotonin reuptake inhibitors (SSRIs), serotonin or nor epinephrine reuptake inhibitors, atypical antidepressants, tricyclic antidepressants, and monoamine oxidase inhibitors. SSRIs are the most widely prescribed drugs since these have effective antidepressant properties. These drugs elevate the serotonin (a chemical in the brain which regulate the mood) level within brain to normal level. These SSRIs have several side effects such as nausea, insomnia, anxiety, restlessness, decreased sex drive, dizziness, weight gain, tremors, sweating, sleepiness or fatigue, dry mouth, diarrhea, constipation, and headaches. This chapter approaches herbs which can also be used so as to enhance the effects of the synthetic antidepressants along with a reduction in their side effects and their delivery through nanofibrous drug-delivery systems and transdermal patches. Nanofibers with sizes less than 100 nm are especially useful in the field of medicine because these nanomaterials replicate components of in vivo cellular environment. Their multiple properties such as large surface-area-to-volume ratio and high porosity provides a mechanism for sustained release of herb extracts in their nano to micro form for the treatment of the diseases.

13.1   INTRODUCTION

The psychiatric conditions accompanied by disturbances in mood rather than that of thought or cognition, feeling of sadness and loneliness are called depression. It may be mild to severe (psychotic) depression accompanied by hallucinations and delusions. Symptoms of depression include emotional symptoms such as feeling of guilt, loss of motivation, low self-esteem, inadequacy, etc. as well as biological symptoms such as loss of appetite, loss of libido, sleep disturbances, retardation of thought and action, etc.[1] Approximately 121 million people worldwide are affected by depression and the number is increasing every day. A study conducted on 89,000 people worldwide shows that depressed people are more in high-income countries such as France, Netherlands, and America (over 30%) and common in India too (almost 36%).[2] Centers for Disease Control and Prevention also revealed that the following group of people are affected more by depression: people between the age of 45 and 64, women (suffer twice more than men), people who never go for high school education, married people, unemployed youth, and uninsured people. Depression can lead to dangerous complications in people suffering from chronic conditions such as heart attack or stroke, diabetes, or Parkinson's disease (Table 13.1). Such people are more susceptible to be affected by depression.[3]

TABLE 13.1   Percentage of Depressed Patients Worldwide.

Chronic diseases	Proportion of depressed patients (%)
Diabetes	33
Parkinson's disease	40
Stroke	40
Cancer	42
Heart attack	45

Depression is the major cause of neurodegeneration. Stress is responsible for depression and neurodegeneration by raising the level of central and peripheral macrophages (Fig. 13.1).[4]

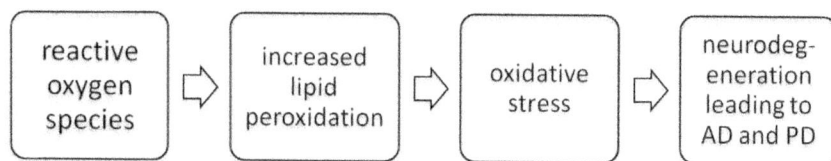

FIGURE 13.1   Mechanism leading to neurodegeneration.

13.2   NEURODEGENERATIVE DISEASES

The most common neurodegenerative diseases are Alzheimer's and Parkinson's disease. In these diseases, various faulty folded variants of physiological proteins get aggregated.

13.2.1   ALZHEIMER'S DISEASE

It is a type of dementia which attacks 30 million people throughout the world.[2] Symptoms of Alzheimer's include loss of memory, judgment, and thinking which prevent the patient from performing daily activities. It is characterized by amyloid plaques, neurofibrillary tangles, and loss of cholinergic neurons. There is synapse loss due to the aggregation of amyloid-beta (α,β) into senile plaques and "tau" protein into neurofibrillary tangles which leads to neurodegeneration and causes Alzheimer's.[5]

On the basis of changes in the brain, Alzheimer's is of three types:

(1) Mild Alzheimer's disease
(2) Moderate Alzheimer's disease
(3) Severe Alzheimer's disease

(1) Mild Alzheimer's Disease

This stage is the diagnostic stage in which the memory worsens and problems like poor judgment, taking longer time to complete daily tasks, having trouble in handling money, getting lost and having some mood, and personality changes occur.[6]

(2) Moderate Alzheimer's Disease

In this stage, damage occurs in areas of the brain that control reasoning, language, sensory processing, and thought. Patients in this stage begin to have problems in recognizing friends and family members. They have problems to do activity of daily life such as getting dressed etc. They may have delusions, paranoia, and hallucinations.[6]

(3) Severe Alzheimer's Disease

This is the final stage; in this stage, shrinkage of the brain tissue occurs due to spreading of plaques and tangles throughout the brain. Patients are unable to communicate and totally depend on others to do daily activities.[6]

It is estimated that around 65.7 million people in 2030 and 115.4 million people in 2050 will suffer from Alzheimer's, if it is not treated.[7]

13.2.2 *PARKINSON'S DISEASE*

It is a chronic and progressive movement disorder. Symptoms of Parkinson's disease include loss of coordination or postural instability, tremor of limbs and jaw, bradykinesia and rigidity of the limbs.[8] Due to the formation of Lewy body inclusions and Lewy dystrophic neuritis, there is a loss of dopamine producing nerve cells in substantia nigra which ultimately causes Parkinson's disease.[9]

Parkinson's disease appears to have five different stages as described (Fig. 13.2).

(1) Stage one:

In this stage, patients usually show mild symptoms such as presence of tremors or shaking in one of the limbs. Also during this stage, Parkinson's patient show some changes including loss of balance, abnormal facial expressions, and poor posture.[10]

(2) Stage two:

In this stage, patients show bilateral symptoms means affecting both sides of the body and both limbs. Patients are unable to walk properly as well as unable to maintain the balance of the body.[10]

(3) Stage three:

It is the more severe stage; in this stage, patients completely lose their physical movements or unable to walk straight or stand properly.[10]

(4) Stage four:

In this stage of the disease, walking is still there, but it is limited and there is rigidity and bradykinesia. Patients are unable to do day to day activities and rely on another person for care. The tremors become lessen for this time.[10]

(5) Stage five:

This is the final stage of Parkinson's disease in which patients are unable to stand and require constant one-on-one nursing care.[10]

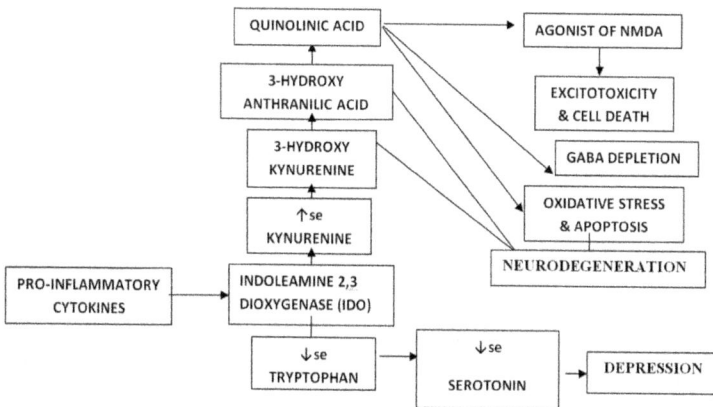

FIGURE 13.2 Mechanism linking neurodegeneration and depression.

13.3   SYNTHETIC ANTIDEPRESSANTS IN NEURODEGENERATION

In humans, there are two zones subventricular zone and subgranular zone, an area in brain (hippocampus) is responsible for learning and memory.[11,12] Due to aging, there is reduction of postsynaptic density in hippocampus resulting in a decrease in long-term potentiation (LTP) and increase in long-term depression which results in major depression.[13,14] SSRIs (selective serotonin reuptake inhibitors) or atypical antidepressants (venlafaxine) in chronic treatment are found to be more beneficial than tricyclic antidepressants (TCAs) because they prevent stress induced LTP.[15,16] In hippocampus and Cornu Ammonis pyramidal cells, cellular plasticity increases due to SSRIs (fluoxetine), while this neuroplastic activity is decreased by TCA due to its anticholinergic activity.[17–19]

Apart from the activity of these synthetic antidepressants, there are some side effects also such as disruption of sleep, digestion, and neurological symptoms like tingling, tics, and zapping sensations in the brain which ultimately aggravates patient difficulty.

Hence, the use of herbal antidepressants which show greater or equal therapeutic effect as compared to synthetic antidepressants with less number of side effects is being preferred.

13.4   HERBS AS CONVENTIONAL THERAPY

Here are some plants which are used as antidepressants, as well as for the treatment of neurodegeneration. The information mentioned in the following yields a descriptive insight into the antidepressant properties of these herbs.

13.4.1   *Hypericum perforatum (ST. JOHN'S WORT)*

13.4.1.1   INTRODUCTION

It is an herbaceous perennial plant, family *Hypericaceae*, commonly known as goat weed or Millepertuis. It is native of England and found in some parts of Europe, Australia and is grown in temperate region of China, Canada, Africa, and the United States. In India, it is found distributed in Western Himalaya up to an altitude of 1000–3000 m. It is conventionally used for treatment of depression as per international studies given in National Center for Complementary and Integrative Health (NCCIH).[20]

13.4.1.2 CHEMICAL CONSTITUENTS

Anthraquinones like hypericin and pseudohypericin, flavanol derivatives, biflavones, proanthocyanidines, xanthones, phloroglucinol derivative hyperforin, and naphthodianthrones.[21]

13.4.1.3 MECHANISM OF ACTION

It inhibits uptake of serotonin, dopamine, and noradrenaline in synapse with almost equal affinity. The polyphenols by mechanism of simple diffusion can cross the blood–brain barrier and hence serve as an active neuroprotective agent.[22,23]

13.4.1.4 USES

For depression and also has antibacterial, antiviral, anxiolytic, and astringent activity.[24]

13.4.2 Ginkgo biloba (GINGKO)

13.4.2.1 INTRODUCTION

It is a plant from family *Gingkoaceae*, tracing its history up to Mesozoic era (150 million years ago) and is shown to have medicinal properties in Chinese system of medicine. It is commonly known as Maiden hair tree or Knew tree. The genus name *Ginkgo* is regarded as *Gin Kyo* in Japanese "silver apricot." It has been commercially cultivated as food crop in the United States, Russia, and Japan.[25]

13.4.2.2 CHEMICAL CONSTITUENTS

Main constituents found in this plant are flavonoids and diterpene lactones like gingkolides A, B, C, J, and M and bilobalide.[25]

13.4.2.3 MECHANISM OF ACTION

Ginkgo biloba extract normalizes stress-elevated alterations in brain cate-cholamines, serotonin, and plasma corticosterone levels.[25] It decreases the production of fatty acids that are produced by degradation of arachidonic acid,[26] and inhibition of phospholipase A2 activity.[27]

13.4.2.4 USES

It has antidepressant, antioxidant, antiplatelet, and anticancer activities.[28]

13.4.3 *Bacopa monnieri* (BRAHMI)

13.4.3.1 INTRODUCTION

Tender herbs of *Scrophulariaceae* family, Bacopa, are grown in wet marshy areas of India, Australia, Africa, Europe, North, and South America. Brahmi is traditionally used in Ayurveda such as Charaka Samhita, Atharva-Veda, and Susrut Samhita as medhya rasayana for treatment of various mental deficits.[29]

13.4.3.2 CHEMICAL CONSTITUENTS

It consists of chemically active constituents like Bacosides A and B (saponin mixture), bacopasaponin C, and bacopasaponin C along with Bacogenin A1 and A2, Hersaponin, Monnierin, and Brahmine are all isomers of jujubogenin. It contains saponins, designated as bacopaside I, II, III, IV, and V. Additional phytochemicals like oroxindin betulinic acid and wogonin have been sequestered from the aerial parts.[29, 30]

13.4.3.3 MECHANISM OF ACTION

Two mechanisms of action have been proposed:
  (i) Bacoside induced membrane dephosphorylation increases production of protein and RNA turnover in the brain.
  (ii) *Bacopa monnieri* enhances hippocampic protein kinase activity causing increased neuronal synthesis along with synaptic activity restoration and nerve impulse transmission.[31]

13.4.3.4 USE

Brahmi is widely used in traditional Indian medicine as a nerve tonic and is thought to improve memory. Alcoholic extract of Brahmi may be used for ameliorating neurodegenerative disorders associated with the irresistible oxidative stress.[30, 32]

13.4.4 *Rosmarinus officinalis* (ROSEMARY)

13.4.4.1 INTRODUCTION

It belongs to family *Lamiaceae*, commonly known as rosemary, romarin, rosemarin, rosmarini, rosemarino, alecrim, and Romero. It is a woody, perennial herb with fragrant and needle-like leaves and white, pink, purple, or blue flowers, native of the Mediterranean region. It is native of Africa, Asia, and Europe.[33]

13.4.4.2 CHEMICAL CONSTITUENTS

Rosemary contains many antioxidants like carnosic acid, rosmarinic acid, and also other bioactive compounds including camphor, caffeic acid, ursolic acid, betulinic acid, rosmaridiphenol, and rosmanol.[34]

13.4.4.3 MECHANISM OF ACTION

Carnosic acid in rosemary is an active compound, responsible for neuroprotective activity. Carnosic acid in rosemary causes stimulation of novel signaling pathway that protects the brain from free radicals, which is commonly seen in neurodegenerative diseases.[34, 35]

13.4.4.4　USES

Rosemary traditionally has been used as an antioxidant, antispasmodic, analgesic, antirheumatic, carminative, cholagogue, diuretic, expectorant, antiepileptic, and for effects on human fertility.[33-35]

13.4.5　Salvia officinalis (SAGE)

13.4.5.1　INTRODUCTION

It belongs to family *Lamiaceae*, known in common terms "sage." Species of Salvia are annual, biennial, or perennial herbs, along with woody shrubs. Most of the species are used as herbs and some for their aromatic foliage. Some species of salvia include *Salvia apiana, Salvia azurea, Salvia divinorum* (psychedelic drug effects), *Salvia hispanica* (high protein content), *Salvia eucantha*, and *Salvia officinalis* (herbal medicine). It is distributed throughout the world. A survey found out that 23% salvia users said that the effects were like yoga, meditation, or trance.[36–38]

13.4.5.2　CHEMICAL CONSTITUENTS

Essential oil contains ingredients such as cineole, borneol, and thujone. Additionally, the ingredients present in the leaf portion include tannic acid, oleic acid, ursonic acid, ursolic acid, cornsole, cornsolic acid, fumaric acid, chlorogenic acid, caffeic acid, niacin, nicotinamide, flavones, flavonoid glycosides, and estrogenic substances.[39]

13.4.5.3　MECHANISM OF ACTION

The oil of this herb is found to show effects on acetylcholinesterase as well as butylcholinesterase.[40] Salvia has potent inhibitory action and quenching effect on lipid peroxidation which enhances the lipid peroxidation defense system of the brain.[37, 41]

13.4.5.4 USES

The leaves of sage have a plethora of biological activities other than antioxidant activity, such as antibacterial, astringent, fungistatic, eupeptic, virustatic, and antihydrotic as well as hypoglycemic effects.[42]

13.4.6 Melissa officinalis (LEMON BALM)

13.4.6.1 INTRODUCTION

Melissa officinalis is commonly known as lemon balm, common balm, or balm mint which is perennial herbaceous plant in mint family *Lamiaceae*, cultivated in Europe, United States, North Africa, Mediterranean regions, and western Asia. It grows up to 1 m (or 28–59 in) tall. The leaves have a mild lemon scent, related to mint. In season, such as summer, small white flowers have lemon-like flavor and are full of nectar. The white flowers attract bees, henceforth the genus name Melissa (Greek for "honey bee").[43]

13.4.6.2 CHEMICAL CONSTITUENTS

The main components of lemon balm include essential oil (0.01–0.25%). This includes 39% citronellal, 33% citral (citronellol, linalool), and geraniol. It also contains some phenols and flavonoids like rosmarinic acid.[44]

13.4.6.3 MECHANISM OF ACTION

Lemon balm possesses acetylcholine receptor activity along with muscarinic and nicotinic binding property in central nervous system.[43] This herb even potentiates mood and cognition.[45]

13.4.6.4 USES

Lemon balm has anxiolytic and sedative or hypnotic actions. It shows soothing and carminative properties also. It has been reported that lemon balm is also used to treat mild-to-moderate Alzheimer's.[44, 45]

13.4.7 Centella asiatica (MANDUKPARNI)

13.4.7.1 INTRODUCTION

Centella asiatica is also known as Centella, gotu kola, Asiatic pennywort, Indian pennywort, Brahmi with family *Apiaceae* or *Mackinlayaceae*. It is a small herbaceous, frost-tender perennial plant, used as a medicinal herb in Ayurveda, Traditional African and Chinese medicine. It grows in tropical marshy areas. It has small fan-shaped green leaves with white or light purple or pink flowers and small oval fruits. The leaves and stem of the plant are used as medicine. It is a perennial plant native of India, China, Japan, Indonesia, South Africa, Sri Lanka, and the South Pacific.[46]

13.4.7.2 CHEMICAL CONSTITUENTS

Photochemical constituents present in *C. asiatica* include β-carotene, β-sitosterol, campesterol, camphor, caempferol, stigmasterol, pentacyclic triterpenoid saponins (centelloids), and flavonoids. But the major activity is due to presence of asiatic acid, madecassic acid, asiaticoside and madecassoside, and several other terpenoids.[47]

13.4.7.3 MECHANISM OF ACTION

It shows neuron protection by inhibiting the activation of apoptotic pathway that is caused due to enzyme caspase 9. But higher concentrations can cause neurocytotoxicity.[47]

13.4.7.4 USES

C. asiatica is used to elevate the antioxidant level in healing wounds. It has been reported that an aqueous extract of this herb enhances cognitive functions.[48]

13.4.8 Polygala tenuifolia

13.4.8.1 INTRODUCTION

They are the large genus of flowering plants belonging to family *Polygala-ceae*. Its roots are used as a traditional Chinese medicine for improving memory and protect cognitive ailment and commonly known by Yaun Zhi.

13.4.8.2 CHEMICAL CONSTITUENTS

Active constituent in this herb is tetrahydrocolumbamine.[49]

13.4.8.3 MECHANISM OF ACTION

Tetrahydrocolumbamine causes inhibition of dopaminergic receptors, D1 and D2 by competitive and noncompetitive inhibition and enhances the cholinergic activity blocked by N-methyl-D-aspartate receptors thus improving memory and behavioral disorders.[49]

13.4.8.4 USES

Polygala tenuifolia is used as an expectorant, tonic, sedative, and for preventing dementia.[50]

13.4.9 Withania somnifera (ASHWAGANDHA)

13.4.9.1 INTRODUCTION

Ashwagandha is also known as winter cherry, Indian ginseng, poison gooseberry, or Asgandh. It belongs to the family *Solanaceae*. This indigenous herb has been found to be grown in India especially in Madhya Pradesh, Uttar Pradesh, plains in Punjab, Gujarat, and Rajasthan. It has been considered as part of rasayanas in Ayurvedic medicinal system since ages for mental wellbeing. Also countries like Congo, South Africa, Egypt, Morocco, Jordan, Pakistan, and Afghanistan are cultivating this herb.[51–55]

13.4.9.2 CHEMICAL CONSTITUENTS

It includes chemical constituents such as steroidal lactones, alkaloids, flavonoids, tannins, etc.[56] It has been found that more than 12 alkaloids, 40 with anolides and many sitoindosides are present in ashwagandha. The other alkaloids are somniferine, somnine, somniferinine, withananine, pseudowithanine, tropine, pseudotropine, 3-*a*-gloyloxytropane, choline, cuscohygrine, isopelletierine, anaferine, and anahydrine.[57]

13.4.9.3 MECHANISM OF ACTION

Ashwagandha extracts show gamma-aminobutyric acid like activity that inhibits nerve cells from overfiring, ultimately reducing anxiety with mood upliftment.[57]

13.4.9.4 USES

Ashwagandha shows different properties such as antitumor, antistress, anti-inflammatory, antioxidant, and hematopoietic and immunomodulatory properties.[58]

13.4.10 *Nardostachys jatamansi* (JATAMANSI)

13.4.10.1 INTRODUCTION

It is a flowering plant of *Valerianaceae* family grown in alpine Himalayas near Kumaon, Nepal, Sikkim, Punjab, South West China at 3000–5000 m and Bhutan; also known as spikenards, nards, nardin, or muskroot due to its aromatic amber color essential oil.[59]

13.4.10.2 CHEMICAL CONSTITUENTS

The roots of the plant contain essential oils that are rich in sesquiterpenes and coumarins. Jatamansone or valeranone is the principal sesquiterpene.[59]

13.4.10.3 MECHANISM OF ACTION

It enhances memory by increasing cholinergic activity with decrease in glutamate levels. It has its role in relieving psychosis, maniac psychosis, syncope, and hysteria[60] and works well in Parkinsonism,[61] memory enhancement,[62] and as an antidepressant.[63] Jatamansi showed its effect by increasing population of D2 receptors. It ultimately showed an increase in number of surviving neuron which defined its activity in Parkinsonism.[63] Jatamansi showed an increase in central biogenic amines and inhibitory amino-acids, thus showing its antidepressant activity.[64]

13.4.10.4 USES

Jatamansi is used to treat mental disorders, insomnia, spasms, blood disorders, palpitations, and convulsions.[65]

13.5 OTHER HERBAL DRUGS USED IN NEURODEGENERATION (TABLE 13.2)

TABLE 13.2 Other Herbal Drugs Used in Neurodegeneration.

Medicinal herb	Chemical constituent	Action
Allium sativum	s-Allyl cysteine	Antioxidant, protects neuronal cells from β-amyloid toxicity and apoptosis, reduces risk of dementia[66]
Asparagus racemosus	Asperagin, shatavarin	Estrogenic activity which prevents neuronal apoptosis. Estrogen enhancing activity of neurotrophins, which ultimately slows down progression of neurodegeneration.[67] Upregulation of expression of m-RNA for NGF, IGF, BDNF, and TRK-A[68]
Saraca indica	Leucopelargonidin, leucocyanidin, quercetin, amyrin	Potentiates GABAergic inhibition in the CNS through membrane hyperpolarization leading to a decrease in the neuron firing in the brain or may be due to direct activation of GABA receptor by the extract [69,70]

TABLE 13.2 *(Continued)*

Medicinal herb	Chemical constituent	Action
Panax ginseng	Ginsenosides Rg1, Rg2, and Rg3	Inhibition of dopamine uptake, increased serotonin in cortex, inhibition of NMDA and non-NMDA receptors thereby decreasing Ca^{+2} over flux in neurons[71]
Curcuma long	Curcumin	Modulation of dopaminergic receptors, cREB, and phospholipase C gene[72]
Allium sepa	Quercetin glycosides like hyperoside, isoquercetin, and rutin	Prevention of transmitter turnover as quercetin is a selective inhibitor of MAO, and hence increase in serotonergic and dopaminergic activities [73]
Piper methysticum	Pyrones, lactones, phytosterols, alkaloids	Potentiation of GABA or benzodiazepine receptors[74]
Valeriana officinalis	Monoterpenes, sesquiterpenes	Inhibits uptake and stimulates release of GABA from synaptosomes, which is Na^+ dependent and Ca^+ independent due to reversal of the neuronal GABA transporter[75,76]
Semecarpus anacardium	Biflavones A, C, A1, A2, tetrahydrorobustaflavone, B(tetrahydromentoflavone)[12]	Shows neuroprotective effect by inhibiting Ach esterase and enhancing the activity of Ach[77]
Piper longum	Piperidine alkaloid named piperine	Inhibitor of MAO-A and MAO-B activity resulting in enhancement of serotonergic and norepinephrinergic neurotransmission along with dopaminergic neurotransmission[78,79]
Flaxseed, hemp, canola, walnuts	Rich in omega 3-polyunsaturated fatty acids, alpha linolenic acid	Inhibitors of proinflammatory cytokines like TNF-α and IL-1β. Suppression of PGE2, thromboxane A2 and histamine and hence lessens the symptoms. Triggers the cAMP cascade and leads to expression of CREB and BDNF[80]
Convolulus pluricaulis	Alkaloid—shankhpushpine; tropane alkaloids, scopoletin	Interaction with adrenergic, dopaminergic, and serotonergic systems[81,82]

CNS, central nervous system; GABA, gamma–aminobutyric acid; NMDA, N-methyl-D-aspartate.

13.6 NANO/MICROTECHNOLOGY-BASED SYSTEMS TO DELIVER HERBAL OR HERBAL BLENDED WITH SYNTHETIC DRUGS

In view of the foregoing, it is ought to be seen that herbal antidepressants have an enormous potential, mainly as adjuncts to synthetic medications, however, most of these extracts have limited utility, most importantly due to dearth of suitable dosage forms. Most of the plant extracts, not only those limited to ones derived from alcoholic extraction, but also those with aqueous extraction, would be of an immense utility if proper dosage forms or delivery techniques are developed, which can enhance their practical utility. Recently, nanotechnology approaches as effective drug delivery techniques have gained momentum, and can also be utilized for delivery of herbal extracts, majority of those being poorly water soluble. Poorly soluble synthetic drugs and herbs can be incorporated during the fabrication of nanofibers to enhance their efficiency. Nanotechnology offers potential applications in biomedical industry for maintaining and promoting health, preventing, and treating diseases. Nanofibers are known to mimic collagen fibrils in the extracellular matrix and their multiple properties include a large surface-area-to-volume ratio, high porosity, improved cell adherence, cellular proliferation, and migration, as well as controlled in vivo biodegradation rates.[83] Moreover, due to their abundant availability, price effective, renewable extracted form, and unique mechanical properties in nanofibrous structures, the nanofibers developed from natural polymers have attracted attention from researchers for their application in medical arena.[84–86]

To fabricate these nonwoven nanofibers, electrostatic spinning which is a process of producing fibers with diameters in the range of 100 nm[90] is used. This process has been described in literature since the 1930s to make nanofibers from a variety of polymers, both natural and synthetic. The electrospinning of nanoparticulate drug-laden polymer nanofibers can be performed out from a homogeneous solution either in melt- or solvent-(s)-based solution. The nano/microfibers offer potential to deliver herbal or herbal blended with synthetic drugs.[87–89]

The dissolution rate of drugs with poor water solubility can be enhanced by nanoparticulate drug-embedded nanofibers. Electrospinning of solutions of drugs in polymers generates nanofibers having very large surface area. This extremely high surface area has deep influence on the bioavailability of a poorly soluble drug, because it is known that the increased surface area could cause increase in dissolution rate. A suitable dosage form, such as oral or parenteral, including aerosols, may be designed by rational selection of polymeric carriers in terms of their physicochemical properties as well as their regulatory status.[90] Other pharmaceutically acceptable excipients may be included to ameliorate the stabilization and/or deagglomeration of the drug nanoparticles. Electrospun pharmaceutical dosage forms can be designed accordingly to deliver rapid, immediate, delayed, or modified drug release such as sustained and/or pulsatile release characteristics.[90]

13.7 CONCLUSION

This review presents a summary of the herbs which are used to treat depression as well as Alzheimer's and Parkinson's disease by curing neurodegeneration of nerve cells. Neurodegeneration associated with depression involves various neurotransmitter systems which become targets for many antidepressant drugs. SSRIs or other antidepressants cure depression but harm the body as well. The purpose of this chapter is to increase the use of herbs as alone or in combination with synthetic drugs to overcome the side effects of the synthetic drugs which ultimately treat the disease by causing less harm to human body. Novel polymer technology is in development as a means to increase the delivery of these drugs, improving the utility.

KEYWORDS

- depression
- nanotechnology
- herbs
- neurodegeneration
- nanofibers

REFERENCES

1. Rang, H. P.; Dale, M. M. *Pharmacology*, 6th ed.; Churchill Livingstone: London, UK, 2016.
2. Bromet, E.; Andrade, L. H; Hwang, I.; Sampson, N. A.; Alonso, J.; de Girolamo, G.; de Graaf, R.; Demyttenaere, K.; Hu, C.; Iwata, N., et al. Cross-national Epidemiology of DSM-IV Major Depressive Episode. *BMC Med.* **2011,** *9*, 90.
3. Richards, D. Prevalence and Clinical Course of Depression: A Review. *Clin. Psychol. Rev.* 2011, *31*(7), 1117–1125.
4. Leonard, B. E.; Myint, A. Inflammation, Depression and Dementia: Are They Connected? *Neurotox Res.* **2006,** *10*(2), 149–160.
5. Nemeroff, C. B. Recent Findings in Pathophysiology of Depression. *Focus J. Lifelong Learn. Psychiatry* **2008,** *4*, 4.
6. Anand, R.; Gill, K. D.; Mahdi, A. A. Therapeutics of Alzheimer's Disease: Past, Present and Future. *Neuropharmacology* **2014,** *76*, 27–50.
7. Sosa-Ortiz, A. L.; Acosta-Castillo, I.; Prince, M. J. Epidemiology of Dementias and Alzheimer's Disease. *Arch. Med. Res.* **2012,** *43*(8), 600–608.
8. National Institute on Aging. US Department Health and Human Services (Internet). Factsheet on Alzhiemer's disease. http://www.nia.nih.gov/alzheimers/publication/alzheimers-disease-fact-sheet (accessed Jul 10, 2017).
9. Rizzo, G.; Copetti, M.; Arcuti, S.; Martino, D.; Fontana, A.; Logroscino, G. Accuracy of Clinical Diagnosis of Parkinson Disease: A Systematic Review and Meta-analysis. *Neurology* **2016,** *86*(6), 566–576.
10. Kakkar, A. K.; Dahiya, N. Management of Parkinson's Disease: Current and Future Pharmacotherapy. *Eur. J. Pharmacol.* **2015,** *750*, 74–81.
11. Krysinska, K.; Sachdev, P. S.; Breitner, J.; Kivipelto, M.; Kukull, W.; Brodaty, H. Dementia Registries Around the Globe and Their Applications: A Systematic Review. *Alzheimers Dement.* **2017,** *13*(9), 1031–1047.
12. Lipsky, R. H. Epigenetic Mechanisms Regulating Learning and Long-term Memory. *Int. J. Dev. Neurosci.* **2013,** *31*(6), 353–358.
13. Erikson, K. I.; Miller, D. L.; Roecklein, K. A. The Aging Hippocampus: Interactions between Exercise, Depression, and BDNF. *Neuroscientist* **2012,** *18*(1), 82–97.
14. Trigunayat, A.; Raghavendra, M.; Singh, R. K.; Bhattacharya, A. K.; Acharya, S. B. Neuroprotective Effect of Withania somnifera (WS) in Cerebral Ischemia—Reperfusion and Long Term Hypoperfusion Induced Alterations in Rats. *J. Nat. Remedies* **2007,** *7*, 234–246.
15. Intlekofer, K. A.; Cotman, C. W. Exercise Counteracts Declining Hippocampal Function in Aging and Alzheimer's Disease. *Neurobiol. Dis.* **2013,** *57*, 47–55.
16. Evans, V. C.; Alamian, G.; McLeod, J.; Woo, C.; Yatham, L. N.; Lam, R. W. The Effects of Newer Antidepressants on Occupational Impairment in Major Depressive Disorder: A Systematic Review and Meta-Analysis of Randomized Controlled Trials. *CNS Drugs* **2016,** *30*(5), 405–417.
17. Lister, J. P.; Barnes, C. A. Neurobiological Changes in the Hippocampus During Normative Aging. *Arch. Neurol.* **2009,** *66*(7), 829–833.

18. Vouimba, R. M.; Munoz, C.; Diamond, D. M. Differential Effects of Predator Stress and the Antidepressant Tianeptine on Physiological Plasticity in the Hippocampus and Basolateral Amygdala. *Stress* **2006**, *9*(1), 29–40.

19. Racagni, G.; Popoli, M. Cellular and Molecular Mechanisms in the Long-Term Action of Antidepressants. *Dialogues Clin. Neurosci.* **2008**, *10*(4), 385–400.

20. Maya Vetencourt, J. F.; Sale, A.; Viegi, A., et al. The Antidepressant Fluoxetine Restores Plasticity in the Adult Visual Cortex. *Science* **2008**, *320*, 385–388.

21. Barnes, J.; Anderson, L. A.; Phillipson, J. D. St. John's Wort (*Hypericum perforatum* L.): A Review of Its Chemistry, Pharmacology and Clinical Properties. *J. Pharm. Pharmacol.* **2001**, *53*, 583–600.

22. Harner, G.; Schulz, V. Clinical Investigation of the Antidepressant Effectiveness of *Hypericum*. *J. Geriatr. Psychiatry Neurol.* **1994**, *7*, 6–8.

23. Panocka, I.; Perfumi, M.; Angeletti, S.; Ciccocioppo R.; Mass M. Effects of *Hypericum perforatum* Extract on Alcohol Intake and on Behavioural Despair: A Search for the Neurochemical Systems Involved. *Pharmacol. Biochem. Behav.* **2000**, *66*, 105–111.

24. Purohit, A. P.; Kokate, C. K.; Gokhale, S. B. *Pharmacognosy*, 48th ed.; Nirali Prakashan: Pune, Maharashtra, 2013.

25. Silva, B. A.; Ferreres, F.; Malva, J.; Dias, A. C. P. Phytochemical and Antioxidant Characterization of *Hypericum perforatum* Alcoholic Extracts. *Food Chem.* **2005**, *90*, 157–167.

26. Mahadevan, S.; Park, Y. Multifaceted Therapeutic Benefits of *Ginkgo biloba* L. *J. Food Sci.* **2008**, *73*, R14–R19.

27. Rodriguez de Turco, E. B.; Droy-Lefaix, M.-T.; Bazan, N. G. Decreased Electroconvulsive Shock-Induced Diacylglycerols and Free Fatty Acid Accumulation in the Rat Brain by *Ginkgo biloba* Extract (EGb 761): Selective Effect in Hippocampus as Compared with Cerebral Cortex. *J. Neurochem.* **1993**, *61*, 1438–1444.

28. Shah, Z. A.; Sharma, P.; Vohora, S. B. Ginkgo biloba Normalises Stress-Elevated Alterations in Brain Catecholamines, Serotonin and Plasma Corticosterone Levels. *Eur. Neuropsychopharmacol.* **2003**, *13*, 321–325.

29. Achliya, G. S.; Barabde, U.; Wadodkar, S.; Dorle, A. Effect of Brahmi Grita, a Pollyherbal Formulation on Learning and Memory Paradigms in Experimental Animals. *Indian J. Pharmacol.* **2008**, *36*(3), 159–162.

30. Singh, H. K.; Dhaan, B. N. Neuropsychopharmacological Effects of the Ayurvedic Nootropic *Bacopa monniera* Linn. (Brahmi). *Indian J. Pharmacol.* **1997**, *29*, s359–s365.

31. Gohil, K. J.; Patel, J. A. A Review on *Bacopa monniera*: Current Research and Future Prospects. *Int. J. Green Pharm.* **2010**, *4*, 1–9.

32. Piyabhan, P.; Wetchateng, T.; Sireeratawong, S. Cognitive Enhancement Effects of *Bacopa monnieri* (Brahmi) on Novel Object Recognition and NMDA Receptor Immunodensity in the Prefrontal Cortex and Hippocampus of Sub-Chronic Phencyclidine Rat Model of Schizophrenia. *J Med Assoc Thai.* **2013**, *96*(2), 231–238.

33. Al-Sereitia, M. R.; Abu-Amerb, K. M.; Sena, P. Pharmacology of Rosemary (*Rosmarinus officinalis Linn.*) and its Therapeutic Potentials. *Indian J. Exp. Biol.* **1999**, *37*, 124–131.

34. Selmi, S.; Rtibi, K.; Grami, D.; Sebai, H.; Marzouki, L. Rosemary (*Rosmarinus officinalis*) Essential Oil Components Exhibit Anti-Hyperglycemic, Anti-Hyperlipidemic and Antioxidant Effects in Experimental Diabetes. *Pathophysiology* **2017**, *24*(4), 297–303.

35. Abdelhalim, A.; Karim, N.; Chebib, M.; Aburjai, T.; Khan, I.; Johnston, G. A.; Hanrahan, J. Antidepressant, Anxiolytic and Antinociceptive Activities of Constituents from *Rosmarinus Officinalis. J. Pharm. Pharm. Sci.* **2015**, *18*(4), 448–459.

36. Baggott, M.; Erowid, F. A Survey of *Salvia divinorum* Users. Erowid Extracts, 2004, 6, 12–14.

37. Cvetkovikj, I.; Stefkov, G.; Karapandzova, M.; Kulevanova, S.; Satović, Z. Essential Oils and Chemical Diversity of Southeast European Populations of *Salvia officinalis* L. *Chem Biodivers.* **2015**, *12*(7), 1025–1039.

38. Zupko, I.; Hohmann, J.; Redei, D.; Falkay, G. G. Antioxidant Activity of Leaves of Salvia Species in Enzyme Dependent and Enzyme-Independent Systems of Lipid Peroxidation and Their Phenolic Constituents. Plant Med. **2001**, 67, 366–368.

39. Kenjerić, D.; Mandić, M. L.; Primorac, L.; Čačić, F. Flavonoid Pattern of Sage (*Salvia officinalis* L.) Unifloral Honey. *Food Chem.* **2008**, *110*(1), 187–192.

40. Perry, N. S.; Houghton, P. J.; Jenner, P.; Keith, A.; Perry, E. K. *Salvia lavandulaefolia* Essential Oil Inhibits Cholinesterase In Vivo. *Phytomedicine* **2002**, *9*(1), 48–51.

41. Savelev, S.; Okello, E.; Perry, N.; Wilkins, R. Synergistic and Antagonistic Interactions of Anticholinesterase Terpenoids in *Salvia lavandulaefolia* Essential Oil. *Biochem. Pharmacol. Behav.* **2003**, *75*, 661–668.

42. Ghorbani, A.; Esmaeilizadeh, M. Pharmacological Properties of *Salvia officinalis* and Its Components. *J. Tradit. Complement Med.* **2017**, *7*(4), 433–440.

43. Miraj, S.; Rafieian-Kopaei, M.; Kiani, S. *Melissa officinalis* L: A Review Study With an Antioxidant Prospective. *J. Evid Based Complementary Altern. Med.* **2017**, *22*(3), 385–394.

44. Akhondzadeh, S. S.; Noroozian, M.; Mohammadi, M.; Ohadinia, S.; Jamshidi, A.; Khani, M. *Melissa officinalis* Extract in the Treatment of Patients with Mild to Moderate Alzheimer's Disease: A Double Blind, Randomised, Placebo Controlled Trial. *J. Neurol. Neurosurg. Psychiatry* **2003**, *74*(7), 863–866.

45. Kennedy, D. O.; Scholey, A. B.; Tildesley, N. T.; Perry, E. K.; Wesnes, K. A. Modulation of Mood and Cognitive Performance Following Acute Administration of *Melissa officinalis* (Lemon Balm). *Pharmacol. Biochem. Behav.* **2002**, *72*, 953–964.

46. Mishra, S. H.; Jayathirtha, M. G. Preliminary Immunomodulatory Activities of Methanol Extracts of *Eclipta alba* and *Centella asiatica*. *Phytomedicine* **2004**, *11*, 361–365.

47. Das, A. J. Review on Nutritional, Medicinal and Pharmacological Properties of *Centella asiatica* (Indian Pennywort). *J. Biol. Active Prod. Nat.* **2011**, *4*, 216–228.

48. Veerendra Kumar, M. H.; Gupta, Y. K. Effect of Different Extracts of *Centella asiatica* on Cognition and Markers of Oxidative Stress in Rats. *J. Ethnopharmacol.* **2002**, *79*(2), 253–260.

49. Yong, J.; Tu, P.-F. Xanthone O-glycosides from *Polygala tenuifolia. Phytochemistry* **2002**, *60*, 813–816.

50. Shen, X. L.; Witt, M. R.; Dekermendjian, K.; Nielsen, M. Isolation and Identification of Tetrahydrocolumbamine as a Dopamine Receptor Ligand from *Polygala tenuifolia* Willd. *Acta Pharm. Sin.* **1994**, *29*, 887–890.

51. Lakshmi, C. M.; Singh, B. B.; Simon, D. Scientific Basis for the Therapeutic Use of *Withania somnifera* (Ashwagandha): A Review. *Alternat. Med. Rev.* **2000**, *5*, 334–346.

52. Kaur, N.; Niazi, J.; Bains, R. A Review on Pharmacological Profile of *Withania somnifera*. *Res. Rev. J. Bot. Sci.* **2013**, *2*, 6–14.

53. Trigunayat, A.; Raghavendra, M.; Singh, R. K.; Bhattacharya, A. K.; Acharya, S. B. Neuroprotective Effect of *Withania somnifera* (WS) in Cerebral Ischemia—Reperfusion and Long Term Hypoperfusion Induced Alterations in Rats. *J. Nat. Remedies* **2007**, *7*, 234–246.

54. Dar, P. A.; Singh, L. R.; Kamal, M. A; Dar, T. A. Unique Medicinal Properties of *Withania somnifera*: Phytochemical Constituents and Protein Component. *Curr. Pharm. Des.* **2016**, *22*(5), 535–540.

55. Dar, N. J.; Hamid, A.; Ahmad, M. Pharmacologic Overview of *Withania somnifera*, the Indian Ginseng. *Cell Mol. Life Sci.* **2015**, *72*(23), 4445–4460.

56. Singh, N.; Bhalla, M.; de Jager, P.; Gilca, M. An Overview on Ashwagandha: A Rasayana (Rejuvenator) of Ayurveda. *Afr. J. Tradit. Complement Altern. Med.* **2011**, *8*(5 Suppl), 208–213.

57. Mehta, A. K.; Binkley, P.; Gandhi, S. S.; Ticku, M. K. Pharmacological Effects of *Withania somnifera* Root Extract on GABAA Receptor Complex. *Indian J. Med. Res.* **1991**, *94*, 312–315.

58. Kulkarni, S. K.; Dhir, A. *Withania somnifera*: An Indian Ginseng. *Prog. Neuropsychopharmacol. Biol. Psychiatry* **2008**, *32*(5), 1093–1105.

59. Ahmad, M.; Yousuf, S.; Khan, M. B.; Hoda, M. N.; Ahmad, A. S.; Ansari, M. A.; Ishrat, T.; Agrawal, A. K.; Islam, F. Attenuation by *Nardostachys jatamansi* of 6-Hydroxydopamineinduced Parkinsonism in Rats: Behavioural, Neurochemical and Immunochemical Studies. *Pharm. Biochem. Behav.* **2006**, *83*, 150–160.

60. Joshi, H.; Parle, M. *Nardostachys jatamansi* Improves Learning and Memory in Mice. *J. Med. Food* **2006**, *9*, 113–118.

61. Prabhu, V.; Karanth, K. S.; Rao, A. Effects of *Nardostachys jatamansi*on Biogenic Amines and Inhibitory Amino-Acids in the Rat-Brain. *Planta Med.* **1994**, *60*, 114–117.

62. Vinutha, J. P. Acetyl cholinesterase Inhibitory Activity of Methanolic and Successive Water Extracts of *Nardostachys jatamansi*. *Indian J. Pharmacol.* **2007**, *23*, 127–131.

63. Singh, A.; Kumar, A.; Duggal, S. *Nardostachys Jatamansi* DC. Potential Herb with CNS Effects. *JPRHC* **2009**, *2*, 276–290.

64. Prabhu, V.; Karanth, K. S.; Rao, A. Effects of *Nardostachys jatamansi* on Biogenic Amines and Inhibitory Amino Acids in the Rat Brain. *Planta Med.* **1994**, *60*(2), 114–117.

65. Srivastava, P.; Yadav, R. S. Efficacy of Natural Compounds in Neurodegenerative Disorders. *Adv. Neurobiol.* **2016**, *12*, 107–123.

66. Borek, C. Garlic Reduces Dementia and Heart-Disease Risk. *J. Nutr.* **2006**, *136*(3 Suppl), 810S–812S.

67. Deshpande, S. B. Protective Role of Estrogen in Neurodegenerative Disorders. *Indian J. Physiol. Pharmacol.* **2000**, *44*, 43.
68. Gabbay, V.; Klein, R.; Katz, Y.; Mendoza, S.; Guttman, L.; Alonso, C. The Possible Role of the Kynurenine Pathway in Adolescent Depression with Melancholic Features. *J. Child Psychol. Psychiatry* **2010**, *51*(8), 935–943.
69. Shepherd, G. M. *The Synaptic Organization of Brain*; Oxford University Press: New York, 2003.
70. Verma, A.; Jana, G. K.; Sen, S.; Chakraborty, R.; Sachan, S.; Mishra, A. Pharmacological Evaluation of *Saraca indica* Leaves for Central Nervous System Depressant Activity in Mice. *J. Pharm. Sci. Res.* **2010**, *2*(6), 338–343.
71. Nah, S. Y. Ginseng Ginsenoside Pharmacology in the Nervous System: Involvement in the Regulation of Ion Channels and Receptors. *Front. Physiol.* **2014**, *19*(5), 98.
72. Kumar, T. P.; Antony, S.; Gireesh, G.; George, N.; Paulose, C. S. Curcumin Modulates Dopaminergic Receptor, CREB and Phospholipase C Gene Expression in the Cerebral Cortex and Cerebellum of Streptozotocin Induced Diabetic Rats. *J. Biomed. Sci.* **2010**, *17*, 43.
73. Sakakibara, H.; Yoshino, S.; Kawai, Y.; Terao, J. Antidepressant-Like Effect of Onion (*Allium cepa L.*) Powder in a Rat Behavioral Model of Depression. *Biosci. Biotechnol. Biochem.* **2008**, *72*(1), 94–100.
74. Jussofie, A.; Schmiz, A.; Hiemke, C. Kavapyrone Enriched Extract from *Piper methysticum* as Modulator of the GABA Binding Site in Different Regions of Rat Brain. *Psychopharmacology* **1994**, *116*, 469–474.
75. Wake, G.; Court, J.; Pickering, A.; Lewis, R.; Wilkins, R.; Perry, E. CNS Acetylcholine Receptor Activity in European Medicinal Plants Traditionally Used to Improve Failing Memory. *J. Ethnopharmacol.* **2000**, *69*, 105–114.
76. Santos, M. S.; Ferreira, F. An Aqueous Extract of Valerian Influences the Transport of GABA in Synaptosomes. *Planta Med.* **1994**, *60*, 278–279.
77. Gil, R. R.; Lin, L. Z.; Cordell, G. A.; Kumar, M. R.; Ramesh, M.; Reddy, B. M.; Mohan, G. K.; Narasimha, A. V.; Rao, A. Anacardoside from the Seeds of *Semecarpus anacardium*. *Phytochemical* **1995**, *39*(2), 405–407.
78. Al-Baghdadi, O. B.; Prater, N. I.; Van der Schyf, C. J.; Geldenhuys, W. J. Inhibition of Monoamine Oxidase by Derivatives of Piperine, An Alkaloid from the Pepper Plant *Piper nigrum*, for Possible Use in Parkinson's Disease. *Bioorg. Med. Chem. Lett.* **2012**, *22*(23), 7183–7188.
79. Wąsik, A.; Antkiewicz-Michaluk, L. The Mechanism of Neuroprotective Action of Natural Compounds. *Pharmacol. Rep.* **2017**, *69*(5), 851–860.
80. Painter, F. M. Neurobehavioural Aspects of Omega 3-Fatty Acids: Possible Mechanisms and Therapeutic Value in Major Depression. *Alternat. Med. Rev.* **2003**, *8*(4), 410–425.
81. Agarwa, P.; Sharma, B.; Fatima, A.; Jain, S. K. An Update on Ayurvedic Herb *Convolvulus pluricaulis Choisy. Asian Pac. J. Trop. Biomed.* **2014**, *4*(3), 245–252.
82. Siddiqui, N. A.; Ahmad, N.; Musthaq, N.; Chattopadhyaya, I.; Kumria, R.; Gupta, S. Neuropharmacological Profile of Extracts of Aerial Parts of *Convolvulus pluricaulis* Choisy in Mice Model. *Open Neurol. J.* **2011**, *8*, 11–14.
83. Lyons, J.; Ko, F. Nanofibers. *Encycl. Nanosci. Nanotech.* **2004**, *6*, 727–738.

84. Kenawy, E.-R.; Abdel-Hay, F. I.; Wnek, G. E. Processing of Nanofibers through Electrospinning as Drug Delivery Systems. *Mater. Chem. Phys.* **2009,** 296–302.

85. Formhals, A. Method and Apparatus for the Production of Fibers. U.S. Patent 2,924, 1938.

86. Verreck, G.; Chun, I.; Peeters, J.; Rosenblatt, J.; Brewster, M. E. Preparation and Characterization of Nanofibers Containing Amorphous Drug Dispersions Generated by Electrostatic Spinning. *Pharm. Res.* **2003,** *20,* 810–817.

87. Langer, R.; Tirrell, D. A. Designing Materials for Biology and Medicine. *Nature* **2004,** *428,* 487–492.

88. Juntaro, J.; Pommet, M.; Kalinka, G.; Mantalaris, A.; Shaffer, M. S. P.; Bismarck, A. *Adv. Mater.* **2008,** *20,* 3122.

89. Ignatious, F.; Baldoni, J. Electrospun Nanofibers in Oral Drug Delivery. *Pharm. Res.* **2010,** *27,* 4.

90. Ignatious, F.; Sun, L. Electrospun Amorphous Pharmaceutical Compositions. WO 2004014304, 2004. Ignatious, F.; Sun, L. Electrospun Amorphous Pharmaceutical Compositions. WO 2004014304, 2004. https://patents.google.com/patent/WO2004014304A2/en (accessed Aug 8, 2018).

PART V
Indigenous Medical Practices

CHAPTER 14

DECOLONIZING KNOWLEDGE: BIOMEDICAL BELIEFS AND INDIGENOUS MEDICAL PRACTICE

RONNIE G. MOORE*

School of Public Health, Physiotherapy and Sports Science and School of Sociology, University College Dublin, Dublin 4, Ireland

*E-mail: Ronnie.g.moore@ucd.ie

ABSTRACT

Critical discussions about medicine and medical practices are cognoscente of the evolution of such practices and the historical and cross-cultural developments of healthcare systems, or arenas. In a seminal text, Charles Leslie outlined some of the key examples in terms of comparative (Asian) healthcare systems. This sets the scene for future generations of researchers to apply a more comparative understanding, not just to Asian medical systems but to any such cross-cultural analysis of medicine and health care. The text also brings into sharp relief the relative merits and potential drawbacks of applying a unified homogenized overarching approach to medical practice. This chapter therefore concerns itself with the idea of healthcare *systems* rather than any notion of a single universally agreed medical practice and the meaning this has for "modern medicine" in the contemporary world in the (post) Industrial West *and* in the so-called developing societies.

Contemporary currents of Western medical thought and practice illustrate a particular cognitive trajectory and scholars have outlined linkages between medical knowledge and dominant (social) ideas in what have been described as "medical cosmologies."[20] In this regard, medical endeavor may also be construed as a sociological and anthropological endeavor.[37]

Medical traditions are born in antiquity and are, by definition, ethnocentric. They are defined by the immediate circumstances and surroundings of individuals in context, that is, the socioeconomic, environmental, and cultural circumstances from which they emerge. We may regard these healthcare systems as profoundly personal and tied to such things as cosmological canopy, belief systems and ritual, organized religion, kinship structures, local topography, indigenous ethno pharmacological practices, food, and lifestyle behaviors. The point here is that when we come to look at such practices historically and cross-culturally, we see common themes, such as how individuals, groups, and societies respond to health chances[1] to relieve specific ailments or conditions. This is context based. We see this through, for example, organizational responses to care, within the family; or in the community; or through national, regional healthcare services; or via the use of indigenous pharmacological substances or ritualistic behavior or performance and symbolic meaning (such as prayer, penitence, or sacred offerings).

However, we also see important variations. Different cultures (and healthcare systems) rely on *specific* knowledge. These are often dependent on local resources and local notions of health beliefs and associated practices. These are derived from, and embedded in, tradition and culture. These beliefs and practices, while they may make sense locally, may not be easily translated to circumstances beyond the immediate environment. The classic anthropological example of this is Evans-Pritchard's now-famous discussion surrounding the transmission of medical (magical) knowledge among the Azande.[11], p 186) We also see trends. For example, dominant ideologies and power structures drive and legitimate practice, thereby giving license to practice and define authenticity. Nowhere is this truer than within the rise of "modern medicine," particularly in the West. This "is embodied in and comes with the day-to-day rational-scientific practices associated with the work of doctors in the hospital or clinic" (Ref. [6], p. xii). Such everyday practices contribute to the (social) construction and reproduction of a particular world view or what some have termed a "biomedical discourse" or "clinical gaze."[12] In the so-called advanced industrial world of the late 18th and early 19th centuries, health care made a profound move from within the community, to the more alienating hospital–clinic-based medicine that linked the "bench, the bedside, and

---

[1]Mortality and morbidity.

the production plant," and this came to characterize modern medicine (Ref. [25], p. 118). This development was tied to wider social, historical processes of the period, such as the growth of towns and cities amid rapid capitalist expansion in the West.[20,32] In addition, medical knowledge and health practice also progressed rapidly in the wake of various (more notably, colonial) conflicts. The world wars were also significant here. We see, for example, the "accelerated and intensified collaboration between biologists, clinicians and industrialists, a development exemplified by the wartime production of penicillin…. and the rapid growth of the pharmaceutical industry" (Ref. [25], p. 117). World War II, in particular, is seen as a key juncture in terms of the "biomedicalization" process.

14.1 "MODERNITY," EUROPEAN ETHNOCENTRISM, AND THE RISE OF "NEW" SCIENCE

As a social scientific concept, "modernity" is problematic. However, the notion is often popularly (loosely) held to mean a kind of evolved development. In this sense, there has been an increasing emphasizes on "modern science" (essentially stemming from the European Enlightenment). Cartesian (1596–1650) philosophy, Newtonian (1642–1727) experimentation and observation, the notion of the body as machine, and later germ theory are central aspects of this approach. "Contributions in science have been made ever since man [sic] acquired the ability to hand on his [sic] experiences with nature; but in the case of medical sciences, at least, such advances as were made down to the 14th century were upon the whole unimportant, and for the most part casual" (Ref. [10], p. 136).

There is now a cultural dominance of science that never existed before. With these developments we see "historical and historiographical relationships, and the diminishing utility of distinctions between science, medicine and technology" (Ref. [33], pp. 97–99). We now talk of "scientific medicine" and with this the emergence of (bio) power. It is no coincidence that the recent burgeoning of biomedicine and the expansion of high-tech, high-spec industries have arisen in tandem.

In contrast, earlier European epochs were characterized by a variety of medical or health practitioners (many of whom were women), and the emphasis was on locally derived experiential knowledge (incorporating locally practiced scientific principles) and holistic medicine. This was organically and community based, and incorporated multiplex features. With the development of increasingly specialized (and arguably more myopic) biomedical knowledge, the relationship, and the power nexus between the patient and the physician began to change. The doctor became subordinate to "medical knowledge" as medicine developed as a key site for scientific research within the clinical setting. "From somewhere in the mid-ninetieth century, doctors did not just evoke 'science,' they increasingly relied on laboratory science" (Ref. [25], p. 117). Crucially, the patient moved from the *object* of care, to the *subject* of care.

The enlightenment as a legitimizing principle for medical practice may therefore be regarded as relatively new. With this, the concept of (personal) *Illness* is declined in relevance and (scientific) *disease*, that is, the physiological and chemical processes became the central focus, while psychosocial, cultural, behavioral, and environmental factors were effectively underplaying or ignored. It is this notion of modern, Western "new" science that underpins the rise, development, expansion, and (colonial and capitalist) exportation of scientific medicine. Biomedicine has come to be regarded as the "one true medicine" in terms of power, authority, significance, prestige, and legitimate practice, whereas traditional indigenous medical systems have largely been ignored, derided as quackery, fraudulent, irrelevant, and/or dangerous. This has given rise to two broad categories: formal and informal medicine.[27] Formal science (involving broad intellectual theorizing) arguably existed in other places and, at other times, predating modern incarnations.[2] Informal science (empirical experimentation, i.e., trial and error) was also commonplace. Arguably, there is a science in discerning edible mushrooms from poisonous *toadstools* (Anglicized).[3]

14.2   BIOMEDICINE AS IMPOSTER?

Historical and ethnographic research problematizes modern medicine as imposter. At the center of the discussion is the notion of what counts as legitimate knowledge, and on the concomitant power structures and associated discourse. In the West, biomedicine, arguably, replaced religion as a key source of power and authority in modern society. This points up

---

[2]In Europe, predating, for example, Roger Bacon (around 1220–1292).
[3]The original German translation being Todestools or "death stools."

historical and cultural processes and begs the question. Why did this not happen at other times, or in other places, such as China or in the medieval Middle East? The period of Enlightenment in the European context forged a whole new way of thinking about the world. The context was that religious ideas and the church were predicted to become less important as new scientific, anthropological, and biological theories began to question the old order of things. Indigenous health beliefs were replaced by new ideas that increasingly utilized new inventions and technology. Superstitious beliefs, it was suggested, have given way to rationality, the observed and the testable. These ideas had even permeated the classical social-science literature. Max Weber, for example, famously espoused the *disenchantment theory* and the seemingly unstoppable rise of rationality. This has even been taken up by contemporary writers of history such as Thomas.[40] A modern scientific biomedical discourse expanded. Ever since, biomedicine has assumed considerable power, authority, and prestige.

The positive aspects of biomedicine today are universally celebrated. But there are now numerous exponents of the shortcomings and failures within biomedicine, and there are growing critical voices calling out the dangers of such pre-eminent, privileged, and guarded knowledge. A key concern remains. What do we regard as authentic medicine? This compels us to consider the relationship between biomedicine and other organic healthcare systems such as folk or indigenous medicine. We therefore need to unpack some critical issues at the heart of the often-abrasive interface between the critical social sciences in medicine and modern, Western dominated notions of "scientific" biomedical practice. The ensuing conflict between lay and professional perceptions of health and healthcare practices in the West, exposed by Parsons, [31] for example, continues to be highlighted by the numerous academic papers on the physician/patient relationship.[18].

The problem is that much of the critique leveled at indigenous medicine and folk medicine holds for biomedicine. For example, the iatrogenic aspects of biomedicine are continually being exposed and, if anything, often present a greater challenge in terms of scope, magnitude, and consequences. Some historical examples include the thalidomide scandal; blood transfusions scandals; various mal practice cases, ranging from misdiagnoses, unintended or willful neglect but also extend to organ marketing[35];

in vitro fertilization misinformation; unnecessary operations[4]; drug trial deaths; to the premeditated murder of patients.[5]

The medical doctrine of *Primum non nocere* is called into question, as modern medicine moves into (arguably idealized and Westernized) notions of body image and body enhancement procedures. The "new science" and biomedicine are not only complicit but also appears to be unashamedly active in promoting these rapidly developing and lucrative markets.

Conflicts are underscored not only by social scientists but also by a range of prominent biomedical physicians. Kleinman[23] crucially points up the significance of a range of alternative healthcare arenas.[6] Others have suggested that biomedicine has made key category errors that have affected the health and human rights of individuals.[38] While yet others question the role, effectiveness, and even morality of biomedical training.

Now, more than a decade after I told Mr Lazaroff's story, what strikes me is not how bad his decision was but how much we all avoided talking honestly about the choice before him. We had no difficulty explaining the specific dangers of various treatment options, but we never really touched on the reality of his disease. His oncologists, radiation therapists, surgeons, and other doctors had all seen him through months of treatments for a problem that they knew could never be cured. We could never bring ourselves to discuss the larger picture about his condition or the limits of our capabilities, let alone what might matter most to him as he neared the end of his life. If he was pursuing a delusion, so were we (Ref. [13], pp. 5–6).

The scientific and biomedical paradigm now dominates globally, and it is this Western centric, privileged, and expert knowledge that is exported to the rest of the world with the associated mantras of "evidence based," "scientific testing," and "randomized controlled trials." And there

---

[4]Dr. Michael Neary carried out 129 of 188 peripartum hysterectomies carried out in an Irish hospital over a 25-year period, needlessly removed 129 women's wombs.

[5]Dr. Harold Shipman was convicted of killing his patients in England.

[6]Kleinman's seminal analysis views health and health care as "a local cultural system composed of three overlapping parts: the Popular, Professional and Folk sectors." The model suggested that the *Popular* sector referred to the lay, culturally specific treatment of sickness. The *Professional* denoted organized healing professions, and the *Folk* captured the specialist, nonprofessional sector encompassing secular and sacred healers. Kleinman identifies overlap and ambiguity between the sectors (see Ref. [24], p. 50). Moore and McClean[27] however suggest that Kleinman's category of folk medicine begs refinement in the West at least. They make the distinction within Kleinman's folk sector as folk medicine being distinctly separate category from CAM and other forms of healing (such as religious healing) and treatment where monetary payment or prestige is involved.[29]

is continued deference to biomedicine as the gold standard by which other healthcare systems are judged.

However, the evidence that the Western scientific paradigm has usurped the role and importance of cosmology, religion, and folk medicine is unconvincing. It would be a mistake to assume that the developing biomedical system meant that there was no reference to magic, superstition or "otherworldliness." Within the British colonial context, the celebrated doctor Livingstone of Africa, physician and Christian, exemplified the West's best efforts to heal both *the person* and *the soul*. With this, we see not just rapid culture contact, but the resultant growth and exportation of a raft of Western ideas, including Western scientific biomedical and cosmological ideology.

There is significant contemporary literature demonstrating that rather than running counter to science, superstition actually continued to operate alongside science. Magical[7] ideas were just as alive in Elizabethan London as in central Africa.[21]

It is argued here that there is a central problem with modern scientific discourse. Current biomedical practice and modernity have eradicated indigenous healing. The recognition of the importance of cosmology and magic in health care may have been eclipsed by the rise of biomedicine[3] but it did not die. The empirical evidence suggests that superstition coexisted and continues to exist with biomedicine. These ideas are profound, ubiquitous, and embedded not only in lay beliefs and religion but are also incorporated into biomedical practice.[27] Biomedicine and folk medicine (often presented as incompatible modalities) are mutually dependent not only in the developing societies but also in high modernity. Biomedical science collides, colludes, and collaborates with indigenous healthcare systems. This is evidenced by historical[21] and by contemporary ethnographic accounts in the non-Western[1] and Western contexts.[27]

(. . .) *ritual healing is not officially referred to as a healing practice and is segregated as 'superstition' (Chin. mí xìn; Tib. mongdé). Yet in practice, medicine and healing have not become scientized in every domain, as the existence of healing Tantrists (ngagpa) or diviners (mopa) or some traditionally oriented senior lineage doctors of Tibetan medicine demonstrates. This does not mean that they are not in contact with Western medicine.*

---

[7]For ease of reading magic hereafter refers to superstition and practices that may not be scientifically explained but may also refer to established practices that might be deemed as indeed scientific, such as taking ancient remedies for illness.

Rather, they mediate between their healing and biomedicine in relation to their patients, some of whom might receive the latter form of treatment.... Sometimes, biomedicine might appropriate 'religious' or rather ritual traits, often glossed as the 'placebo effect' in the literature. For example, multicolored biomedical pharmaceuticals might have a color-based effectiveness and might be placed in front of an altar or Buddha image .... and pertains to a cultural logic of healing in which 'medicine' and 'religion' are intertwined and not juxtaposed. Sometimes, however, they just exist side by side (Ref. [1], p. 161).

Within the Western context, folk and alternative medicines have become revitalized in recent years. These systems are not as some believe, "New Age" medicine, but have coexisted with the rise of biomedical science.

The noted decline in importance of the established church and the dominance of biomedicine do not mean that people are less spiritual. Modernity has never really been without magical sentiment. In fact we now see a multiplicity of spiritual inspired expression in the form of New Age Movements, some of these have a Christian flavor but others that do not. The likelihood is that these will proliferate and compete for state recognition and resources (as CAM[8] currently do), and the state will seek to enforce regulation and control. This is not, as Kuhling suggests, 'New Age re-enchantment' in a post-Celtic Tiger Ireland (Cited in Cosgrove et al, 2012:201–220), since disenchantment did not happen![28] Another central problem is that while Western scientific biomedicine attempts to debunk other (historical and/or culturally unacceptable) forms of knowledge as "fake" or quackery, it appropriates and uses such practices that cannot be considered to be scientific. The most extreme example of this is what anthropologists often refer to as witchcraft or magic. In modernity, this is reframed by biomedicine as placebo/nocebo.

The expansion of biomedicine as an ideology and practice also coincided with the great historical efforts of many European states in their drive for self-identity and nationalism and for colonial growth and domination. This also raises a number of important questions in regard not only just epistemological concerns but also in terms of sociopolitical and economic factors and to what science means for (Western and non-Western) societies. The postcolonial experience of India is an exemplar of how the ideological power of science (and thereby biomedicine) has

---

[8]Complementary and alternative medicine (CAM).

come to remain dominant even when the British Empire receded. In this regard, India in the immediate postcolonial phase offers a useful example of both the potency of Western biomedical ideology and the problematic nature of biomedicine set in this context (since it derides other healthcare systems). While the postcolonial experiences of countries are as diverse as the nations, ethnic groups, and peoples involved, some commentators have asked, "Where is the post-colonial history of science?" (Ref. [2], p. 360). After all, in the immediate postcolonial period, Nehru regarded science, "as heroic" (Ref. [2], p. 363). It is seen as a gift from the British, as a positive legacy, having qualities that had the potential to liberate a postcolonial India from backwardness. It was believed that Western science would contribute to the possibility of a new, modern, international, self–defined, and assured nation state. As developing societies incorporate more and more biomedical features this raises important questions in relation to continued or *nouveau* colonialism[9]? (The) "Introduction of allopathic drug [sic] during British era and neglecting Indian traditional medicine by British ruler (sic) are responsible for significant erosion of Indian traditional medicine" (Ref. [34], p. 2).

There are also concerns in relation to attempts to biomedicalize, folk or alternative healthcare systems.

In China today, the theoretical distinctions made in public health arenas and by different official representatives of biomedicine, Tibetan medicine and Chinese medicine alike, all belong to a global modern discourse that aims at legitimizing and professionalizing these systems and their medical practices by using biomedical standards (Ref. [1], p. 161).

Orthodox medicine in the West also demands that alternative folk practices be subjected to scientific testing.[36]It should also be remembered that in Western professional medicine, scientific hegemony and practice are relatively new.[10] Surgeons, apothecaries, and physicians (formerly apprenticeships) came together in 1858 in Britain banning all other practitioners outside the new profession. The new medical profession established itself professionally in relation to a cash nexus economy and in so doing lost its personalized and community-based nature. It largely treated those who could best afford it (Ref. [29], p. 38). In contrast, Chinese, **Ayurvedic,**

---

[9]Tibet, for example, began to embrace biomedicine in the 1980s.
[10]Darwin's "On the Origin of Species" was belatedly published in 1859 and in 1858. A formal Act in Britain brought together of apothecary, surgery, and physicians, formalizing medical care and thereby created a monopoly for Western scientific knowledge and medical practice.

Unani, Sidda, Amchi, and Folk medicines provide significant examples of important complex systems where organic and indigenous medical practices exist that display a different and self-sustained logic base tied to community beliefs and expectations, yet may also be viewed as scientific in terms of efficacy and in how treatments are observed and practiced (although some of these buy into or "compliment" biomedicine to some degree or other). These, however, do tend to be more personalized or bespoke in nature.

In modernity, these ancient systems largely fall outside the orbit of the new biomedical science and they are associated with industries in the West. Middle Eastern medicine (e.g., Avicenna's medical cannons) is not referenced within Western medical discourse. Biomedicine appears to trump all other healthcare systems and historical medical practices. While the annual William Harvey[11] Day is celebrated at the oldest biomedical hospitals in England (St Bartholomew and the Royal London Hospitals), there is no such praise, pomp, or ceremony for the writings of Avicenna.[12]

As a medical system, biomedicine goes largely unquestioned in its training, its effectiveness in treating aliments and conditions and in helping to control and manage pain. At the same time, indigenous health beliefs and practices (in traditional, so-called "developing," "traditional," and "modern societies") are largely dismissed off hand (in the West at least) as inherently nonscientific. Folk or indigenous medicine remains "odd," "irrelevant," "iatrogenic," and "dangerous" (as are its practitioners). Such informal medical systems are viewed as the remnants or survival of a superstitious past that are best forgotten.

These positions have largely defined medical systems in the modern era, particularly in the industrial or postindustrial West. Biomedicine became so dominant as to mask Western folk medical practices and remove virtually all traces from official discourse. However, contrary to concerted attempts to remove, make illegal, or to do down organic healthcare systems in the West, there is no compelling evidence to show that such beliefs and practices have been eradicated anywhere. Comparative literature illustrates that, biomedicine, did not hold a complete monopoly over or displace other healthcare practices in either modern or modernizing societies. Even in the most hostile environments such as the former Soviet Union, these practices appear to have remained and coexisted.[27] As various historical

---

[11]William Harvey (1578–1657).
[12]Avicenna (Ibn Sina, around 980—1037).

and contemporary anthropological data suggest, it is difficult to dispel the use and significance of folk medicine in advanced or "post-Industrial" societies. And it is the non-discussion of these other systems that remains the biggest "elephant in the room." Within the biomedical establishment, we observe public disavowal (yet, for many practitioners, private belief in, and/or acceptance of the role of informal healthcare practices) offers itself as an ardent critique of biomedical ideology. The evidence suggests that it is intermingled with and even dependent on other systems. The evidence suggests a contingency and fluidity between biomedicine and other healthcare systems in the West,[28] and in developing nations.[1]

14.3 DEMOCRACY AND ACCOUNTABILITY

The contemporary significance of this is the rise in the recognition of the failings in biomedical health practice in the West and in the reluctance in replacing trusted indigenous practices with biomedicine. In the West, patient dissatisfaction is fast becoming a problem for biomedicine. Affordable computer technology and the Internet revolution have helped accelerate the democratization of knowledge, including medical knowledge.

Public concern and lay uneasiness with many aspects of biomedical practice have begun to undermine the epistemological superiority accorded to biomedicine, has led to the rise of patient activism, and have helped reinvigorate folk, complementary, and alternative medicine (CAM).[7,30] Some have argued that this has also made alternative medicine more acceptable, "increasing accountability and the legitimacy afforded to patients' wishes in Western Medicine and the increasing acceptance of some 'alternative' practices" (Ref. [33], p. 98). The literature points to increased public awareness in new (modern) forms of risk and a realist perspective in relation to the benefits and limits of biomedicine. A canon of literature has emerged[4,8,26,39] and risk, trust, and health chances have now emerged as dominant themes in the sociology/anthropology of health and public health.[5,22]. Public understanding of science and medicine is now fast becoming a commanding feature and is currently afforded a high consideration in research, including biomedical research.[14,15]

14.4   THE FUTURE OF HOLISTIC HEALTH CARE

While biomedicine has been interpreted as offering respectability to emerging nations, the scientific foundations it claims, as well as its efficacy, are questioned not just in the developing societies. Health care in the West is, in truth, characterized by eclectic medical practices.[9,16,17,19,30] Much of the recent literature discusses how different epistemologies and practices intersect and coexist. Moore, for example, illustrates with ethnographic work conducted in Ireland, showed the importance of "the cure" or "the charm." It is widely believed that some individuals with "the charm" have the ability to cure an illness or multiple illnesses. This knowledge is largely secret and hidden, only discussed at times of crisis, but it is well understood locally and utilized when necessary by many ordinary people, professionals, including a wide range of health professionals. In Ireland, this has its roots in pagan health belief systems, and it transcends both the religious and social class divide.

I have an open mind on them, because I have seen them work both in my professional capacity and in our private life…. I remember the doctor sending me to an old man who lived more or less like a hermit in an old shack and the doctor said to me. "You may go down and do the best you can, …. for that man has shingles, and just get the clothes off him and treat him with Gentian Violet". So on my way home that evening I called and I really never saw anything like it in my whole professional career…. He says, "Will you quit worrying nurse. I'm going for the charm tonight". I said to myself. Oh, does he think he is going to get ride of this in a day or two. But quite honestly, within a week he was completely cured and I couldn't see it in a month. (Madge, Senior Community Nurse, in Ref. [27], p. 117).

The ethnographic evidence shows that even those trained in biomedicine referred people to curers. In reality, ordinary people when faced with health problems will utilize whatever resources are available, that are trusted and seen to work, or at the very least offer solace or hope. This includes practices that may be regarded as more occult:

Illness can affect all levels of the body—the individual, social, environmental and cosmological—even though one might need at times more attention than the other. In times of crisis and depending on the local situatedness, to cover all options and levels at the same time might be simply the most efficacious. Therefore, mantra and 'syringe' do not exclude each other, and ritual healing can play an equally important role in patients' health-seeking behaviour alongside the influence of institutionalized medical practice and public health policies (Ref. [1], p. 177).

These practices are more personal and holistic in nature and include bioscience as one aspect of the caring process.

14.5 CONCLUSION

While closing this chapter, I hoped to illustrate not only the acceptance, importance, and centrality of enduring local, more holistic indigenous health systems but also their resilience in the face of modernity and amid powerful historical forces, ideological discourse, and authority. In returning to Leslie's text, we should note not only the importance between different healthcare systems but also the overlap of medical practice between various healthcare systems in various contexts. This discussion illustrates, for example, how informal, folk, and holistic medicine and biomedicine do not simply coexist, but importantly, have historically been and remain codependent on one another.[27] As in the case of the nascent state of India, biomedical practices, that appear modern and progressive, may rather have degenerative consequences and this is a warning to other such nations and cultural configurations.

Similarly, it should be recognized that, in the West, folk and alternative medicine is experiencing a serious revival, and this is currently stimulated discussion and debate within biomedicine about the role and salience of these alternative systems. In response, some have sought to medicalize (and therefore control) indigenous healing practices. Others highlight the importance and the (pragmatic, functional, social, and spiritual) value of alternative healthcare resources. One thing is clear. The discussion points to medical pluralism as the norm rather than the exception for health care for most people in the modern world. Progressive biomedical commentators call for a tentative understanding of alternative medical practices with a view to some kind of accommodation since the alternative, the *status quo*, is clearly problematic for both biomedicine and folk medicine.

KEYWORDS

- medicine
- science
- indigenous
- anthropology
- colonial
- cross-cultural

REFERENCES

1. Adams, V., Schrempf, M.; Craig, S. *Medicine Between Science and Religion: Explorations on Tibetan Grounds*; Berghahn: New York, Oxford, 2010.
2. Arnold, D. Nehruvian Science and Postcolonial India. *Isis* **2013,** *104* (2), 360–370.
3. Bakx, K. The Eclipse of Folk Medicine in Western Society. *Sociol. Health Illness*, **1991,** *13* (1) 20–38. DOI:10.1111/1467-9566.ep11340307.
4. Beck, U. *Risk Society. Toward a New Modernity*; Sage: London, 1992.
5. Barrett, R.; Moore, R. G.; Staines, A. Blood Transfusion in Ireland: Perceptions of Risk, A Question of Trust. *Health Risk Soc.* **2007,** *9* (4), 375–388.
6. Bunton, R.; Petersen, A., Eds. *Foucault, Health and Medicine*, Routledge: London, 2002.
7. Cant, S.; Sharma, U. Alternative Health Practices and Systems. In *Handbook of Social Studies in Health and Medicine*; Albrecht, G., Fitzpatrick, R., Scrimshaw, S., Eds.; Sage: London, 2000; pp 426–439.
8. Douglas, M. *Risk and Blame: Essays in Cultural Theory*; Routledge: London, 1992.
9. Eisenberg, D. M.; Kaptchuk, T. J.; Laine, C.; Davidoff, F. Complementary and Alternative Medicine—An Annals Series. *Ann. Intern. Med.* **2001,** *135* (3), 208–208.
10. Erlanger, J. The Past and the Future of the Medical Sciences in the United States. *Science* **1922,** *55* (1415), 135–145.
11. Evans Pritchard, E. E. *Witchcraft, Oracles and Magic among the Azande*; Clarendon Press: Oxford, 1976.
12. Foucault, M. *The Birth of the Clinic. An Archaeology of Medical Perception*; Tavistock: London, 1973.
13. Gawande, A. *Being Mortal: Illness, Medicine and What Matters in the End;* Profile Books: London, 2014.
14. Gobat, N. H.; Gal, M.; Francis, N.; Hood, K.; Watkins, A.; Turner, J.; Moore, R.; Webb, S. A. R.; Butler, C. C.; Nichol, A. Key Stakeholder Perceptions about Consent to Participate in Acute Illness Research: A Rapid, Systematic Review to Inform epi/Pandemic Research Preparedness. *Trials* **2015,** *16* (1), 1.
15. Gobat, N.; Gal, M.; Butler, C. C.; Francis, N. A.; Anthierens, S.; Bastiaens, H.; Godycki-ćwirko, M.; *et al.* Public Attitudes Towards Research Participation

During an Infectious Disease Pandemic: A Qualitative Study Across Four European Countries. *Lancet* **2016**, *388*, S51.

16. Hand, W. D. The Folk Healer: Calling and Endowment. *J. Hist. Med. Allied Sci.* **1971**, *26* (3), 263–275.

17. Hand, W. D. *Magical Medicine: The Folkloric Component of Medicine in the Folk Belief, Custom, and Ritual of the Peoples of Europe and America: Selected Essays of Wayland D. Hand*. Univ. of California Press: Berkeley, 1980.

18. Heritage, J.; Maynard, D. W. Problems and Prospects in the Study of Physician–Patient Interaction: 30 Years of Research. *Annu. Rev. Sociol.* **2006**, *32*, 351–374.

19. Hufford, D. J. Folk Medicine and Health Culture in Contemporary Society. *Prim. Care* **1997**, *24* (4), 723–741.

20. Jewson, N. D. The Disappearance of the Sick-Man from Medical Cosmology, 1770–1870. *Sociology* **1976**, *10* (2), 225–244.

21. Kassell, L. *Medicine and Magic in Elizabethan London*. Clarendon Press: Oxford, 2005.

22. Kawachi, I.; Kennedy, B. P.; Lochner, K.; Prothrow-Stith, D. Social Capital, Income Inequality, and Mortality. *Am. J. Public Health* **1997**, *87* (9), 1491–1498.

23. Kleinman, A. *Patients and Healers in the Context of Culture: An Exploration of the Borderland between Anthropology, Medicine and Psychiatry*; University of California, Press: Berkeley, 1980.

24. Leslie, C., Ed. *Asian Medical Systems: A Comparative Study*; University of California Press: Berkeley, 1977.

25. Löwy, I. Historiography of Biomedicine: "Bio," "Medicine," and in Between. *Isis* **2011**, *102* (1), 116–122. DOI:10.1086/658661.

26. Luhmann, N. *Risk: A Sociological Theory*. Routledge: New York, 2002.

27. Moore, R. G.; McClean, S., Eds.; *Folk Healing and Health Care Practices in Britain and Ireland: Stethoscopes, Wands and Crystals*. Berghahn: New York, Oxford, 2010.

28. Moore, R. Beyond Religion, Science and Secularism: Health Beliefs and Complex Diversity in the North of Ireland. *RECODE, Online Working Paper No. 23*; 2014. http://www.recode.fi.

29. McClean, S.; Moore, R. Money, Commodification and Complementary Health Care: Theorising Personalised Medicine within Depersonalised Systems of Exchange. *Soc. Theor. Health* **2013**, *11* (2), 194–214.

30. McQuaide, M. M. The Rise of Alternative Health Care: A Sociological Account. *Soc. Theor. Health* **2005**, *3* (4), 286–301.

31. Parsons, T. *The Social System*; Routledge & Kegan Paul: London, 1951.

32. Pickstone, J. V. Sketching Together the Modern Histories of Science, Technology, and Medicine. *Isis* **2011**, *102* (1), 123–133. DOI:10.1086/657506.

33. Pickstone, J. V.; Warboys, M. Focus: Between and Beyond 'Histories of Science' and 'Histories of Medicine. *Isis* **2011**, *102* (1), 97–101 (The University of Chicago Press). http://www. Jstor.org/stable/10.1086/658658 (accessed Dec 20, 2016).

34. Sen, S.; Chakraborty, R. Revival, Modernization and Integration of Indian Traditional Herbal Medicine in Clinical Practice: Importance, Challenges and Future. *J. Tradit. Complement. Med.* **2017**, *7* (2), 234–244.

35. Scheper-Hughes, N. Parts Unknown Undercover Ethnography of the Organs-Trafficking Underworld. *Ethnography* **2004**, *5* (1), 29–73.

36. Sharma, U. Using Alternative Medicine. *Health Visitor* **1991,** *64* (2), 50–51.
37. Sigerist, H. E. Preface to Volume IV. The History of Medicine and the History of Science. An Open Letter to George Sarton, Editor of Isis. *Bull. History Med.* **1936,** *4,* 1.
38. Szasz, T. *The Myth of Mental Illness: Foundations of a Theory of Personal Conduct.* Secker: London, 1961.
39. Sztompka, P. *Trust: A Sociological Theory*; Cambridge University Press: Cambridge, 1999.
40. Thomas, K. *Religion and the Decline of Magic*; Penguin: London, 1973.

CHAPTER 15

SPINAL PHYSIOLOGY RECOVERY OR RUSSIAN ALTERNATIVE TO CHINESE ACUPUNCTURE

KLIMENKO M. MIKHAILOVICH*

Academy of Medical Technology, OOO Scientific Industrial Enterprise "Exergy," Lenina Prospect Bld. 120, Apt. 131, 650023 Kemerovo, Russia

*E-mail: Leonardo-co@yandex.ru

ABSTRACT

For more than 2000 years, the method of Chinese acupuncture has been used for the treatment of spinal disorders. About 20 years ago, on the failures of Chinese medicine, a Russian method emerged. This method became the basis for the development of new medical technologies in the treatment of spine and comorbidities.

15.1 INTRODUCTION

Each human body is designed with a strong health potential. If we use at least half of it, we would live without knowing what pain is. This is pointed out by ancient knowledge about diseases treatment, which was groped for many thousands of years. From the depths of the centuries, we gained a unique opportunity to recover our health naturally.

There are several methods of pain management. Today, among them, the only popular is acupuncture or needle therapy (or reflexotherapy), which is an ancient practice of Chinese medicine born several thousands of years ago, very far from China. Its root is in interruption of pain impulse and endorphin rush into blood. Apart traditional needle therapy, there's used acupressure, which is a kind of acupuncture that includes rubbing, fire acupuncture, applications with metal plates, Su Jok therapy, and others. The Chinese believe that needles open the holes for illness to go out and fire kills the illness.

It should seem that the Chinese system created meets completely the requirements of the treatment process. Considering this, it was quite unexpected to hear in a private discussion from a Chinese high-level officer that he had 3 milliards of diseased spines. This statement is rather factually accurate (as judged by health condition of Chinese workers and entrepreneurs living in Russia as well as, then again, of Urumchi residents in China).

In the 1980s, an ability of our body was discovered, which was when working with spine via paravertebral zone, patients could release their acute spine pains. Then, a method of biomechanical therapy of patient's spine for relaxation of paravertebral muscles with no drug or other exterior help was developed. Besides this, it was noticed that application of medications or other exterior help (acupuncture, manual therapy, etc.) negated the treatment effectiveness and remission sustainability. Further research upon acute and chronical pains management and following-up of patients during remission has led to development of a system of therapeutic maneuvers named autokinesiotherapy (AKT), which is sometimes called Russian Alternative (as worded by the Ministry of Health of the Russian Federation—M. M. Klimenko massage and gymnastic method). While using this method, between the patient and the physician, a mutual understanding is established, risk of unwanted side effects is reduced, and medical malpractice is mitigated. The major part of responsibility for the treatment success is automatically taken by the patient himself. The physician gets more time to analyze the patient's condition and to correct the therapeutic approach. Such direct care design has led to the state when some nosologies considered incurable started responding to the treatment, and some nosologies showed contradictions to the existing concepts of the diseases. Beside this, on the one hand, the new system outlined a few negative developments when physicians abuse medicinal treatment with analgesics and hormones replacing organism's functions and causing unwanted side effects. On the other, patients, having experienced the method's effectiveness, started using the method independently from any assistance of specialists (especially in the locations where medical attendance is not much available). This reflects the current state of the medicine where some specialists do not want to implement more effective treatment methods.

15.2   STUDY MATERIALS AND METHODS

The main apparatus for research on AKT is the complex KUMP-01 (complex of devices for vertebral massage-01).[1] The main method of AKT is in working with spine with the help of the massage and gymnastic instrument (MGI), which has more than 100 variants of manipulations. The use of MGI ranges from recovery of normal physiological spine curvatures and motor patterns to intensification of metabolic processes in our body.

For logging of the study results, a spirometer, a visual analogue scale (VAS) a scoliometer, "Diton" (an apparatus for identification of preinsult and precrisis states), a thermovision display device "Svit," a video camera "Panasonic," and a dynamic pain display (DPD) were used.

15.2.1   STUDY METHOD

The study method consists of two parts.

The first part of the method is based on instrumental measurements of changes in physiological parameters of organism while working on the complex KUMP-01. Upon the procedures, the following measurements were made:

- Changes in lung volume under influence of MGI on breast with the help of spirometer;
- Changes in motor pattern under the influence of MGI with the help of video camera "Panasonic";
- Changes in spine and obliquity of pelvis with the help of scoliometer;
- Synchronic measurements of arterial blood pressure in hands and legs before, during, and after the procedure with the help of the apparatus "Diton";
- Changes of skin cover temperature upon the procedure with the help of a thermovision display device "Svit";
- Pain measurements on VAS and DPD.

Upon the procedure on KUMP-01, the spinal column is unloaded in vertical plane of the body and the intensity of compression state of the nerve roots is lowered. The complex KUMP-01 is designed to provide the patient simultaneously with the following[2]:

1.   Influencing on the spinal columns meridians (according to Chinese terminology);
2.   Manual influence on intervertebral joints and physiological curvatures;
3.   Microexercises for intervertebral joints;
4.   Exercises for pectoral and pelvis arches;
5.   Massage for muscles of neck, spine, pelvis, legs, abdomen, and chest;
6.   Imitation of cupping treatment;
7.   Optimization of blood, lymph, liquor, and tissue fluid flow.

So, namely, the combinations of the abovementioned effects cause therapeutic effects in the form of

1.   Recovery of normal physiological curvatures of the spinal column.
2.   Recovery of natural reflexes.
3.   Recovery of natural temperament.
4.   Psychosomatic immunity.

The second part of the study shows some comparisons of AKT with the method of Chinese acupuncture and European neurology as well as an analysis of the results received.

15.3   RESULTS AND DISCUSSIONS

The research was conducted on the patients suffering with spinal pains (in spine, hands and legs) who could not be helped in traditional medical institutions. Such patients were classified as having neuroorthopedic pathologies which reflected the essentials of spinal column diseases more completely. The patients were going around the circles, their pains caused scoliosis, and scoliosis caused pains, what, most likely, was the very reason of all failures when treatment was held separately by neurologists and orthopedists. Nevertheless, already while the first procedure, the patients showed comorbidities, which did not match with the terms of neuroorthopedic pathologies. Upon the current healthcare system, such patients should have been sent to rheumatologists, pulmonologists, nephrologists, and other specialists. Nut, as the main problems, was in the spinal column, we invited these specialists to follow these patients mutually and simultaneously on the complex KUMP-01 on each nosology. It means, on the complex KUMP-01 patients received treatments on several nosologies simultaneously. At that, the treatment procedures for the spinal column were also well influencing their comorbidities. Consequently, in the practical use of the AKT method, we have gained good effects on more than 50 nosologies. The list of the nosologies is provided in Table 15.1. To maintain everything clear and not to introduce any new nosology, we completed Table 15.1 in accordance with common standards of pathologies classification.

TABLE 15.1   Pathology.

1.	In the field of neuroorthopedic pathologies
1.1.	Diagnostics preclinical developments
1.2.	Correction of postural disorder, "computer scoliosis"
1.3.	Correction of functional scoliosis
1.4.	Correction of morphological scoliosis
1.5.	Correction of the spinal column's "depression"
1.6.	Correction of chest deformation (costal humpback, carnitines)
1.7.	Stopping of acute pain in degenerative disk disease (scapulohumeral periarthritis, sciatic nerve impaction, repetitive stress injury, intercostal neuralgia)
1.8.	Stopping of chronical pains for degenerative disk disease
1.9.	Stopping of pains of pelvic organs
1.10.	Rotational deformations of the spinal column complicated with forth level of kyphoscoliosis deformation, right and left-sided gibbuses, deflation of shoulder bone
1.11.	Relaxation of cramps
1.12.	Correction of listhesis
1.13.	Prevention of recurrence of degenerative disk diseases
1.14.	Compensation of cardiac syndrome
1.15.	Treatment of stenocardia
1.16.	Stopping of carpal syndrome

TABLE 15.1 *(Continued)*

1.17.	Treatment of plexopathy
1.18.	Treatment of neuropathy
1.19.	Treatment of vegetovascular dystonia
1.20.	Treatment of hydrocephaly
1.21.	Treatment of unstable spinal column
1.22.	Compensation of vertebral arteria syndrome (vegetovascular dystonia, brain blood supply disturbance)
1.23.	Treatment of infantile cerebral paralysis
1.24.	Stopping neurasthenic syndrome
1.25.	Rehabilitation of patients after surgery
1.26.	Prevention
2.	In the field of rheumatic pathologies
2.1.	Compensation of rheumatoid arthritis attack (polyarthritis)
2.2.	Stopping of chronic pain for scapulohumeral periarthritis
2.3.	Stopping of pain for deforming arthrosis
2.4.	Treatment of knee-joints arthritis
3.	In the field of somatic pathologies
3.1.	Prevention of ischemic strokes
3.2.	Stopping of ischemic stroke
3.3.	Fallot's tetrad
3.4.	Stabilization of hemodynamical parameters (arterial tension) on normal figures
3.5.	Restoration of reproductive functions in women
3.6.	Restoration of sexual potency
3.7.	Treatment of cystitis
3.8.	Prevention of renal diseases
3.9.	Stopping of cochvestibular syndrome
3.10.	Treatment of gastroptosis
3.11.	Treatment of hyperhidrosis (hydrosis)
3.12.	Prevention of somatic diseases
3.13.	Treatment of dysmenorrhea
4.	In the field of autoimmune diseases
4.1.	Treatment of bronchial asthma
4.2.	Relaxation of bronchospasm while working with paravertebral zone

TABLE 15.1 *(Continued)*

4.2.	Treatment of ankylosing spondylitis (Bekhterev's disease)
4.3.	Treatment of allergic rhinitis
5.	In the palliative care
5.1.	Pain relief for oncological diseases
5.2.	Rehabilitation after clinical death
5.3.	Treatment of patients with paraparesis and tetraparesis
5.4.	Improvements in the course of somatic comorbidities including:
5.4.1.	Bronchitis
5.4.2.	Pneumonia
5.4.3.	Cardiovascular insufficiency
6.	Spinal cord injuries
6.1.	Compression fractures
6.2.	Tailbone fracture
6.3.	"Vertical crash"

As it is shown in Table 15.2, on the complex KUMP-01, the patient's body responds to the procedures positively and more actively than while treatment with widespread methods. We could not find any explanation to this phenomenon. That's why, to explain the results received there were developed some hypothesizes (suggestions) that could explain the therapeutic effects gained. We will show the actuality of some hypothesizes by comparing the contemporary vision of nosologies with the results of treatment on KUMP-01.

1. Upon acute pain, the patient is immobilized and treated with analgesics.
   Hypothesis: While working with KUMP-01, the movements are used that support peristaltic processes in muscles providing spasm management and improving liquor drainage from the spinal canal. At that, each movement is accompanied with endorphins rush from the hippocampus. Consequently, to manage pains, human body has two processes—cerebrospinal fluid drainage and endorphins production in hippocamp. At that, there's no necessity to use analgesics that replace endorphin, and, in some cases, narcotic analgesics withdrawal is possible.

2. According to a published data, if somewhere in body members a pain arises, then in the brain, pain centers are formed. But in the complex KUMP-01, patients controlled pains by influencing the spinal column and, in most cases, during the first procedure. It is also proved by control of phantom limb pain that disturbed the patient especially in change of weather.

   Hypothesis: The pain centers are in the spinal cord or the mechanism of pain development is out of all relation to pain centers formation.

3. In the treatment on the complex KUMP-01, the left and the right parts of the body respond to the influence independently, especially in terms of hemodynamical parameters. At that, it was determined that within the age range of 20–94, the normal pressure should be 120/70 mmHg ± 10 points, and, at any deviation from these figures, it is necessary to search for a pathology not only in the cardiovascular system. At the equalization of systolic pressure on the left and right hands, sciatic nerve entrapment syndrome disappeared.

   Hypothesis: In unanimity of our organism, the left and the right sides of our body live independently.

   This fact clearly explains the reasons of gibbus in girls' puberty.

   Hypothesis: Gibbus formed in puberty of girls is caused by malfunction of paired organs, ovaries, against a background of connective tissue dysplasia.

4. The complex KUMP-01 was designed to control the spinal pains. At that, it was noticed that normal physiological curves of the spinal column were automatically restored. This was accompanied by scoliosis correction. Deformity of physiological curves caused pains return, consequently, all other types of lordosis were considered as disturbance.

   Hypothesis: Any deviation from physiologically normal curves of the spinal column, both lumbar and cervical, causes fatigue supertension of muscles, in the first place, of the paravertebral zone and launches the mechanism of disks pathology development, and the discomfort in the localities of supertension indicates this long before the clinical manifestation of the disease. It follows that in presence of discomfort in spine, the patient cannot be considered in remission.

Due to this hypothesis, a preventive regime against recurrence of degenerative disk diseases was developed and extended the application range of the complexes KUMP-01 up to the level of training device, which made possible to provide the treatment domiciliary.

5. In the formation of lordosis, on the complex KUMP-01, the patient automatically controls pains both in root compression and disk dehydration independently and, without the use of medicaments, restores physiological curves of the spinal column.

    Hypothesis: Disk deformation predisposes pain, but its development is going according other laws, and this pain can be controlled in presence of both disk deformation and disks dehydration, at any age as well.

6. In controlling spinal pains of the patients suffering from bronchial asthma and exercising on the complex KUMP-01, the increase of vital lungs volume for from 15% to 40% was noticed. At that, the bronchial asthma attack proceeded more easily or disappeared completely. Some patients acquired the ability to control asthma attacks independently by moving shoulders.

    Hypothesis: A bronchial asthma attack is a defensive reaction of organism that most often occurs because of allergens. Because of our life style, lumina in bronchi are narrow, the reaction to allergens makes it narrower, spasms are summed up, and asphyxia occurs. Influencing the spinal column, we release the spasm of the bronchial tree, which is formed due to our life style, bronchi spread up to the normal state and the spasm against the allergen becomes a normal defensive reaction of organism. So, we can trace the dependence of bronchial asthma attack on the state of the spinal column

7. According to clinical observations of pain control in body members, there arose a hypothesis of changes of the spinal column state and formation of pain in paravertebral zone.

    Hypothesis: As hands and legs pains are controlled on the complexes KUMP-01, generally, by influencing only one spinal zone, then the pain develops in spinal column, irradiates into members, and is controlled by the change of the cerebrospinal fluid drainage regime.

8. In treatment of cramps, they use a hypothesis of calcium and magnesium deficiency in the organism and, consequently, assign a

related drug therapy. Exercises on KUMP-01 stop cramps within several minutes; at that, there is no possibility to change magnesium or calcium content.

Hypothesis: Cramps are caused by increased liquor pressure in the spinal canal and practically do not depend on calcium or magnesium content in the organism.

9. The spinal column does not remain unchanged throughout life as form of its separate elements and the spinal column changes with age not only because of physical activity but also physiological processes depending on motor activity and nutrition of the patient.

   Hypothesis: A nerve root that is responsible for a certain part of the organism starts giving signals about a problem occurred and shows the information, about itself, but we feel it as pain in the part of the organism, for which it is responsible.

On the ground of the hypothesis developed, some researches were undertaken in terms of the spinal column state and its development metamorphosis, which provided the basis for 50 designed treatment methods that are most adequate to physiological state of the spinal column. This allowed to increase effectiveness of treatment of the spinal column and provided possibility to manage somatic diseases by influencing the spine. Today, more than 200,000 patients have received treatment. Effectiveness of some of the methods reaches 95%. Now, there is a real opportunity to provide a real help in disorders that are believed to be cureless.

Below, there are some examples of the practical use of AKT as compared to Chinese acupuncture and European neurology, as well as the differences in views in terms of the pathologies treatment, which occurred while working with AKT. Table 15.2 represents an example of cramps treatment.

TABLE 15.2 Comparison of Treatment Methods.

Cramps (cramps in legs)		
Chinese acupuncture	**European neurology**	**AKT**
There is applied the method of strong (braking) influence. In *this method*, stimulation is strong, intensive, long lasting, with gradually increasing deep effect on small quantity of points or a small zone. In the affected zone, the patient feels aches, spreading, warmth, electrical current irradiating to the periphery or to the center as well as to the sides. One influence usually covers from 2–3 to 4–6 points. This method is called relaxing, sedating, hypotensive, analgesic. The session lasts 15–20 min	Drug treatment gives limited improvement of health state, which is accompanied with occurrence of problems in digestive tract Manual influence and massage procedures last 20–30 min. The cramps control effect is instable	While working with AKT, cramps stop within 3–5 min during the first procedure in 95% of the patients. Influence is made by the method of reclination for 15–30 s. 30% of the patients feel discomfort on the next day, which is stopped with the help of AKT within 5–7 min Hypothesis: The pathology is connected to increased pressure in spinal canal because of disorder of liquor drainage
Length of treatment is up to 10 sessions. Some patients show fear of needles. The treatment course may be repeated for 2–3 times. Remission length is not predictable	Length of treatment may reach from 2–3 weeks to 6 months. Recurrence is possible	Usually, 1–4 procedures are sufficient to stop the cramps. Remission depends on the life style and may last for from 6 months up to 1–2 years
Most often, it is applied in occurrence of hyperfunctions in organs and systems, paroxysms, cramps, and pains. The cause of hyperfunction is usually not specified, but covered with Eastern philosophy	The main cause is explained as microelements deficiency in the organism	It is impossible to specify the influence of microelements deficit on occurrence of cramps, as the patient stopped the cramps earlier than the microelements content changed
Treatment expense for overall time		
200 min	More than 2 weeks	20 min

Table 15.3 shows the example of intercostal neuralgia treatment.

TABLE 15.3 Comparison of Treatment Methods.

Intercostal neuralgia		
Chinese acupuncture	**European neurology**	**AKT**
Points of the Heart Meridian

The *Chi Chuan* point is located on the level of plica axillaries, at the lower end of large muscle of chest and the inner end of the biceps muscle of arm. It is used to treat pericarditis, intercostal neuralgia, and hysteria | Intercostal neuralgia or thoracalgia means a pathological process occurring because of pressure, inflammation, or irritation of intercostal nerves. To release the pain, syndrome several physiotherapeutic methods are used: UHF iontophoresis with Novocain, reflexotherapy with influencing on special zones of skin cover responsible for sensibility of intercostal nerves, needle therapy, vacuum therapy, pharmacopuncture with injection of medicines in acupuncture points, magnet therapy, and laser treatment. The complex of therapeutic interventions often include local treatment—creams, balms with pain killing, warming and anti-inflammatory effect, having relaxing and warming influence and indirectly lowering pain limits with agents consisting of insect poisons. Pepper plaster also releases muscles and lowers pain syndrome | The patient is laid down on MGI, then, by changing the height of MGI, they influence the spinal column until the pain releases. Acute pains are stopped during the first procedures lasting for up to 30 min. Chronical pains are stopped within 10–20 procedures. Length of remission depends on life style and may reach from 3 months to 1 year. If discomfort reappears, the procedures are repeated for 3–7 times until the complete disappearance of the symptoms. Drug support is not used

Hypothesis: Increased pressure in spinal canal because of disorder of liquor drainage causes intercostal neuralgia |
Unsustained remission	Unsustained remission	Sustained remission
Treatment expense for overall time		
Unpredictable	Unpredictable	From 20 to 30 days

15.3.1 LONG-LASTING SUBACUTE PERIOD IN DEGENERATIVE DISK DISEASE

Patients came to our medical center after neurologists referred them to psychotherapists for "regulation of a pain center formed in brain."[3] Working with AKT stopped pain during the first procedures in 85% of patients. Sustained remission was gained after 20–30 procedures. There was no known sign of presence and influence of a pain center in brain on pains in spinal column. There was a necessity of rehabilitation after the influence of side effects from medicaments taken earlier (especially reoperine).

15.3.2 IN ACUTE PERIOD

Pains were stopped during the first procedure in 90% of the patients with degenerative disk disease, both lumbar and cervical, and polyregional as well.[3] At that, the influence was directed to thoracic section and lower part of pelvis only. After stopping acute pains, the influence zone was enlarged; consequently, the length of acute state was decreased as compared to medical treatment. This served as an argument to suppose that every even very small movement of muscles is accompanied with adequate endorphin rush resulting in pain relief.

The use of AKT suggests considering the degenerative disk disease as a system disease without dividing it into regions. This conclusion is proved by the fact that while influencing on only one section of the spinal column, pain stops sustainably in all other sections, and, accordingly, division of the spinal column into sections makes no sense.

Figure 15.1 shows an example of sequestration. During the first procedure, the patient managed to control acute pain. During the fifth procedure, the patient entered the remission mode, pain stopped, but full recovery of motor pattern in legs did not occur.

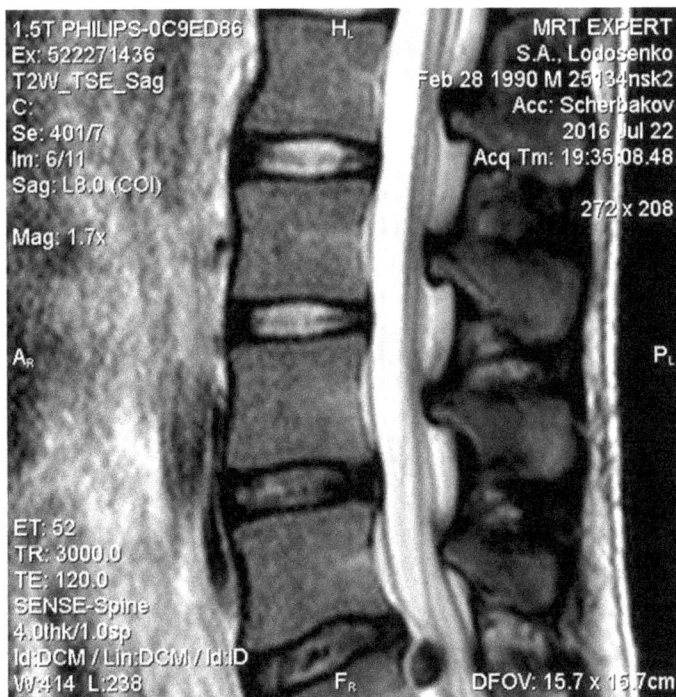

FIGURE 15.1   The example of sequestration.

15.3.3   ORTHOPEDIC PATHOLOGIES

The most effective orthopedic pathology was treatment of birth trauma with hip joints dislocation and incomplete dislocation by influencing on sacral joints.[4] There was no drug treatment or physical therapy led. Motor stereotypes of legs recovered for 85–90% after 2 months.

15.3.4   CORRECTION OF SCOLIOTIC SPINE

It was led intensively, 1 h of exercise per day with increasing load during 1 or 2 months and lasted for up to 1 year and more in compensator regime. Physical therapy was refused.

15.3.5 CORRECTION KYPHOSCOLIOSIS

After surgical treatment of kyphoscoliosis of 3–4 grade, long-term effects were accompanied with pains in spine and unpredictable deformations.[5] For pain control and correction of reappearing deformations, some training devices were developed based on KUMP-01, which led the gibbus correction process out the limits of medical care into sports and health mode. Today, these training devices are working in 12 countries around the world including the United States, Canada, Germany, and Israel. Working with AKT let to a necessity to divide these disorders in terms of their etiology into two groups:

1. The first group—deformation in young girls in puberty.
2. The second group—long-lasting static load of "deliberate computer workers" and lovers to sit crookedly.

This division was made because gibbus is well corrected without surgery in female patients at the age of from 50 to 60 after menopause. The correction period is 1–2 years. It should be noted that correction of scoliosis of 4 up to 1 grade is well managed in 40% of the children. 30% of the children show imperceptible correction. But even these humble results should not be ignored as the quality of life of the patients after their work with AKT independently on the correction results is much higher than before and after surgery, especially in long-term period. It is proved by video recordings on a video camera "Panasonic."

15.3.6 SOMATIC PATHOLOGIES

While treatment of the spinal column on KUMP-01, the patients noticed disappearance of symptoms of somatic nosologies and their overall health improved.[6]

This served as an argument to follow the changes in patients with somatic pathologies, while working with the spinal column. In the following subsections, a few examples of most common nosologies are given.

15.3.7   UROLOGY

One of the most common somatic nosologies is cystitis. As practice showed, working with paravertebral zone during 10–15 procedures calms the process and causes remission. Influence effectiveness reaches 90%, at that parallel use of drug treatment in the control groups of patients did not affect the treatment results. This does not match the common vision of cystitis as just a virus and parasitic pathology. According to data received from urologists, recently, the occurrence of pathological irritation of urinary bladder increased.

15.3.8   GYNECOLOGY

In treatment of dysmenorrhea (menstrual cramps) chronical pains are stopped after 5–7 procedures, acute pains are stopped during the first procedure.

Hypothesis: Increased pressure in spinal canal because of disorder in liquor drainage causes pains in dysmenorrhea.

15.3.9   RESTORING OF FEMALE REPRODUCTIVE FUNCTIONS

Here are some extracts from patient's charts provided by a gynecologist–endocrinologist from the city of Omsk.

Female patient: L.A., born in 1976. Diagnosis: primary sterility (for 7 years); chronical pyelonephritis, regularly recurring form. The patient received a preparatory treatment course with the use of homeopathic medicines and phytopreparations as well as the course of AKT from the 5th to 16th day of menstrual cycle during 3 months. During the treatment pregnancy came.

Female patient: M.O., born in 1975. Diagnosis: secondary sterility (for 9 years); genital endometriosis, common form of the second severity level, adenomyosis, endometriotic left ovarian cyst, chronical enterocolitis. Against a background of a regular course of AKT pregnancy came. Timely delivery. Cesarean section (considering the patient's anamnesis). The baby is healthy.

Female patient: A.O., born in 1978. Diagnosis: primary sterility (for 6 years); Scoliosis of second level, menstrual cycle disorder, amenorrhea.

The patient had a preparatory course with the use of homeopathic medicines and phytopreparations, as well as the course of AKT from the 5th to 16th day of menstrual cycle during 4 months. During the treatment pregnancy came. No pathologies. Timely normal delivery. The baby is healthy.

Female patient: C.A., born in 1985. Diagnosis: menstrual cycle disorder, amenorrhea. State after because of toxic goiter. Against a background of homeopathic medicines, hiruditherapy and courses of AKT—the menstrual cycle recovered.

Female patient: M.A., born in 1979. The patient came with the following diagnosis: primary sterility (for 3 years); menstrual cycle disorder, resistant ovary syndrome. Has been observed in the clinic since 2002. Menstrual cycle recovered. In 2004 and 2010—two timely deliveries. The patient uses homeopathic medicines, a course of AKT once per 3 months.

The procedures without the use of homeopathic medicines and phytopreparations, only on the complexes KUMP-01, restoring of reproductive functions occurred. Today, more than 3000 women in Russia with primary and secondary infertility have become moms. Upon the use of KUMP-01 at the early stages of pregnancy, no toxicosis is observed.

Hypothesis: Increased pressure in spinal canal because of disorder in liquor drainage causes hyperfunctions of pelvic organs and vasospasms. Beside releasing vasospasms, due to liquor pressure release, blood flow increases, and leads to normal physiological state of pelvic organs.

15.3.10 PULMONOLOGY

Spirometry tests led in a sports group of Greco-Roman wrestling showed that after intensive trainings, maters of sports, who used AKT, demonstrated increase of vital lungs volume by 15%.

Spirometry measurements in patients leading sedentary lifestyle and in patients with restricted mobility, as well as in children in nurseries, showed that the use of AKT increases vital lungs volume by 40%. This proves that such patients are predisposed to disorders because of hypoxia. This served as an argument for treatment of the spinal column in patients with broncho-obstructive disorders.

In 1996, a female patient came to us, at the age of 68, with neuroorthopedic pathology and bronchial asthma. The patient needed antiasthmatic medicines every morning and evening. After treatment of the spinal column, she no more needed to take the medicines in the evenings. It was determined that AKT, beside increasing the vital lungs volume, potentiates the effect of medicines, which allows lowering the medicines doses. Consequently, motivated research was led in terms of the use of AKT in treatment of the spinal column in patients with comorbidity—bronchial asthma. The results of the research showed therapeutic effects, with the help of which the disorder severity decreases essentially, and some patients acquire capability to control the bronchial asthma attacks independently. Below are some of the effects:

1. Destruction of bronchospasm.
2. Occurrence of precursors.
3. Capability to control bronchospasms.
4. Psychological stability.
5. Reduction (decreasing) of an expressiveness of asthenoneurotic developments.
6. Decrease of spastic stricture development threat.
7. Disappearance of sputum, recovery of olfaction (recovery of receptors, dilution of sputum).
8. Destruction of bronchospasm's dependence on exterior causes. Destruction of the stimulus–spastic stricture relationship.
9. Decrease of allergic process reactivity.
10. Increase of incubation interval length.
11. Deboosting of speed of development of a bronchospasm.
12. Immunity to allergens.
13. Replacement of a bronchospasm by a respiratory dyspnea attack.
14. Reduction of drugs consumption.

The study results are recorded on a videocassette.

15.3.11   RHEUMATOID PATHOLOGIES

When Bekhterev's disease is early diagnosed, with the use of AKT (the patient is 16), it is possible to receive regress of the disorder. Adult patients can stop the disease and prevent its development, at that, creatinine remains on normal parameters. Regular use of AKT helps to improve essentially the quality of life of the patients, which is unobtainable with other treatment methods including drug treatment.

It was determined that the longer the patient with Bekhterev's disease is treated with medicines, the less is the effectivity of the use of AKT, especially if the medicine treatment causes intolerable concentrations of creatinine.

More than 20 years ago, orthopedic complexes KUMP-01 have been successfully tested for the treatment of degenerative spine diseases. Use of the complex permitted to stop acute pain in one procedure at 90% of patients. Among the rest 10% of the patients, someone had spondylosis, listhesis, and Forestier's disease—ossification of the anterior longitudinal ligament. Deeper examination of patients with spondylosis led to the detection of Bekhterev's disease of patients. Moreover, the patients' disease has developed after the "abuse" of treatment at radon springs. All patients had formed "suppliant's" posture: marked kyphosis of the thoracic spine, significantly decreased chest excursion. The limited mobility of patients' spine was marked in the sagittal and frontal planes. The overall disease pattern was supplemented by limited rotation.

The state of health of one of the patients is shown in Figure 15.2.

As you can see at the picture, the patient suffers from pathology of hip joints that leads to crossing legs against a background of the "suppliant's" posture.

During the treatment at the KUMP complexes, a restoration of normal physiological curvatures occurs, as the main impact of the device is accented on the spine. In addition, there is a restoration of natural mobility of vertebral joints.

The use of KUMP complexes by patients with Bekhterev's disease stopped pain within 5–8 treatment procedures.

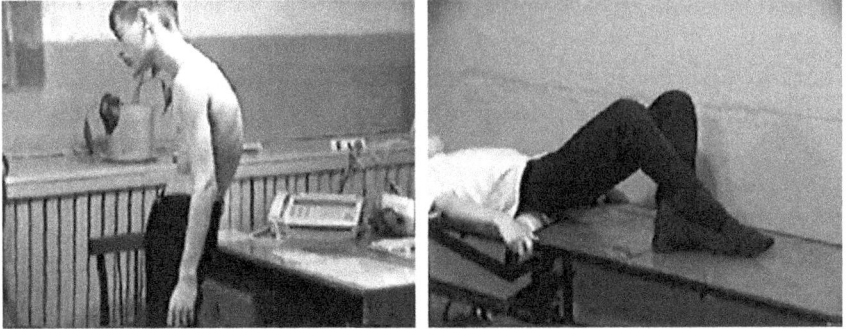

FIGURE 15.2   Patient's condition before treatment.

Patient's condition after 9 months of treatment at the KUMP complexes is shown in Figure 15.3.

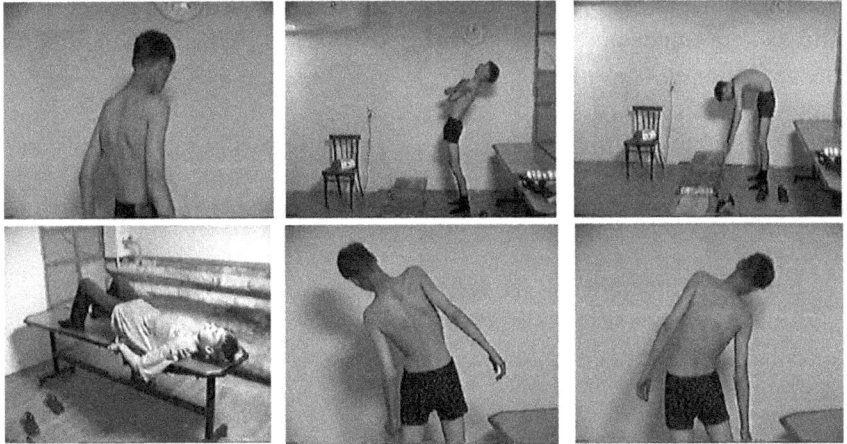

FIGURE 15.3   Patient's condition after 8 months of treatment.

"Suppliant's" posture recovered to a small stoop, spine mobility recovered significantly in frontal and sagittal planes, convergence of crossing legs offset, and hip joints mobility recovered (Fig. 15.3).

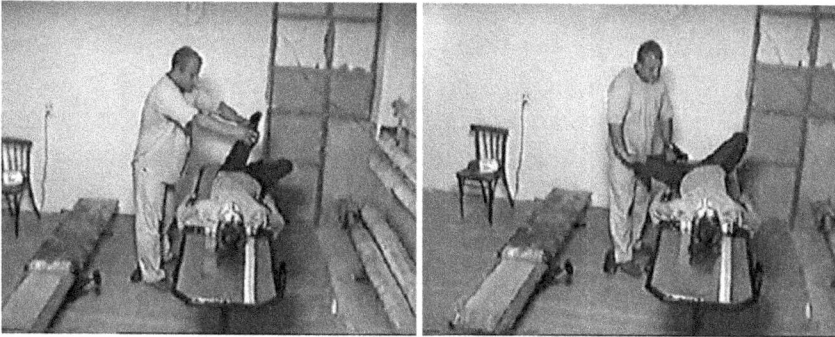

FIGURE 15.4 Examination of sacroiliitis.

Intensification of lymph flow and blood flow during the procedure permitted to abandon completely anti-inflammatory drugs. A restoration of vertebral joints mobility eliminated the occurrence of pain.

Figure 15.4 shows two types of KUMP complexes: the professional one, where the surgeon is examining joints mobility, and the device for home use, where the patient does exercise every morning for 30 min.

Figure 15.5 shows the patient's condition in 3 years. Stoop is not observed; the mobility of the intervertebral joints is satisfactory.

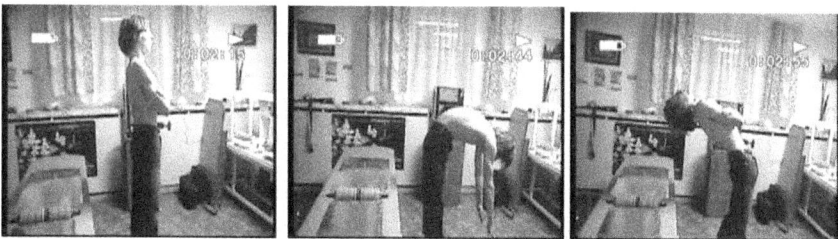

FIGURE 15.5 Patient's condition 3 years after treatment.

Conducted studies have shown that a patient suspends progression of the disease and, in some cases, reaches the regression process. With KUMP complexes, the doctor is able to provide a real help to the patient. In this case, the patient using the complex develops the medical load significantly greater than with chiropractic or massage treatments, and the heart load does not exceed the load during normal walking. Using home complexes allows the patient to return to normal life and improves quality of life.

Currently, using of home complexes became a part of everyday life for several tens of patients.

There is a hypothesis that this disease is caused by viruses. Today, some infectious agents are identified that may pretend to be etiological factors. The most probable hypothesis states that these diseases develop on the background of immunodeficiency.

15.3.12 RHEUMATIC ARTHRITIS (POLYARTHRITIS)

Sustained results were received in treatment of rheumatic arthritis—a chronical systemic inflammatory disorder of connective tissue with progressing damage of mostly peripheral (synovial) movable joints in the form of symmetrical progressing erosive destructive polyarthritis referring to disorders with unknown etiology. Treatment was provided for a patient with spinal pains, after stopping the pains, it was needed to recover the joints mobility in hands and legs as the patient drug allergy against all known preparations and herbal mixtures. Deformation of the joints considerably decreased but did not disappear completely, the cementation level of ankles lowered. And without questions, of course, the quality of life of the patient improved. But, the state achieved requires support in the form of morning exercises, though less intensive than in Bekhterev's disease.

The study results are recorded on a videocassette.

15.4 CONCLUSION

The conclusions are stated in Table 15.4.

TABLE 15.4 Conclusions.

Chinese acupuncture	Russian alternative
1 The main principle of Chinese acupuncture is a mediated influence on the central nervous system (generally, on the spinal cord)	The main principle of AKT is direct influence on the spinal cord roots and direct pressure influence on both spinal and abdominal meridians

TABLE 15.4 *(Continued)*

Chinese acupuncture	Russian alternative
2	The main result of treatment is depressure of hyperfunctions of organs and systems, cramps, spasms, and pains	The main result of the treatment is decrease of liquor pressure, depression of activation of nervous system, and restoration of physiologically optimal mode of organs functions
3	Associated results—there are two types of influence on biologically active points: *method* of strong (braking) and weak (activating) influence	Associated results. It increases metabolic processes in organism and depresses allergic and toxic processes and reactions
4	The patient receives procedures successively	The patient receives all procedures simultaneously
5	The patient is passive in needle therapy, massage, and manual influence	The patient is active during all procedures on the complex KUMP-01
6	The patient cannot adequately respond to disease recurrence and needs the help of the specialist	The patient can adequately respond to disease recurrence and is able to manage it without the help of the specialist
7	Exercises help to maintain the life tonus of the patient	Procedures on AKT allow not only maintaining life tonus of the patient but also identify a hidden development of pathologies long before their clinical manifestation
8	Specialist's training is a complicated and long-lasting process, which may take more than 1 year and require continual improvement of knowledge	During the treatment on AKT, the patient learns needed treatment methods, usually within 1–2 months, independently on education. Specialists can be trained for half a year. Regular improvement of knowledge is desired
9	Reflexotherapy has existed for more than 5000 years, Chinese variant has existed for about 2000 years, AKT has existed for about 20 years, but in terms of treatment of nosologies related to depression of hyperfunction of organs and systems, paroxysms, spasms and pains, and, especially, in Bekhterev's disease, AKT may be preferable	
10	Effective treatment of several nosologies is not possible without restoration of normal physiology of the spinal column	

KEYWORDS

- physiology
- acupuncture
- alternative
- KUMP-01
- neurology
- orthopedics
- rheumatology
- somatic diseases

REFERENCES

1. Klimenko, M. M.; Kretov, B. K. Massage and Gymnastic Table. Applicant and Patentee Scientific Industrial Enterprise "Exergy"-94002344/14, Appl. 18.01.1994, Publ. 20.06.1996 Bull. No. 17. Patent No. 2,062,084, Russian Federation MPK7 A47B9/00, A61G12/00.

2. Klimenko, M. M.; Kretov, B. K. The Method of Pain Relief in the Spinal Column. Applicant and Patentee Scientific Industrial Enterprise "Exergy"-92012929/14 Appl.: 21.12.1992 Publ. 10.04.1999 Bull. No. 10. Patent No. 2,128,492, Russian Federation МПK7 A61H23/00.

3. Klimenko, M. M.; Subbotin, A. V.; Duda, E. E.; Strazhnikov, V. N. Management of Vertebrogenic Pain Syndrome with the Method of Auto-Kinesiotherapy. *Int. J. Immunorehabil.* **1996,** *2,* 144.

4. Duda, E. E.; Klimenko, M. M.; Strazhnikov, V. V.; Grachev, V. V. In *Auto-Kinesiotherapy as a Biophysical Method of Diagnosing and Treatment of Orthopedic Disorders,* Proceedings of the International Conference; Sports Medicine Specialists Association, Novosibirsk, 2001; pp 24–25.

5. Klimenko, M. M.; Isakova, O. P. Spinal Pains Relief in the Treatment of Broncho Obstruction with the Method of Auto-Kinesiotherapy. *In the Collected Volume "Pain Palliative Help",* 2002, 99.

6. Krasilnikova, S. V.; Klimenko, M. M.; Pedder, V. V. In *Rehabilitation of the Patients with Ankylosing Spondylitis (Bekhterev's Disease) Using KUMP Orthopedic Complexes,* Proceeding of Eighth Russian National Congress, Saint-Petersburg, 2003; pp 206.

CHAPTER 16

MEDICAL EMERGENCY RESPONSE SERVICES IN THE STATE OF KERALA—EVALUATION REPORT

BINOY SURENDRA BABU[1*], K. RANJITHKUMAR[2],
JITENDAR SHARMA[3,4], and S. REGI RAM[2]

[1]*Directorate of Health Services, Trivandrum 695312, Kerala, India*

[2]*Division of Health Management, School of Medical Education, Mahatma Gandhi University, Kottayam 686008, Kerala, India*

[3]*Division Health Care Technology and Innovations, National Health System Resource Centre, New Delhi, India*

[4]*Andhra Pradesh Medtech Zone, Visakhapatnam, Andhra Pradesh, India*

Corresponding author. E-mail: drbinoysbabu@gmail.com

ABSTRACT

A study conducted to assess the effectiveness of the medical emergency service response provided in two districts, Thiruvananthapuram and Alappuzha, in the state of Kerala with reference to the service provided by 108 Ambulance.

16.1 INTRODUCTION

Emergency Medical Services (abbreviated to the initialism EMS in some countries) are a type of emergency service dedicated to provide out-of-hospital acute medical care, transport to definitive care, and other medical transport to patients with illnesses and injuries which prevent the patient from transporting themselves.

EMS may also be locally known as a first aid squad, emergency squad, rescue squad, ambulance, squad ambulance service, ambulance corps, or life squad.

The goal of most EMS is to either provide treatment to those in need of urgent medical care, with the goal of satisfactorily treating the presenting conditions, or arranging for timely removal of the patient to the next point of definitive care. This is most likely an emergency department at a hospital. The term emergency medical service evolved to reflect a change from a simple system of ambulances providing only transportation, to a system in which actual medical care is given on scene and during transport. In some developing regions, the term is not used, or may be used inaccurately, since the service in question does not provide treatment to the patients, but only the provision of transport to the point of care.

The first use of the ambulance as a specialized vehicle, in battle, came about with the ambulances volunteers designed by Dominique Jean Larrey (1766–1842), Napoleon Bonaparte's chief physician Larrey was present at the battle of Spires, between the French and Prussians, and was distressed by the fact that wounded soldiers were not picked up by the numerous ambulances (which Napoleon required to be stationed two-and-half miles back from the scene of battle) until after hostilities had ceased and set about developing a new ambulance system. Having decided against using the Norman system of horse litters, he settled on two- or four-wheeled horse-drawn wagons, which were used to transport fallen soldiers from the (active) battlefield after they had received early treatment in the field. These "flying ambulances" were first used by Napoleon's Army of the Rhine is 1793. Larrey subsequently developed similar services for Napoleon's other armies and adapted his ambulances to the conditions, including developing a litter which could be carried by a camel for a campaign in Egypt.

The first known hospital-based ambulance service operated out of Commercial Hospital, Cincinnati, Ohio (now the Cincinnati General) by 1865. This was soon followed by other services, notably the New York service provided out of Bellevue Hospital which started in 1869 with ambulances carrying medical equipment, such as splints, a stomach pump, morphine, and brandy, reflecting contemporary medicine.

The earliest emergency medical service was reportedly the rescue society founded by Jaromir V. Mundy, Count J.N. Wilczek, and Eduard Lamezan-Salins in Vienna after the disastrous fire at the Vienna Ring Theater in 1881. Named the "Vienna Voluntary Rescue Society," it served as a model for similar societies worldwide.

In 1971, after release of the National Highway Traffic Safety Administration's study, "Accidental Death and Disability: The Neglected Disease of Modern Society," a progress report was published at the annual meeting, by the then president of American Association of Trauma, Sawnie R. Gaston M.D. Dr. Gaston reported the study a "superb white paper" that "jolted and wakened the entire structure of organized medicine." This report was the "prime mover" and made the "single greatest contribution of its kind to the improvement of EMS." Since then a concerted effort has been undertaken to improve emergency medical care in the prehospital setting. Such advancements included Dr. R Adams Cowley creating the country's first statewide EMS program, in Maryland.

Service providers

- Government Ambulance Service
- Fire or Police Linked Service
- Volunteer Ambulance Service
- Private Ambulance Service
- Combined Emergency Service
- Hospital-based Service
- Charity Ambulance
- Company Ambulance

16.2 REVIEW OF LITERATURE

In India, EMS is a relatively new concept, where the most dominant model is the EMRI (Emergency Management and Research Institute) services.

(1) EMRI "108" Model (Comprehensive EMS model)

The most widespread Emergency Response Model in India is the "108" Emergency service managed by EMRI.

The "108 Ambulance Service" is a public–private-partnership model between state governments and EMRI, and the service provides complete prehospital emergency care from event occurrence to evacuation to an appropriate hospital. The concept of "108 Ambulance" aims at reaching the patients/sites within 20 min in urban areas and 40 min in rural areas and that the aim is to shift the patient to the nearest hospital within 20 min after reaching him/her. The emergency transportation is conducted in a state-of-the-art ambulance, which is provided free. The transportation is coordinated by a state-of-the-art emergency call response center, which is operational 24-h a day, 7 days a week. In addition, the call to the number "108" is a toll-free service accessible from landline or mobile. The ambulances have been designed with a uniquely Indian perspective, and it includes space for the patient, paramedic in the back, and also bench seat for family members. EMRI ambulance fleet includes basic life support (BLS) and advanced life support (ALS) ambulances. The ALS ambulances are available with cardiac monitor and defibrillator in addition to the basic provisions of a BLS ambulance.

The emergency response services (ERS) implemented by EMRI also includes trained human resources from the call center staff to support staff in ambulances. Each ambulance has three pilots (drivers) and three EMTs who work in pairs of two for every 12-h shift with a break in every fourth day. For every 15 ambulances, there is one operation executive and one fleet executive. Above them, there is one district manager and one administrative officer, for every district.

One of the key functions that EMRI performs is to recruit private hospitals who would participate in the ERS, and this would imply cashless service for the first 24 h till the patient is stabilized. For this purpose, EMRI has signed MOUs with large number of hospitals to formalize an understanding that the hospital would not refuse admission if a patient is brought to it.

(2) Janani Express Scheme (non-EMS, merely transportation model)

The *Janani Express* scheme is a public–private-partnership model, where the contract is signed between the government (at the district/block level) and the private vehicle provider who is generally a local transporter. The *Janani Express* is basically a vehicle (four wheeler—Jeep/Tata Sumo/Mahindra) hired locally for a period of 1 year, to ensure provisioning of 24-h transport availability at the field level (Block level) in order to bring the pregnant women to the health institutions. Transport is made available in the area served by a government hospital, CHC, and PHC. The Rogi Kalyan Samitis (RKS) of the concerned health facility plays a vital role in all issues related to the contracted vehicle and all reimbursements and the monitoring and control of the scheme is with the respective RKS. There is also the provision of performance-based incentives to the transport agency.

(3) Bihar Model: "102" and "1911" (mix of EM and basic transportation model)

In Bihar, the ambulances and respective hospitals are connected through a toll-free number—"102." In addition to this, doctors are also empaneled, who would provide services on conference call and also would visit the patients who needed immediate doctor's assistance (using another toll-free number—"1911"). The calls can be transferred from 102 to 1911. Details of the empaneled ambulances and hospitals are provided to the control room operated by IT managers who would contact the ambulance at the time of emergency. The State Health Society of Bihar (SHSB) under National Health Rural Mission (NRHM) is the nodal agency for 102 control room. The SHS, along with District Health Society (DHS), has district wise empaneled list of ambulances (who are functional at that point of time) with their driver contact details and also enrolled ambulances from interested not-for-profit NGOs.

(4) West Bengal Ambulance PPP Model (non-EMS, merely transportation model)

Another model of emergency transport is contracting out of the management and operation of Ambulance services to various NGOs/CBOs/Trusts under PPP arrangement in West Bengal. In this PPP model, the state government procured and equipped ambulances and handed them over to selected NGOs, keeping the ownership with itself. This was facilitated by entering into agreements with various NGOs/CBOs/Trusts by the respective District Health and Family Welfare Samiti (DHFWS) for a 5-year period. These NGOs then operate the ambulance in the designated area on a user-fee basis. The DHFWS fixes the user charges, and these can be retained by the NGOs for meeting the recurring expenditure. The monitoring of the program is done by Block Health and Family Welfare Samitis.

(5) Referral Transport System in Haryana (trauma/highway ambulance)

To reduce the maternal and neonatal deaths the Government of Haryana has launched a unique scheme to provide referral transport service branded as "*Haryana Swasthya Vahan Sewa* No. 102" on November 14, 2009. All the 21 districts of Haryana are covered under the scheme.

The scheme offers (1) transportation from the site of accident or home or any other place to nearest appropriate medical facility in case of medical need, and (2) transportation from a medical facility to a higher medical facility. Free transportation services are provided to pregnant women, victims of road side accident, patients belonging to BPL or notified slums, postnatal cases in case of emergency (till 6 weeks after delivery), neonates in case of emergency (till 14 days after birth), freedom fighters, and ex-defense personnel. For all other categories of patients, user fees are charged which amounts to Rs. 7/km.

The scheme is run by the government in collaboration with District Red Cross Societies and toll-free telephone number "102" installed at each district control room for easy access to the public. There exists a 24 × 7 control room in each district hospital, for receiving the calls and monitoring of ambulances through GIS/GPS. There is a common pooling of ambulances belonging to the Health Department as well as those owned or operated by the District Red Cross Societies. The operating cost for ambulances run by District Red Cross Society is reimbursed to them by the government.

16.2.1   EMRI MODEL IN KERALA

Management of emergencies is of serious concern to the state of Kerala, especially in the light of increasing road accidents, health-related problems, outbreak of diseases and unexpected natural disasters, etc. While 45% of the emergencies are owing to road accidents, 55% are health-related emergencies. Cardiac problems, pregnancy problems, suicides, asthma attacks, snake bites, etc. are medical emergencies needing immediate intervention. It is an established fact that effective emergency response will significantly reduce deaths, disabilities suffering from length of hospital stay, etc. The critical concept in trauma is "golden hour," which means to say more than 50% of all accident mortality takes place within the first hour. It is highly significant, in this context, to establish ERS in the state of Kerala on a large scale.

So far in the state of Kerala, no concentrated effort has ever been put in to meet emergency management requirements. A number of emergency services that have been either in existence or worked sometime in the past have been mainly serving single dimensional interests, be it corporate hospital or limited context interests of social organization which run them. Though the state made some efforts to make available EMS to people under various schemes, the desired results could not be achieved.

Therefore, a project titled Kerala Emergency Medical services Project (KEMP) has been initiated in the state hiring the service of an expert organization under the notion of public–private partnership. KEMP is an Emergency Management System which is established scientifically through a network of sophisticated ambulances connected and controlled with an Emergency Response Center having single seamless solution including Computer Technology Integration, Voice Logger system, Geographic Information System maps, Geographic positioning System, Automatic Vehicle Tracking and Mobile Communication technology. The project has been conceived by the Engineering division of the State chapter of NRHM. Police help, ambulance help, and Medical assistance are provided under one roof to make the venture successful.

This Emergency Medical Service can be availed by any person through a toll-free number 108. The project was launched initially in the district of Thiruvananthapuram on May 19, 2010 and on April 20, 2012 in Alappuzha district.

A fleet of Advance Life Support Ambulances will be parked in different strategic locations in the district to provide 24 × 7 prehospital emergency response ambulance service accessible to all. The ambulance will have sophisticated equipment to tackle all kinds of emergencies, medicines, and consumables required for stabilizing the life of the patient including oxygen. All the ambulances will be monitored and controlled through a 24 × 7 Emergency Response Center (control room) with the help of GPS and GPRS network. This prehospital emergency service is accessible to all the people of Thiruvananthapuram through a toll-free number 108. When a call is received, the nearest ambulance will be located by the control room and will be dispatched immediately to the location with the help of the information provided by the caller and with Geographic Information System. In case of road traffic accidents, the patient will be taken to the nearest government hospital to stabilize the patient depending upon the condition of the patient. In case of other emergencies, the patient will be admitted to any hospital of their choice and may be charged only if they opt for a private hospital. This rate for transport to a private hospital will be finalized later. The service under KEMP will be available for only prehospital emergency and not for shifting the patient from the hospitals. This service will also be not available for transferring dead bodies.

M/s Ziqitza Health Care, Mumbai, who was qualified as the successful bidder through a tender process has been awarded the contract for operating the KEMP project in Thiruvananthapuram district. The control room for KEMP has been established in Technopark.

The KEMP Advance Life Support Ambulance is designed to handle all types of emergencies including Trauma, cardiac, labor emergencies, etc. Equipment were also provided for handling such emergencies. The trauma and life-saving medical equipment meet the CEN 1789 European Safety Standards for medical transportation vehicles. This European Standard specifies requirements for the design, testing, performance, and equipping of road ambulances used for the transport and care of patients. The ALS ambulances also have extraction tools which is very important in emergency ambulances, because in many a time, the mangled debris had to be cut open to save the life of people.

The interior of the ambulances are made of seamless medical grade fiber reinforced polymer (FRP) panels and joint-less medical grade polyurethane antiabrasive epoxy flooring which is antistatic, antibacterial, antifungal, antiskid, and antifire. This type of interiors is easy to clean and maintain sterile and hygienic.

The major medical equipment on board are defibrillator and patient monitor with automated external defibrillation and telemetry facility, ventilator which is driven pneumatically and easy to transfer along with patient, fetal monitor, syringe pump, pulse oxymeter, battery-operated suction apparatus, nebulizer, needle destroyer, glucometer, BP apparatus, etc.

The trauma equipment available in the ambulances are autoloading patient trolley which can be loaded in the ambulance effortlessly with a single person, scoop stretcher which is useful in shifting patients with multiple injuries and spine injuries and helps in shifting the patient keeping the spine intact, spine board which helps in providing adequate support to an injured patient during transfer, folding wheel/stair chair to carry the patient, where the trolley cannot be taken, splints for immobilizing particular parts especially long bone fractures, cervical collar to avoid irreparable damage to the patient in the case of cervical fracture and spinal brace to stabilize and immobilize spine during an injury.

Proper storage spaces for medical equipment, medicines, and consumables including refrigerated medicine cabinet are available. Each ambulance has two bulk oxygen cylinders which are capable of storing more than 12,000 L of oxygen. All ambulances are fitted with solar panel to charge the battery when the ambulance remains stationary.

Rescue tools necessary for extrication of a victim in a crash, fire, and other situations like Bolt cutter, Crowbar, Axe, Spade, High tensile rope, Hacksaw blade with frame, wrench, screw driver, vise grip pliers, hammer, wrecking bar, folding shovel, mastic knife, pruning saw, spring loaded center punch, double action tin snips, gauntlets, heavy duty shoring cribbing blocks of various sizes, 5 kg fire extinguisher, rescue blanket which have been proven in saving lives when victims were stuck up in emergency are available in each ambulance.

The ambulances are also fitted with rhombus-shaped light bar with integrated high-intensity public address system and exterior reflective stickers prominently indicating emergency. The doors of all ambulances open 270 degrees enabling quick patient transfer in public places.

16.3   OBJECTIVES AND METHODOLOGY

- To assess the effectiveness (timeliness) in responding to medical emergencies.
- To understand further on patterns of use and equity issues.
- To examine HR issues related to service delivery.

16.3.1   DATA COLLECTION

The study is conducted in two districts in the state of Kerala (Thiruvananthapuram and Alappuzha). The evaluation conducted in two phases, involves both qualitative and quantitative methods. This involved conducting exit interview in hospitals (government as well as private), using structured questionnaires provided by NHSRC.

16.3.2   SAMPLING PLAN AND SELECTION OF RESPONDENTS

Cross-sectional collection of sampling was done. The respondents were selected from various government and private hospitals. The total sample size was 207 (total in both districts including respondents using and not using 108 ambulance services).

Hospitals selected for the study

District	Hospital category	Name and address	Sample
Thiruvananthapuram	**Public health institutions**		
	Apex Referral Hospital	Medical College Hospital, Thiruvananthapuram	30
	First Referral Unit	Taluk Hospital, Varkala	20
	First Referral Unit	CHC Kesavapuram, Thiruvananthapuram	
	First Referral Unit	CHC Kanyakulangara, Thiruvananthapuram	
	Maternity Hospital	SAT Hospital, Thiruvananthapuram	
	Private health institutions		
	Private Medical College	Sree Gokulam Medical College, Venjaramoodu, Thiruvananthapuram	50
	Private Hospital	PRS Hospital, Killipalam Thiruvananthapuram	
	Private Hospital	SP Fort Hospital, Thiruvananthapuram	
Alappuzha	Public health institutions		
	Apex Referral Hospital	TD Medical College Hospital, Vandanam, Alappuzha	30
	First Referral Unit	Taluk Hospital, Cherthala	20
	First Referral Unit	General Hospital, Alappuzha	
	First Referral Unit	CHC, Trikunnapuzha	
	Maternity Hospital	W&C Hospital, Alappuzha	
	Private health institutions		
	Private Hospital	KVM Hospital, Cherthala	50
	Private Hospital	Sahrudaya Hospital, Alappuzha	
	Private Hospital	Huda Trust Hospital, Haripadu	

In each district, around 100 interviews were done. The Apex government hospital, other government hospitals, and private hospitals are three categories of hospitals which are potential sites for meeting casualties and interviewing their attendants. Minimum 30 interviews conducted at each category of hospital, while remaining 10 interviews done at any of the given category hospitals collectively or at different hospitals. The respondent may be the attendant of the patient in the casualty/ward (for cases transferred toward). Interviews were conducted over 5–7 days, with the timing spread across morning (09.00–11.30 h), afternoon (15.00–17.30 h), evening (19.00–21.00 h), and late night (01.00–04.00 h). The proportions of sample to be spread across these four timeframes were based on informed guesses about the proportion of cases coming in these hours in consultation with the doctors in the health facility/casualty.

Proper research protocol and research ethics were followed while interviewing the casualty patients/their attendants. The health authorities in the district and the hospital (including the casualty department/ward) were informed in writing and personally, before starting the survey. The Duty Medical Officer (DMO) in the casualty was also briefed about the purpose and methodology. Patient/attendant's permission was taken before starting the interview and their convenience in spending time in answering the questions was respected. Ideally, those patients were approached in the casualty who had been attended by the DMO/emergency technician, is relatively stabilized, and is waiting to be either shifted to a ward/referred to higher referral institution or discharged.

16.4 ANALYSIS AND INTERPRETATIONS

16.4.1 BACKGROUND CHARACTERISTICS OF THE PATIENT

TABLE 16.1   Age Group.

Age group (in years)	Using 108		Not using 108	
	No. of respondents	Percentage	No. of respondents	Percentage
0–10	2	1.94	2	1.92
11–20	6	5.83	18	17.31
21–30	17	16.50	37	35.58

TABLE 16.1 *(Continued)*

Age group (in years)	Using 108		Not using 108	
	No. of respondents	Percentage	No. of respondents	Percentage
31–40	13	12.62	9	8.65
41–50	25	24.27	12	11.54
51–60	20	19.42	7	6.73
61–70	8	7.77	10	9.62
Above 70	12	11.65	9	8.65
Total	103	100	104	100

TABLE 16.2 Gender.

Gender	Using 108		Not using 108	
	No. of respondents	Percentage	No. of respondents	Percentage
Male	77	75	39	37.50
Female	26	25	65	62.50
Total	103	100	104	100

Among the sample those who are using 108 services 75% are males and 25% are females, while those who are not utilizing the service 37.5% are males and 62.5% females (Tables 16.1 and 16.2).

TABLE 16.3 Place of Residence.

Place of residence of the patient	Using 108		Not using 108	
	No. of respondents	Percentage	No. of respondents	Percentage
Urban	23	22.33	20	19.23
Peri-urban	10	9.71	4	3.85
Rural	70	67.96	80	76.92
Total	103	100	104	100

Among the 108 users and nonusers majority belongs to the rural area, 67.96 and 76.92%, respectively (Table 16.3).

TABLE 16.4 Distance of House from the Hospital.

Distance (in km)	Using 108		Not using 108	
	No. of respondent	Percentage	No. of respondent	Percentage
≤10	29	28.16	38	36.54
11–20	22	21.36	34	32.69
21–30	25	24.27	16	15.38
31–40	17	16.50	5	4.81
41–50	7	6.80	6	5.77
51–60	3	2.91	4	3.85
>60	0	0	1	0.96
Total	103	100	104	100

Majority of the patients who availed 108 service resided within a radius of 10 km from the hospital. About 24.27% resided between 21 and 30 km and 21.36% resided between 11 and 20 km (Table 16.4).

In the case of patient not using 108 service, 36.54% of the patients resided within a diameter of 10 km from the hospital, 32.69% are residing in between 11 and 20 km.

TABLE 16.5 Social Category.

Social category	Using 108		Not using 108	
	No. of respondents	Percentage	No. of respondents	Percentage
SC	17	16.50	1	0.96
ST	1	0.97	2	1.92
Others[a]	85	82.52	101	97.12
Total	103	100	104	100

[a]Includes Hindu, Christian, Muslim, etc.

TABLE 16.6   Economic Status.

Economic status	Using 108		Not using 108	
	No. of respondents	Percentage	No. of respondents	Percentage
BPL	62	60	49	47
APL	41	40	55	53
Total	103	100	104	100

60% of the respondents of 108 users are of BPL, but among not utilizing 108 service, majority belongs to APL category (53%) (Tables 16.5 and 16.6).

TABLE 16.7   Clinical Diagnosis of the Emergency.

Clinical diagnosis of the emergency	Using 108		Not using 108	
	No. of respondents	Percent	No. of respondents	Percent
Abdominal pain	3	2.91	4	3.85
Allergic reactions	3	2.91		0.00
Injury/burn	47	45.63	29	27.88
Cardiac/cardiovascular	16	15.53	4	3.85
Diabetes	3	2.91	2	1.92
Disasters	1	0.97		0.00
Epilepsy	3	2.91	1	0.96
Fever (infections)	2	1.94	1	0.96
Normal delivery	1	0.97	13	12.50
Obstetric emergency	8	7.77	35	33.65
Respiratory	3	2.91	4	3.85
Stroke	4	3.88	2	1.92
Others[a]	9	8.74	9	8.65
Total	103	100.00	104	100

[a]Fainting, management of bed ridden patients, etc.

The study revealed that among the 108 ambulance users, the clinical diagnoses of the emergency category injury/burn was the major one comprising of 45.63% followed by cardiac/cardiovascular emergency

(15.53%). The study among the group of patients not using 108 ambulance services revealed that 33.65% of cases fall in the emergency category "Obstetric emergency" which is the major category (Table 16.7).

TABLE 16.8   Type of Trip.

Type of trip	Using 108		Not using 108	
	No. of respondents	Percent	No. of respondents	Percent
Fixed earlier	1	11.11	12	25
Emergency call	8	88.89	36	75
Total	9	100	48	100

Among the respondents only nine patients who utilized 108 service responded to the question on whether the trip was fixed earlier or it was an emergency call, of which a great majority (88.89%) was emergency calls, which include obstetric emergency cases (Table 16.8).

Among the category of patients not utilizing 108 ambulance service, 48 patients responded to the question on whether the trip was fixed earlier or it was an emergency call. Among these respondents 75% of the cases were emergency call and the rest 25% were preplanned.

TABLE 16.9   Reason for Fixing the Call.

Reason	Using 108		Not using 108	
	No. of respondents	Percent	No. of respondents	Percent
High risk delivery case	8	88.89	36	75
Normal full term case	1	11.11	12	25
Total	9	100	48	100

Of the obstetric emergency cases that were transported using 108 ambulance service 88.89% were identified as high risk delivery cases and 11.11% were normal booked case at full term. Among the obstetric emergency cases that did not avail 108 ambulance facility 75% of the cases were identified as high risk delivery cases and 25% were normal booked case at full term (Table 16.9).

TABLE 16.10   Time of Developing Complication (in Pregnancy Case).

Time	Using 108		Not using 108	
	No. of respondents	Percent	No. of respondents	Percent
After the labor pain had started	6	86	45	93.75
During transportation	1	14	3	6.25
Total	7	100	48	100

TABLE 16.11   Location of the Patient When the Call Was Made.

Location	Using 108		Not using 108	
	No. of respondents	Percent	No. of respondents	Percent
Home	36	34.95	78	75
Workplace	5	4.85	5	4.81
Other hospital/clinic	43	41.75	4	3.85
Road/in transport	16	15.53	16	15.38
Public place	1	0.97	1	0.96
Field	1	0.97	0	0
Others[a]	1	0.97	0	0
Total	103	100	104	100

[a]Relative's home.

The study shows among the users of 108 service, 41.75% of the cases were at other hospital/clinic when the call was made followed by location at home with 34.95%. This shows that more cases are utilized for shifting patient from one hospital to another, that is, referral cases (Tables 16.10 and 16.11).

The study among patients utilizing services other than 108 ambulance revealed that 75% were at home when the call was made. The nearest highest score is road/in transport which consists of 15.38% only.

TABLE 16.12 Decision to Call the Vehicle.

Decision to call	Using 108		Not using 108	
	No. of respondents	Percent	No. of respondents	Percent
Self (patient)	2	1.94	15	14.42
Family members/friends/colleagues, etc.	67	65.05	80	76.92
Police	5	4.85	1	0.96
Doctor/paramedical personnel	20	19.42	4	3.85
Others[a]	9	8.74	4	3.85
Total	103	100	104	100

[a]People who gathered there.

Most of the decision to call the 108 ambulance was by family members, friends, or colleagues. This consists of 65.05% of the total sample. In certain cases, doctors or paramedical personnel made the call—19.42% (Table 16.12).

Most of the decision to call other vehicles/ambulance was by family members, friends, or colleagues. This consists of 76.92% of the total sample.

TABLE 16.13 Reason for Making the Call.

Reason for making the call	Using 108		Not using 108	
	No. of respondents	Percent	No. of respondents	Percent
Medical emergency needing attention in a hospital	76	73.79	70	72.92
Pregnant woman in labor	4	3.88	15	15.63
Shift from one hospital to another	23	22.33	11	11.46
Total	103	100	96	100

Majority of the reasons to call 108 ambulance service is coming under the category medical emergency needing attention in a hospital, that is, 76 (Table 16.13).

Majority of the reasons to call other vehicle/ambulance is coming under the category medical emergency needing attention in a hospital of the questionnaire, that is, 70. Other categories like shifting patients from one hospital to another and for delivery comprise of 15 and 11, respectively.

TABLE 16.14 Police Case.

Police case	Using 108		Not using 108	
	No. of respondents	Percent	No. of respondents	Percent
Yes	14	13.59	8	7.69
No	89	86.41	96	92.31
Total	103	100	104	100

Among the 108 users, 13.59% of the cases were police cases, and 86.41cases were not police cases, while among the patients utilizing other services 7.69% of the cases were police cases and 92.31% were not (Table 16.14).

TABLE 16.15 Police Accompanying.

Police accompanying	Using 108		Not using 108	
	Frequency	Percent	No. of respondents	Percent
Accompanied and with the patient after admission	1	7.14	1	12.5
Accompanied but left later	5	35.71	1	12.5
Did not accompany	8	57.14	6	75
Total	14	100	8	100

Of the 13.59% cases that availed 108 service had police accompanying patient, and in one case the police was with the patient even after admission. The rest of the eight cases had no police accompanying them (Table 16.15).

Survey among the patients who utilized other services revealed that in six cases police did not accompany the patient. In one case police had accompanying them, and in one case, the police was with the patient even after admission.

16.4.2 MODE OF TRANSPORT

TABLE 16.16 Mode of Conveyance of Patient to the Hospital (for Patients Utilizing Services Other than 108 Ambulance).

Mode of conveyance of patient	No. of respondents	Percent
Own/employer's transport	29	27.88
Hired private transport/taxi/auto	60	57.96
Police vehicle	2	1.92
Other government run ambulance	1	0.96
Private ambulance services	11	10.58
Others[a]	1	0.96
Total	104	100

[a]Third party.

In the survey among the patients who utilized services other than 108 ambulance, 57.96% were transported to the hospital by hired private transport vehicle and 27.88% by own or employer's vehicle. Other ambulance service was utilized by 10.58% patients only (Table 16.16).

TABLE 16.17 Awareness of "108" Ambulance (for Patients Utilizing Services Other than 108 Ambulance).

Awareness of "108" ambulance service	No. of respondents	Percent
Yes	89	86
No	15	14
Total	104	100

Awareness of 108 ambulance service was conducted among the second group, of which, 86% were aware of the service and 14% were not aware of 108 ambulance service (Table 16.17 and Fig. 16.1).

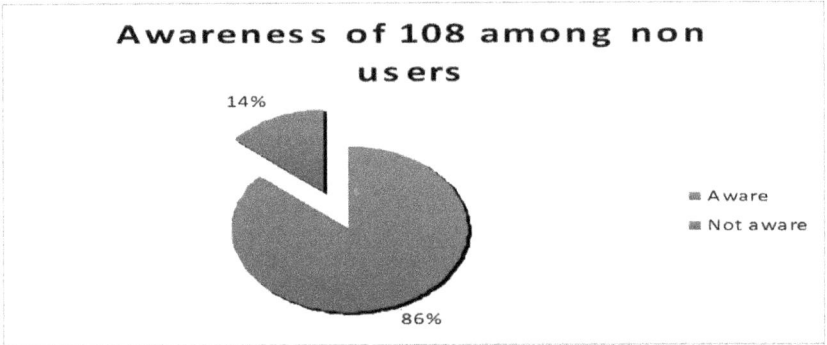

FIGURE 16.1   **(See color insert.)** Awareness of 108 among nonusers.

TABLE 16.18   Tried Calling "108" Ambulance Service (for Patients Utilizing Services Other than 108 Ambulance).

Called 108 ambulance	No. of respondents	Percent
Yes	6	6.74
No	83	93.26
Total	89	100

Survey among the patients utilizing other service providers revealed that a good majority had awareness of 108 ambulance service, only 6.747% of patients tried calling this service and the rest of 93.26% did not try for the same (Table 16.18).

TABLE 16.19   Result of Calling 108 Ambulance Service (for Patients Utilizing Services Other than 108 Ambulance).

Result	No. of respondents	Percent
Call did not connect	4	67
Call connected but dispatch of ambulance was denied	2	33
Total	6	100

Among those who tried calling 108 ambulance service, four of them did not get connection and the rest two calls were connected but dispatch of ambulance was denied (Table 16.19).

TABLE 16.20   Accompanying the Patient.

Anyone accompanying the patient during transportation	Using 108		Not using 108	
	No. of respondents	Percent	No. of respondents	Percent
Accompanying	103	100	103	99.04
Not accompanying	0	0	1	0.96
Total	103	100	104	100

All patients were accompanied with someone in the 108 ambulance (Table 16.20).

TABLE 16.21   Accompanying Person.

Accompanying person	Using 108		Not using 108	
	No. of respondents	Percent	No. of respondents	Percent
Family members/friends/colleagues	100	97.09	103	96.26
Police	6	0	2	1.87
Medical/paramedical personnel	103	0	1	0.93
Others	3	2.91	1	0.93
Total	103	100	106	100

Among the accompanying persons of the 108 users, a majority of 97.09% of cases had their family members accompanying them. All cases were accompanied by the medical/paramedical personnel, that is, emergency medical technicians in all 103 cases.

Stabilization care	Using 108		Not using 108	
	No. of respondents	Percent	No. of respondents	Percent
Provided	101	98.06	1	0.96
Not provided	2	1.94	103	99.04
Total	103	100	104	100

Of the other services, 99.04% of the patients were not provided with stabilization care (Table 16.21).

TABLE 16.22   Stabilization Care Provider.

Stabilization care provider	Using 108		Not using 108	
	No. of respondents	Percent	No. of respondents	Percent
Family members/friends/colleagues	0	0	1	100
Medical/paramedical personnel	101	100	0	0
Total	103	100	1	100

In 108 service, 99.03% of the stabilization care was provided by trained medical/paramedical personnel in the ambulance (Table 16.22).

The stabilization care provided in the above case of respondents not using 108 service was by the family member of the patient.

TABLE 16.23   Point of Arrival of Ambulance (for 108 Users).

Point of arrival of ambulance	No. of respondent	Percent
Site of emergency	87	84.47
Pick up point	16	15.53
Total	103	100

84.47% of the 108 service reached the site of emergency and only 15.53% of the ambulance reached up to the pick-up point (Table 16.23).

TABLE 16.24   Time Taken by Patients to Reach Pick-Up Point (for 108 Users).

Time taken to reach pick-up point (in min)	No. of respondents	Percent
Less than 5	1	6
5–9	3	19
10–15	8	50
16–20	4	25
Total	16	100

50% of the patients took between 10 and 15 min to reach the pick-up point and 25% took 16–20 min and the rest of the cases reached the pick-up point within 10 min (Table 16.24).

TABLE 16.25 Expense to Reach Pick-Up Point (for 108 Users).

Expense to reach pickup point (in Rs.)	No. of respondents	Percent
No expense	3	18.75
1–100	5	31.25
100–150	6	37.50
Above 150	2	12.50
Total	16	100

Of the 16 patients who were picked up from the pick-up point 37.50% had to spend between Rs. 100 and 150 and 31.25% patients had to spend less than Rs. 100, and Rs. 12.50% patients had to spend above Rs. 150. The remaining 18.75% patients did not incur any expense to reach the pick-up point. They were transported free of cost by neighbors or friends (Table 16.25).

TABLE 16.26 Time Taken for Ambulance to Reach the Emergency Site.

Time taken (in min)	Using 108		Not using 108	
	No. of respondents	Percent	No. of respondents	Percent
Less than 10	68	66.02	87	83.65
11–20	29	28.16	8	7.69
21–30	5	4.85	7	6.73
Above 30	1	0.97	2	1.92
Total	103	100	104	100

TABLE 16.27 Time Taken from Emergency Site/Pick-Up Point to Hospital.

Time taken (in min)	Using 108		Not using 108	
	No. of respondents	Percent	No. of respondent	Percent
Less than 10	17	16.50	18	17.31
11–20	31	30.10	26	25
21–30	23	22.33	30	28.85
31–40	11	10.68	7	6.73
41–50	14	13.59	9	8.65
Above 50	7	6.80	14	13.46
Total	103	100	104	100

30.10% of the cases were transported from the emergency site/pick-up point to the hospital by 108 ambulance service between 11 and 20 min and 22.33% between 21 and 30 min (Fig. 16.2, Tables 16.26 and 16.27).

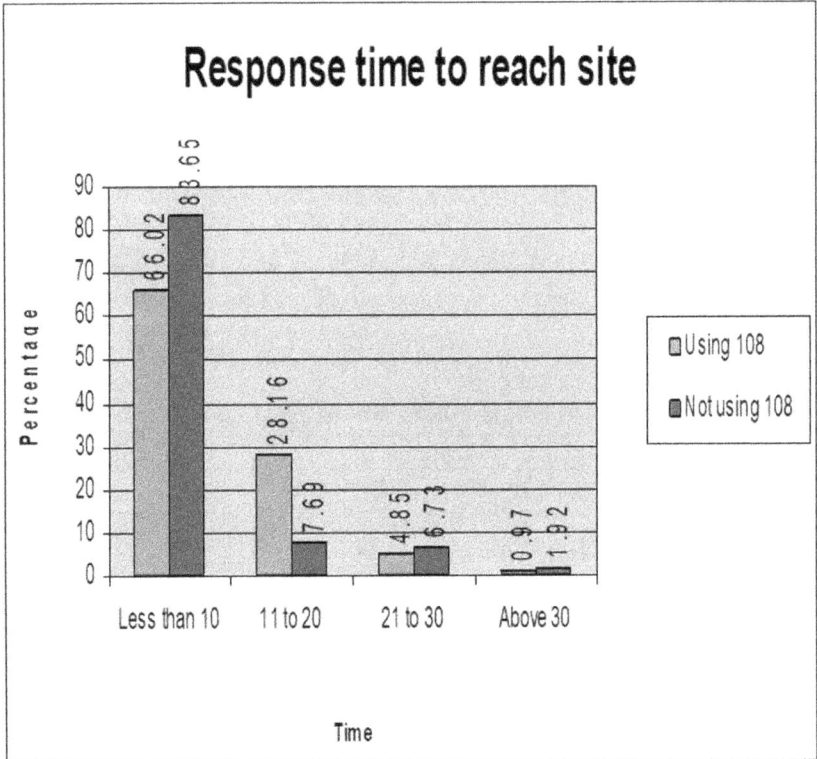

Response time to reach site

FIGURE 16.2   (See color insert.) Time taken by ambulance to reach the emergency site.

In the case of patients using other services, 28.85% of the patients were transported from the emergency site to the hospital between 21 and 30 min and 25% between 11 and 20 min, followed by 17.31% within 10 min (see Fig. 16.3).

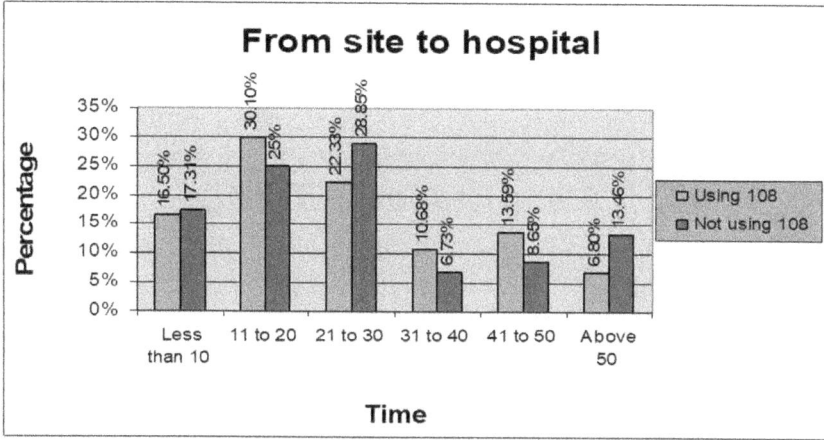

FIGURE 16.3   **(See color insert.)** Time taken for transporting patient from emergency site to hospital.

TABLE 16.28   Mean Response Time by the Vehicle.

Mean response time (in min)	Using 108		Not using 108	
	No. of respondents	Percent	No. of respondents	Percent
Less than 20	20	19.42	35	33.65
21–40	42	40.78	34	32.69
41–60	27	26.21	16	15.38
61–80	12	11.65	11	10.58
81–100	2	1.94	5	4.81
Above 100	0	0.00	3	2.88
Total	103	100	104	100

The total time in reaching the emergency site/pickup point and taking the patient to the hospital for 108 ambulances were between 21 and 30 min for 40.78% of the patients and 26.21% between 41 and 60 min. 19.42% cases took less than 20 min (Table 16.28).

In the case of patients using other services, the mean turnaround time was less than 20 min for 33.65% of patients and between 21 and 40 min for 32.69% of respondents (see Fig. 16.4).

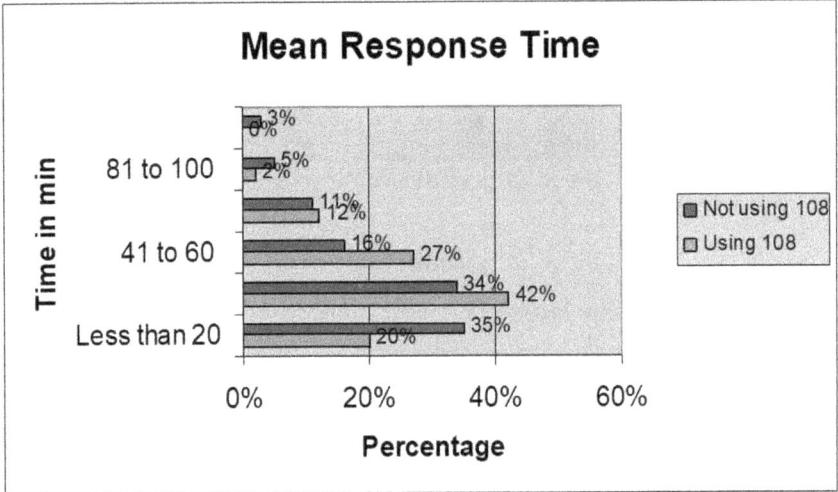

FIGURE 16.4   (See color insert.) Mean response time of the vehicle.

TABLE 16.29   Dropping Point at the Hospital.

Dropping point at the hospital	Using 108		Not using 108	
	No. of respondents	Percent	No. of respondents	Percent
In the general OPD	2	1.94	23	22.12
In the casualty/emergency	101	98.06	81	77.88
Total	103	100	104	100

TABLE 16.30   Time Taken by the Hospital Personnel to Attend the Patient.

Time taken by the hospital personnel to attend the patient (in min)	Using 108		Not using 108	
	No. of respondents	Percent	No. of respondents	Percent
0–15	103	100	98	94.23
15–30			4	3.85
More than 30			2	1.92
Total	103	100	104	100

All cases taken to the hospital by 108 service were attended within 15 min of arrival (Tables 16.29 and 16.30).

94.23% of the patients transported by other services were attended by medical/paramedical personnel within 15 min and 3.85% between 15 and 20 min and 1.92% more than 30 min.

TABLE 16.31 Attended by Qualified Physician or Not (for Category Who Utilized Services Other Than 108 Service).

Attended by qualified physician in the hospital	No. of respondents	Percent
Yes	104	100
Total	104	100

All the patients were attended by qualified personnel (Table 16.31).

TABLE 16.32 Condition of Patient.

Condition of patient (stabilized or not)	Using 108		Not using 108	
	No. of respondents	Percent	No. of respondents	Percent
Yes, under treatment	90	87.38	100	96.15
No, but under treatment	12	11.65	4	3.85
No, referred on to some other facility	1	0.97	0	0
Total	103	100	104	100

While conducting the interview 87.38% of the patients of the user of 108 service category were stabilized and were under treatment. In other cases, the data were collected from the bystanders (Table 16.32).

While conducting the interview 96.15% of the category of patients who utilized other services were stabilized and were under treatment. In other cases, the data were collected from the bystanders.

TABLE 16.33 "108" Transportation.

"108" Transportation	Using 108		Not using 108	
	No. of respondents	Percent	No. of respondents	Percent
Offered	1	100	0	0
Not offered	0	0	0	0
Total	1	100	0	0

TABLE 16.34   Satisfaction with the Service.

Satisfaction level	Using 108		Not using 108	
	No. of respondents	Percent	No. of respondents	Percent
Unhappy	0	0	1	8.33
Not satisfied	0	0	1	8.33
Cannot say	0	0	2	16.67
Somewhat satisfied	0	0	3	25
Satisfied	51	49.51	5	41.67
Very satisfied	52	50.49	0	0
Total	103	100	12	100

There is a high satisfaction level with 108 ambulance service among the respondents, of which 50.49% are very satisfied and 49.51% are satisfied (Tables 16.33 and 16.34).

The satisfaction level was assessed from the patients who used other ambulance service for transportation. Out of them, 41.67% were satisfied and 25% were somewhat satisfied, 8.33% were not satisfied, and 8.33% were unhappy with the service. The satisfaction level is represented in Figure 16.5.

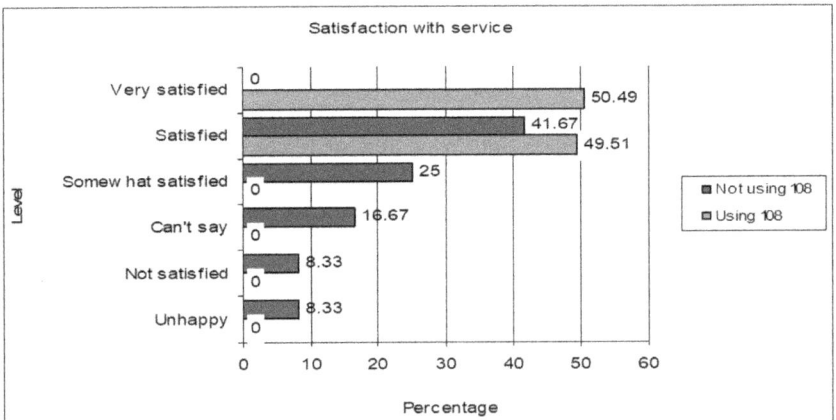

FIGURE 16.5   (See color insert.) Satisfaction with the service.

TABLE 16.35   Expenditure.

Expenditure while transportation	Using 108		Not using 108	
	No. of respondents	Percent	No. of respondents	Percent
Incurred	18	17.48	63	61
Not incurred	85	82.52	41	39
Total	103	100	104	100

82.52% of the patients did not incur any expenditure while being transported to the hospital by 108 ambulance service, but 17.48% of the patients incurred some expense during transportation to hospital by means of hiring vehicle to reach the pick-up point (Table 16.35).

61% of the patients of the category of respondents who were not transported by 108 ambulance incurred expense during transportation to the hospital and 39% did not incur any expense. This may be either they utilized their own vehicle or may have utilized friends' or family members' vehicle free of cost.

TABLE 16.36   Total Expenditure.

Total expenditure while transporting (in Rs.)	Using 108		Not using 108	
	No. of respondents	Percent	No. of respondents	Percent
Less than 500	18	100	47	75
501–1000	0	0	7	11
Above 1000	0	0	9	14
Total	18	100	63	100

The expenditure incurred for the above category of users of 108 ambulance was less than Rs. 500 (Table 16.36).

Among the users of other services, 75% of the category who incurred expenditure during transportation had spent amount less than Rs. 500, whereas 14% incurred expense above Rs. 1000.

TABLE 16.37   Category of Expenditure.

Expenditure—category wise	Using 108		Not using 108	
	No. of respondents	Percent	No. of respondents	Percent
(a) Transport/vehicle hiring				
Less than Rs. 500	18	100	45	61.64
501–1000	0	0	8	10.96
Above 1001	0	0	8	10.96
(b) Medical consumables				
Less than Rs. 500	0	0	1	1.37
Above 1001	0	0	1	1.37
(c) Others				
Less than Rs. 500	0	0	10	13.7
Total	18	100	73	100

The breakup of expenditure incurred for the above category for 108 user was less than Rs. 500, which is for vehicle hiring to reach the pick-up point (Table 16.37).

The breakup of the above category for users of other service shows that 61.64% of the patients had to spend less than Rs. 500 for vehicle hiring and 13.7% on other expense.

TABLE 16.38   Deposit Sought by the Hospital.

Deposit sought by the hospital	Using 108		Not using 108	
	No. of respondents	Percent	No. of respondents	Percent
No (not sought)	103	100	104	100
Total	103	100	104	100

16.4.3   CHOICE OF AMBULANCE SERVICE (PATIENTS NOT USING 108 AMBULANCE)

TABLE 16.39   Awareness about Ambulance Service.

Awareness about ambulance service in the state/ city	No. of respondents	Percent
Aware	89	85.58
Not aware	15	14.42
Total	104	100

Of the total 104 respondents, 85.58% were about ambulance service in the state/city (Tables 16.38 and 16.39).

TABLE 16.40   Knowledge of Ambulance Service.

Type of ambulance services aware of	No. of respondents	Percent
108 Ambulance	89	70
Other government run ambulance	10	8
Other privately operated ambulance service	29	23
Total	128	100

70% of the respondents had knowledge of 108 ambulance services (Table 16.40).

TABLE 16.41   Rating of Best Ambulance Service.

Rating of best ambulance	No. of respondents	Percent
108 Ambulance	68	65.38
Other government run ambulance	2	1.92
Other privately operated ambulance service	3	2.88
Information not available	31	29.81
Total	104	100

Even though the respondents had to avail other services during emergency, 65.38% of them rated 108 ambulance service as the best (Table 16.41).

TABLE 16.42   Reason for Rating the above as Best.

Reason for rating	No. of respondents	Percent
Very quick service	57	43.18
Well-equipped ambulance	30	22.73
Ambulance staff friendly and competent	5	3.79
Guidance by call center	1	0.76
Links with good hospitals	1	0.76
Service is free	36	27.27
Any other reason	2	1.52

The reason for rating 108 ambulance service according to 43.18% was very quick service and according to 27.27% service was free, and according to 22.73% it was well equipped (see Fig. 16.6 and Table 16.42).

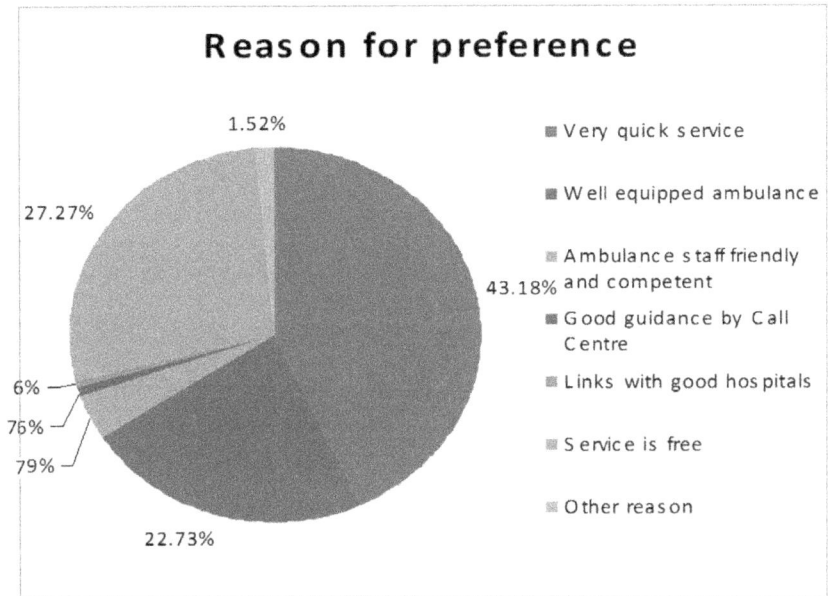

Reason for preference

1.52%

27.27%

6%
7[6]%
79%

22.73%

43.18%

- Very quick service
- Well equipped ambulance
- Ambulance staff friendly and competent
- Good guidance by Call Centre
- Links with good hospitals
- Service is free
- Other reason

FIGURE 16.6   **(See color insert.)** Reason for preference.

1. Choice of Hospital

TABLE 16.43   Choice of Hospital (for Users of Other Services).

Choice of hospital made by	No. of respondents	Percent
Patient or their family members	97	89.81
Ambulance driver	3	2.78
Referring doctor/clinic	7	6.48
Police	1	0.93
Total	108	100

Choice of hospital was made mainly by patient or family members which consists of 89.81% of the sample (Table 16.43).

TABLE 16.44   Reason for Choosing the Hospital.

Reason for choosing the hospital	Using 108	Not using 108
	No. of respondents	No. of respondents
Referred by treating doctor in other hospital/clinic	0	7
Suggested by the vehicle/ambulance operator	13	5
Directed by police	0	2
Guided by the call center of the ambulance operator	2	0
Nearest hospital from the site of emergency	18	47
Treatment is free/low cost	44	20
Known hospital/hospital staff	16	20
Other reasons[a]	30	29
Total	123	130

[a]Opinion by third parties, friends, etc.

One of the major reasons for choosing a particular hospital is lower cost of treatment or treatment free of cost. Other reasons include being the nearest hospital. This was followed by other personal reasons comprising 30 respondents. Certain options together may the reason like nearest hospital and acquaintance of hospital staff. In the case of patients who utilized other service, the major reason for the choice of hospital is hospital being the nearest hospital (Table 16.44).

16.5   SUGGESTIONS BY THE RESPONDENTS

- Majority of the users suggested that the present condition should be maintained and the service should be made available to other districts also.
- Among the patients who utilized other services, majority opined that people are not much aware of 108 service. People do not know it is a free emergency service.
- The users suggested that return trip from hospital should also be provided for bedridden patients.

- The female users suggested of maintaining a female paramedical staff during transportation of female patients.
- There was a grievance among the users that the ambulance personnel were reluctant to take the patient to private hospitals. This may due to the fact that the drivers are afraid of being suspected by their higher officials for some underhand dealings with the private hospital management or some other malpractices.

16.6   FINDINGS AND RECOMMENDATIONS

Major findings of the study are as follows:

- Regarding time taken for ambulance/vehicle to reach the site 66.02% cases, the 108 ambulance reached the site of emergency within 10 min and 28.16% within 11–20 min. Whereas in the case of users of other services in 83.65% of the cases the vehicle/ambulance reached the site of emergency within 10 min and 7.69% within 11–20 min and 6.73% between 21 and 30 min.
- In the case of 108 users, 30.10% of the cases were transported from the emergency site/pick-up point to the hospital by 108 ambulance service within 20 min and 22.33% within 30 min. In the case of other services, 28.85% of the patients were transported from the emergency site to the hospital within 30 min and 25% within 20 min followed by 17.31% within 10 min.
- There is a high satisfaction level with 108 ambulance service among the respondents of which 52% are very satisfied and 51% are satisfied.
- Regarding awareness about ambulance service, a vast majority (92.31%) was aware of an ambulance service.
- Awareness of 108 ambulance service among the category of patients who utilized other services also revealed that majority (67%) were aware of this service.
- Majority (93.15%) of the respondents rated 108 ambulance service as the best and the reason for this is very quick service, well-equipped ambulance, and also free of cost service.
- 108 service are mainly utilized by the rural population (67.96%).

Recommendations

1. Throughout the survey among the nonusers of 108 ambulance service, it was found that many are still not aware of this service. Some of them even did not know this service is free of cost. So, awareness should be spread among the community about this service.
2. Based on the survey, a majority of rural population are utilizing ambulance services. So, more services should be made available especially among the rural areas.
3. There is a high satisfaction rate among the 108 users. Respondents were of the opinion that the present status should be maintained and the service should be spread to other districts in the state.
4. Reluctance from some drivers and personnel to take the patient to private health facility was also observed.

16.7 CONCLUSION

The goal of most EMS is to either provide treatment to those in need of urgent medical care, with the goal of satisfactorily treating the presenting conditions, or arranging for timely removal of the patient to the next point of definitive care. The term emergency medical service evolved to reflect a change from a simple system of ambulances providing only transportation, to a system in which actual medical care is given on scene and during transport. In India, EMS is a relatively new concept, where the most dominant model is the EMRI services. The most widespread Emergency Response Model in India is the "108" emergency service managed by EMRI. The concept of "108 ambulance" aims at reaching the patients/sites within 20 min in urban areas and 40 min in rural areas and that the aim is to shift the patient to the nearest hospital within 20 min after reaching him/her.

The patients in the modern world are well informed and educated. They demand and expect the healthcare system to give timely and qualitative treatment. They look for timely accessibility and responsiveness when they require the service of health care. Perceived quality go hand in hand with professional, personal, and financial satisfactions. Now people are ready to pay for qualitative services.

The study titled "Medical Emergency Response Services in the State of Kerala" revealed that the service provided by the ambulance services in the state of Kerala is highly satisfactory, especially with the service of 108 ambulances. The primary objective of the study was to analyze the effectiveness of ambulance services in responding to emergency. This can be concluded by stating that 108 ambulance services maintained a rather quick response in transporting patients to the hospital as compared to other services.

Even though the service provided is excellent, there is lack of awareness among the community on the service provided by "108" ambulances. The services provided can be improved by providing more facilities and the service of medical personnel as followed in the developed countries.

The ultimate aim of emergency service is to provide quick and timely service to the community so that a life can be saved. These services should also reach to all the population even to far rural area. The investment required is very high in extending the services to the rural area as well as providing more facilities, which can be a burden to the government. So, public–private participation may be devised to meet the expense of infrastructure development so that emergency care is not compromised due to lack of fund.

ACKNOWLEDGMENTS

The review of EMRI model of Emergency Response Services (ERS) was commissioned by the National Health Systems Resource Center (NHSRC), a resource center for National Health Rural Mission (NRHM), Ministry of Health and Family Welfare, Government of India, New Delhi. This review is to validate the data presented by EMRI in the first phase of the study, understand the patterns of use, equity issues and quality of service delivery, and estimate the efficiency and effectiveness of ERS which helps to recommend to the Ministry of Health and Family Welfare, Government of India and State Governments on utilization, requirements, effectiveness, and efficiency of operations, financing arrangements, and governance mechanisms and institutional frameworks.

Division of Health Management (DHM) thanks Sri Dr. T. Sundara-raman, Executive Director and Dr. Jitendra Kumar Sharma, Sr. Consul-tant and Division Head, Healthcare Financing, NHSRC for considering

Division of Health Management to be a part of the Evaluation of Medical Emergency Response Services in the State of Kerala. DHM also takes this opportunity to thank Dr. Beena, State Mission Director, NRHM; Dr. Jameela, Director of Health Services, Kerala; and Dr. Geetha, Director of Medical Education, Kerala for providing help in conducting the evaluation. Mr. Tushar Mokashi, Consultant, NHSRC had provided us with good guidance and support in completion of this project and we thank him for the same. We also take this opportunity to thank Medical Superintendents of all government hospitals and the management of hospitals in the private sector for their support in this evaluation.

Regi Ram S.

APPENDIX-1

Schedule Identification Code ☐☐☐☐☐
Review of Emergency Response Service (ERS) in the State of Kerala
by
National Health Systems Resource Centre
(Technical support agency under NRHM, Ministry of Health & FW, Govt. of India)

HOSPITAL (CASUALTY) PATIENT INTERVIEW SCHEDULE

(For patients not using the "108" ambulance)
Date of Interview: ___ ___ / ___ ___ / 2013   Investigators'   name:
_____
Name and location of Hospital: _____
_____
Category of Hospital: Public.....(1)   Private.....(2)   NGO/Trust Hospital.....(3)

1. **Background Characteristics of the Patient**
   1.1 Age of the Patient (in completed years)
       years

1.2 Sex of the Patient
Male   1
Female   2
1.3 Place of Residence of the patient
Urban   1
Peri-urban 2
Slum 3
Rural   4
Information not available   9
1.4 Residential Address of the patient
1.5 How far is the place of residence of the patient from this hospital?
(Rounded off to nearest km)
km
1.6 Social category of the patient
SC 1
ST 2
Others 3
(Specify_____)
1.7 Economic category of the patient
BPL 1
APL 2

2. Type of Emergency

2.1 What is the type of emergency the patient is facing? *(as per the respondent)*
Abdominal pain 01
Allergic reactions..02
Injury/burn 03
Cardiac/cardiovascular 04
Diabetes 05
Disasters 06
Epilepsy 07
Fever (infections) 08
Neonatal emergency (up to 1 month) 09
Pediatric emergency (up to 12 years).................. 10
Normal delivery 11
Obstetric emergency 12

Respiratory   13

Stroke   14

Others   88

→ *(Specify:* _____ *)*

2.2 What is the clinical diagnosis of the type of emergency the patient is facing? *(as per the hospital records...check with the attending doctor/paramedic)*

Abdominal pain 01   →Skip to question 2.6

Allergic reactions............... 02   →Skip to question 2.6

Injury/burn 03   →Skip to question 2.6

Cardiac/cardiovascular 04   →Skip to question 2.6

Diabetes 05   →Skip to question 2.6

Disasters 06   →Skip to question 2.6

Epilepsy 07   →Skip to question 2.6

Fever (infections) 08   →Skip to question 2.6

Neonatal emergency 09   →Skip to question 2.6

(upto 1 month)

Pediatric emergency............ 10   →Skip to question 2.6

(upto 12 years)

Normal delivery in labor.... 11

Obstetric emergency 12

Respiratory 13   →Skip to question 2.6

Stroke 14   →Skip to question 2.6

Others 88   →*(Specify:* _____ *)*

2.3 Whether the trip was fixed earlier or it was an emergency call.

Fixed earlier 1

It was an emergency call...2

2.4 What was the reason for fixing up the call?

Because the lady was an identified high risk delivery case (for example twins) 1

It was just a normal booked case at full term................................2

2.5 Was the call made for complication developed after the labor pains had started or the complications developed during transportation?

After the labor pains had started...1

During transportation...2

2.6 Where did the emergency occur? Give address of the place. (Mention village, block, district or ward)

Home	1	Address: _____
Workplace	2	_____
Other Hospital/Clinic	3	_____
Road/in transport	4	_____
Public place	5	_____
Field	6	
Others	8	→(Specify:_____)
Information not available	9	

2.7 Who decided to call ambulance/vehicle?

Self (patient) 1

Family members/friends/colleagues ... 2

Police 3

Doctor/paramedical personnel 4

Others .... 8 → (Specify: _____)

Information not available..................... 9

2.8 What was the reason for which the call was made?

Medical emergency needing attention in a hospital.... 1

Shift from one hospital to another............................ 2

For delivery.. 3

Non-emergency.. 4

2.9 Is this a Police case?

Yes 1

No .... 2 → skip to question 3.1

2.10 Is the Police accompanying the patient to the hospital?

Yes, they are still with the patient 1

Police had accompanied but left later 2

No, they did not accompany the patient 3

3. Mode of Transport

3.1 How did the patient come to the hospital?

Own/employer's transport 1

Hired private transport/taxi/auto .. 2

Police vehicle 3

Other Government run ambulance 4

Private Ambulance Services 5

Others .... 8 → (Specify: _____)

Information not available..................... 9

3.2 Have you heard of "108" Ambulance service?
Yes 1
No .... 2 → skip to question 3.6
3.3 Did you try calling "108" Ambulance service for transporting the patient to this hospital?
Yes 1
No .... 2 → skip to question 3.6
3.4 When you tried to call "108," what happened?
Call did not connect .... 1 → skip to question 3.6
Call connected but could not complete the call .... 2 → skip to question 3.6
Call connected but dispatch of ambulance was denied .... 3 → skip to question 3.6
Call connected and dispatch was assured 4
3.5 If ambulance dispatch was promised on call, what happened?
Arranged an alternative transport before the Ambulance came .... a
Ambulance came but refused to take the patient .... b
Ambulance wanted to take the patient to some other hospital c
Ambulance asked for money .... d
Other reason ....e
Specify (_____)
3.6 Was there anyone accompanying the patient during transportation?
Yes 1
No .... 2 → skip to question 3.10
3.7 Who was accompanying the patient during transportation?
Family members/friends/colleagues ...a
Police .... b
Medical/paramedical personnel c
Others .... d →   *(Specify: ____)*
Information not available................... 9
3.8 Was the patient given stabilization care during transportation?
Yes 1
No .... 2 → skip to question 3.10
3.9 Who provided the stabilization care to the patient during transportation?
Family members/friends/colleagues ...   a
Police ....   b
Medical/paramedical personnel   c

Others .... d →   *(Specify:_____)*

Information not available...................   *9*

3.10 Whether the patient stabilized is out of danger?

Yes, under treatment .... 1 → skip to question 3.12

No but under treatment .... 2 → skip to question 3.12

Yes, but referred on to some other facility.......3

No, referred on to some other facility.............4

3.11 Was "108" transportation offered?

Yes 1

No 2

3.12 What was the time taken for the ambulance/vehicle to reach the site of emergency after calling?

⬜⬜⬜ minutes

3.13 What was the time taken for the ambulance/vehicle to reach the hospital from the site of the emergency?

⬜⬜⬜ minutes

3.14 Where did the vehicle drop the patient in this hospital?

At the general parking 1

In the general OPD 2

In the Casualty/Emergency 3

Others .... 8 →   *(Specify: _____)*

Information not available *9*

3.15 After the patient reached the hospital, within how much time did the medical/paramedical staff of the hospital attend to the patient?

0–15 min........................... 1

15–30 min......................... 2

30 min to 1 h 4

More than 1 h................... 5

Information not available.........   *9*

3.16 Has the patient been attended to by qualified personnel in this hospital?

(Observe and Check with the attending doctor/paramedical staff)

Yes 1

No 2

Information not available.........   *9*

In case the patient has come to this hospital by an Ambulance

3.17 How satisfied are you with the ambulance service that the patient availed for reaching this hospital?

-3	-2	-1	0	1	2	3

(Very unhappy) (Unhappy) (Not satisfied) (Cannot say) (Somewhat
satisfied) (Satisfied) (Very satisfied)

4. Out-of-Pocket Expenditure

4.1 Was any expenditure incurred while transporting the patient to the hospital?

Yes 1

No 2   →   skip to question 4.4

Information not available........ 9   →   skip to question 4.4

4.2 What was the total amount of expenditure incurred while transporting the patient to the hospital?

Total expenditure incurred: Rs. ⬚⬚⬚⬚⬚

4.3 What was the expenditure incurred on while transporting the patient to the hospital?

a. Transport/vehicle hiring: Rs. ⬚⬚⬚⬚⬚

b. Medical consumables: Rs. ⬚⬚⬚⬚⬚

c. Others: Rs. ⬚⬚⬚⬚⬚ → *(Specify: _____)*

4.4 Did this hospital/hospital staff ask for payments for starting the treatment of the patient?

Yes 1

No 2   →skip to question 5.1

Information not available........ 9   →skip to question 5.1

4.5 How much amount did the hospital/hospital staff ask for payments (as advance) for starting the treatment of the patient?

Rs. ⬚⬚⬚⬚⬚⬚

5. **Choice of Ambulance service (Only to the individuals where such a service exists)**

5.1 Have you heard of any ambulance service in your state/city?

Yes 1

No 2   →   skip to question 6.1

5.2 What ambulance services you have heard of?

"108" ambulance .... a

Other Government run ambulance .... b

Other privately operated ambulance service ... c → *(Specify:___)*

5.3 Of the above mentioned ambulance service, which one would you rate as the best?

"108" ambulance 1

Other Government run ambulance 2

Other privately operated ambulance service ...   3

(Specify: _____)

Information not available.............................   9 →

skip to question 6.1

5.4 Why did you rate the above ambulance service as the best?

Very quick service ....   a

Well-equipped ambulance ....   b

Ambulance staff friendly and competent   c

Good guidance by Call Center ....   d

Links with good hospitals ....   e

Service is free ....   f

Any other reason ....   g   → *(Specify:*

_____*)*

Information not available.............................   9

6. Choice of Hospital

6.1 Who made the choice?

I or my family members .... a

Ambulance driver named it .... b

Paramedic named it c

Call center named it .... d

Referring doctor/clinic named it .... e

Police named it .... f

6.2 Why was the patient brought to this hospital?

Referred by treating doctor in other hospital/clinic ...... a

The vehicle/ambulance operator brought us here .... b

Police brought us here c

Guided by the call center of the ambulance operator ... d

This was nearest hospital from the site of emergency .. e

Treatment is free/low cost, in this hospital .... f

This hospital/hospital staff was known to us .... g

Any other reason .... h → *(Specify: ___)*

Information not available...............................9

6.3 Any suggestions for better and responsive ambulance service:

End the interview thanking the respondent

***

APPENDIX-2

Schedule Identification Code
Review of Emergency Response Service (ERS) in the State of Kerala
by
National Health Systems Resource Centre
(Technical support agency under NRHM, Ministry of Health & FW,
Govt. of India)

Hospital (Casualty) Patient Interview Schedule
(For patients using the "108" ambulance)

Date of Interview: ___ ___ / ___ ___ / 2013   Investigators' name: _____

Name and location of Hospital: _____
Category of Hospital: Public....(1) Private....(2) NGO/Trust Hospital....(3)

1. Background Characteristics of the Patient
1.1 Age of the Patient (in completed years)
     ☐☐ years

1.2 Sex of the Patient

Male 1

Female 2

1.3 Place of Residence of the patient

Urban 1

Peri-urban 2

Slum 3

Rural 4

Information not available 9

1.4 Residential Address of the patient

_____

_____

_____

1.5 How far is the place of residence of the patient from this hospital? (rounded off to nearest km)

 ☐☐ km

1.6 Social category of the patient

SC 1

ST 2

Others .... 3 *(Specify_____)*

1.7 Economic category of the patient

BPL 1

APL 2

2. Type of Emergency

2.1 What is the type of emergency the patient is facing? *(as per the respondent)*

Abdominal pain 01

Allergic reactions................................ 02

Injury/burn 03

Cardiac/cardiovascular 04

Diabetes 05

Disasters 06

Epilepsy 07

Fever (infections) 08

Neonatal emergency (up to 1 month) ... 09

Pediatric emergency (up to 12 years)... 10

Normal delivery 11

Obstetric emergency 12

Respiratory 13

Stroke 14

Others .... 88 → *(Specify: ____)*

2.2 What is the clinical diagnosis of the type of emergency the patient is facing? *(as per the hospital records...check with the attending doctor/paramedic)*

Abdominal pain .... 01 → Skip to question 2.6

Allergic reactions.............................. 02 → Skip to question 2.6

Injury/burn .... 03 → Skip to question 2.6

Cardiac/cardiovascular .... 04 → Skip to question 2.6

Diabetes .... 05 → Skip to question 2.6

Disasters .... 06 → Skip to question 2.6

Epilepsy .... 07 → Skip to question 2.6

Fever (infections) .... 08 → Skip to question 2.6

Neonatal emergency (up to 1 month) ... 09 → Skip to question 2.6

Pediatric emergency (up to 12 years)... 10 → Skip to question 2.6

Normal delivery in labor.................... 11

Obstetric emergency 12

Respiratory .... 13 → Skip to question 2.6

Stroke .... 14 → Skip to question 2.6

Others .... 88→ *(Specify: _____)*

2.3 Whether the trip was fixed earlier or it was an emergency call.

Fixed earlier   1

It was an emergency call...................... 2 → Skip to question 2.5

2.4 What was the reason for fixing up the call?

Because the lady was an identified high risk delivery case (for example twins) 1

It was just a normal booked case at full term................................2

2.5 Was the call made for complication developed after the labor pains had started or the complications developed during transportation?

After the labor pains had started..1

During transportation..2

2.6 Where was the patient when the call was made?

Home	1	Address: _____
Workplace	2	_____
Other Hospital/Clinic	3	_____
Road/in transport	4	_____
Public place	5	_____
Field	6	
Others	8 →	*(Specify:* _____ *)*
Information not available	9	

2.7 Who decided to call ambulance/vehicle?

Self (patient)	1
Family members/friends/colleagues ...	2
Police	3
Doctor/paramedical personnel	4
Others	8 → *(Specify:* _____ *)*
Information not available.....................	9

2.8 What was the reason for which the call was made?

Medical emergency needing attention in a hospital	1
Pregnant woman in labor	2
Shift from one hospital to another	3
Non-emergency	4

2.9 Is this a Police case?

Yes	1
No	2 → skip to question 3.1

2.10 Is the Police accompanying the patient to the hospital?

Yes, they are still with the patient	1
Police had accompanied but left later	2
No, they did not accompany the patient	3

3. Mode of Transport

3.1 Was there anyone accompanying the patient during transportation?

Yes 1	
No .... 2 → skip to question 3.5	

3.2 Who was accompanying the patient during transportation?

Family members/friends/colleagues ...	a
Police	b
Medical/paramedical personnel	c

Others .... d → *(Specify:_____)*
Information not available.......... 9
3.3 Was the patient given stabilization care during transportation?
Yes 1
No .... 2 → skip to question 3.5
3.4 Who provided the stabilization care to the patient during transportation?
Family members/friends/colleagues ...   a
Police ....   b
Medical/paramedical personnel   c
Others ....   d → *(Specify: _____)*
Information not available...................   9
3.5 Did ambulance come to
Site of emergency   .... 1 → skip to question 3.9
Or pick up point   2
3.6 What was the time taken by you to reach the pickup point?
☐☐☐ minutes
3.7 How did you reach the pickup point? (Mode of transport)
_____
3.8 How much money did you spend on reaching from the point of emergency to the pickup point?
☐☐☐☐ Rs.
3.9 What was the time taken for the ambulance to reach the site of emergency after calling?
☐☐☐ minutes

3.10 What was the time taken for the ambulance to reach the hospital from the site of the emergency?
☐☐☐ minutes
3.11 Where did the vehicle drop the patient in this hospital?
At the general parking   1
In the general OPD   2
In the Casualty/Emergency   3
Others ....   8 → *(Specify: _____)*
Information not available 9
3.12 After the patient reached the hospital, within how much time did the medical/paramedical staff of the hospital attend to the patient?
0–15 min...........................   1

    15–30 min........................   2
    30 min to 1 h   4
    More than 1 h...................   5
    Information not available.........   9

3.13 Whether the patient stabilized is out of danger?
    Yes, under treatment   1   →   skip to question 3.15
    No but under treatment   2   →   skip to question 3.15
    Yes, but referred on to some other facility   3
    No, referred on to some other facility   4

3.14 Was "108" transportation offered?
    Yes   1
    No   2

3.15 How satisfied are you with the ambulance service that the patient availed for reaching this hospital?

-3	-2	-1	0	1	2	3

(Very unhappy) (Unhappy) (Not satisfied) (Cannot say) (Somewhat satisfied) (Satisfied) (Very satisfied)

4.   Out-of-Pocket Expenditure

4.1   Was any expenditure incurred while transporting the patient to the hospital?
    Yes   1
    No ....   2 → skip to question 4.4
    Information not available........   9 → skip to question 4.4

4.2   What was the total amount of expenditure incurred while transporting the patient to the hospital?
    Total expenditure incurred: Rs. ⬚⬚⬚⬚⬚

4.3   What was the expenditure incurred on while transporting the patient to the hospital?
    a. Transport/vehicle hiring: Rs. ⬚⬚⬚⬚⬚
    b. Medical consumables: Rs. ⬚⬚⬚⬚⬚
    c. Others: Rs. ⬚⬚⬚⬚⬚ → *(Specify: ___)*

4.4   Did this hospital/hospital staff ask for payments for starting the treatment of the patient?
    Yes   1
    No ....   2 → skip to question 5.1
    Information not available........   9 → skip to question 5.1

4.5 How much amount did the hospital/hospital staff ask for payments (as advance) for starting the treatment of the patient?
Rs.

5. Choice of Hospital

5.1 Why was the patient brought to this hospital?

The vehicle/ambulance operator brought us here ....   a
Police brought us here ....   b
Guided by the call center of the ambulance operator ...   c
This was nearest hospital from the site of emergency ..   d
Treatment is free/low cost, in this hospital ....   e
This hospital/hospital staff was known to us ....   f
Any other reason ....   g   →
(Specify: _____)
Information not available..   *9*

6. Any suggestions for better and responsive ambulance service:

End the interview thanking the respondent
***

KEYWORDS

- **emergency medical services**
- **108 ambulance service**
- **emergency response**
- **EMRI**
- **ERS**

BIBLIOGRAPHY

1. Sundararaman, T.; Chakraborty, G.; Nair, A.; Mokashi, T.; Ved, R. Publicly Financed Emergency Response and Patient Transport Systems under NRHM, Andhra Pradesh and Gujarat, 2008.
2. *Study of Emergency response Service—EMRI Model—Phase I Study MOHFW, National Rural Health Mission (2005–12)*; Ministry of Health and Family Welfare, Government of India: New Delhi, 2007.
3. *MOHFW, Directory of Innovations Implemented in the Health Sector*; Ministry of Health and Family Welfare and Department for International Development (DFID): New Delhi, 2008. https://mohfw.gov.in/documents/publications

INDEX

For Product Safety Concerns and Information please contact our EU
representative GPSR@taylorandfrancis.com
Taylor & Francis Verlag GmbH, Kaufingerstraße 24, 80331 München, Germany

9 781774 634059